Methods in Molecular Biology

Series Editor
John M. Walker
School of Life and Medical Sciences
University of Hertfordshire
Hatfield, Hertfordshire, UK

For further volumes:
http://www.springer.com/series/7651

For over 35 years, biological scientists have come to rely on the research protocols and methodologies in the critically acclaimed *Methods in Molecular Biology* series. The series was the first to introduce the step-by-step protocols approach that has become the standard in all biomedical protocol publishing. Each protocol is provided in readily-reproducible step-by-step fashion, opening with an introductory overview, a list of the materials and reagents needed to complete the experiment, and followed by a detailed procedure that is supported with a helpful notes section offering tips and tricks of the trade as well as troubleshooting advice. These hallmark features were introduced by series editor Dr. John Walker and constitute the key ingredient in each and every volume of the *Methods in Molecular Biology* series. Tested and trusted, comprehensive and reliable, all protocols from the series are indexed in PubMed.

Immune Mediators in Cancer

Methods and Protocols

Edited by

Ivana Vancurova and Yan Zhu

Department of Biological Sciences, St. John's University, Queens, NY, USA

Humana Press

Editors
Ivana Vancurova
Department of Biological Sciences
St. John's University
Queens, NY, USA

Yan Zhu
Department of Biological Sciences
St. John's University
Queens, NY, USA

ISSN 1064-3745 ISSN 1940-6029 (electronic)
Methods in Molecular Biology
ISBN 978-1-0716-0246-1 ISBN 978-1-0716-0247-8 (eBook)
https://doi.org/10.1007/978-1-0716-0247-8

Cover Illustration: Ovarian cancer cells grown in a 3D culture.

This Humana imprint is published by the registered company Springer Science+Business Media, LLC, part of Springer Nature.
The registered company address is: 233 Spring Street, New York, NY 10013, U.S.A.

Preface

It is the expression of various immune mediators in tumor cells that dictates the crosstalk between tumor cells and immune cells and determines cancer cell survival, proliferation, invasion, and tumor progression. These immune mediators include a variety of cytokines and chemokines, their receptors, as well as the recently identified immune checkpoints and their ligands. Knowledge of the quantitative and qualitative nature of these immune mediators is critical for early cancer diagnosis, but also for our understanding of the mechanisms regulating cancer progression. However, analysis of these immune mediators in tumor cells and tissues faces many challenges that include the low abundance, the need to distinguish between active and latent forms, and the need to measure multiple mediators in a single assay. This volume provides a comprehensive collection of classic and cutting-edge methodologies, as well as bioinformatics and genome editing approaches that are used to quantify immune mediators and analyze their function and biological activity in cancer cells and tissues.

The chapters are divided into four main parts. The first part focuses on the detection of immune mediators in cancer cells and tissues, biopsies, and blood samples, using assays that measure the total levels of mediators regardless of their biological activities. These assays include immunoblotting, ELISA, flow cytometry, and immunohistochemistry. In addition, the complexity of immune responses has led to the development of multiplex technologies that allow for the simultaneous detection of large numbers of proteins in small volumes. Thus, the first part also includes the Luminex multiplex assays that allow the simultaneous measurement of multiple mediators in small sample volumes with time- and cost-saving advantages.

However, since the aforementioned assays cannot distinguish between biologically active and inactive molecules, bioassays are used to measure the different biological activities of various cytokines, chemokines, and immune checkpoints. These bioassays include analysis of cytokine-induced cancer cell invasion, migration, ability to grow and proliferate in 3D culture spheroids, autophagy, ferroptosis, and isotype switching. Moreover, the second part includes approaches used for blocking the cytokine biological activity by using DNA aptamers, as well as methods used for probing cytokine-induced metabolic changes in cancer cells.

Often, there is a need to analyze the intracellular levels of various immune mediators or the mechanisms regulating their expression and signaling in cancer cells and tumor microenvironment. The third part includes protocols for the analysis of cytokines and immune checkpoints by immunoblotting and flow cytometry, as well as protocols for quantitative analysis of their promoter occupancy by using chromatin immunoprecipitation, and for the analysis of gene polymorphisms and alternative splicing. In addition, the third part includes chapters focusing on the use of microscopic and optogenetic approaches to analyze interactions of cancer cells with tumor microenvironment and to manipulate signaling pathways.

Recent advances in DNA and RNA sequencing and proteomic technology have led to the generation of a large number of datasets. Bioinformatical analyses of those datasets can provide valuable information for studying the function and biological activities of immune mediators in cancer cells and tissues. The fourth part includes some of the bioinformatical tools used for phylogenetic analyses and identification of long non-coding RNAs to expand our knowledge of immune mediators' genes and their regulation. This part also includes protocols for gene knock-out and knock-in in cell-based models through genome editing.

There is no best method, since each has its own merits and limitations. Choosing the right method depends on the sample, purpose of the assay, and the available instrumentation. Often, using combined information from several different approaches can yield the most accurate knowledge of the quantitative and qualitative nature of immune mediators' expression and regulation. The reliability of the protocols has been tested in laboratories around the world. Each chapter is appended by notes that navigate through the protocol and serve as a troubleshooting guide. We hope that this book will be useful to not only biochemists, molecular biologists, cancer biologists, and immunologists but also physician-scientists working in the field of immunology and cancer research.

We would like to thank all the authors for their enthusiastic help and support in assembling this volume; we realize that in the highly competitive environment of academic research, many scientists are reluctant to commit their time to writing book chapters and method articles. We also would like to express our sincere gratitude to the series editor, Dr. John Walker, and the outstanding staff of Humana Press for their support, help, and encouragement.

Queens, NY, USA

Ivana Vancurova
Yan Zhu

Contents

Part IV Bioinformatics and Genome Editing Approaches

Contributors

EHAB M. ABO-ALI • *Department of Pharmaceutical Sciences, College of Pharmacy and Health Sciences, St. John's University, Queens, NY, USA*

GUOQIANG BAO • *Laboratory of Emergency Medicine, The Feinstein Institute for Medical Research, Manhasset, NY, USA*

MADHURA BHAGWAT • *Department of Biological Sciences, St. John's University, Queens, NY, USA*

DEON BURITIS • *Department of Biological Sciences, St. John's University, Queens, NY, USA*

KIERSTEN P. CARTER • *Department of Anatomy and Structural Biology, Albert Einstein College of Medicine, Bronx, NY, USA*

WEIQIANG CHEN • *Laboratory of Emergency Medicine, The Feinstein Institute for Medical Research, Manhasset, NY, USA*

CONG-QIU CHU • *Division of Arthritis and Rheumatic Diseases, Oregon Health & Science University, Portland, OR, USA; Section of Rheumatology, VA Portland Health Care System, Portland, OR, USA*

DIANNE COX • *Department of Anatomy and Structural Biology, Albert Einstein College of Medicine, Bronx, NY, USA; Gruss-Lipper Biophotonics Center, Albert Einstein College of Medicine, Bronx, NY, USA; Department of Molecular and Developmental Biology, Albert Einstein College of Medicine, Bronx, NY, USA*

BETSY DEZA • *Department of Biological Sciences, St. John's University, Queens, NY, USA*

VIKAS V. DUKHANDE • *Department of Pharmaceutical Sciences, College of Pharmacy and Health Sciences, St. John's University, Queens, NY, USA*

MARIA FARESJÖ • *Department of Natural Science and Biomedicine, School of Health and Welfare, Jönköping University, Jönköping, Sweden*

VITALAY FOMIN • *Department of Biological Sciences, Columbia University, New York, NY, USA*

JULIAN J. FREEN-VAN HEEREN • *Department of Hematopoiesis, Sanquin Research-Amsterdam UMC Landsteiner Laboratory and Oncode Institute, Amsterdam, The Netherlands*

BIJAYA GAIRE • *Department of Biological Sciences, St. John's University, Queens, NY, USA*

QI GAO • *Department of Rheumatology and Immunology, The First Bethune Hospital, Jilin University, Changchun, China*

PENG GUO • *Department of Anatomy and Structural Biology, Albert Einstein College of Medicine, Bronx, NY, USA; Gruss-Lipper Biophotonics Center, Albert Einstein College of Medicine, Bronx, NY, USA; Analytical Imaging Facility, Albert Einstein College of Medicine, Bronx, NY, USA*

MAREN HÜLSEMANN • *Department of Anatomy and Structural Biology, Albert Einstein College of Medicine, Bronx, NY, USA; Gruss-Lipper Biophotonics Center, Albert Einstein College of Medicine, Bronx, NY, USA*

LOUIS HODGSON • *Department of Anatomy and Structural Biology, Albert Einstein College of Medicine, Bronx, NY, USA; Gruss-Lipper Biophotonics Center, Albert Einstein College of Medicine, Bronx, NY, USA*

MD. FARUK HOSSAIN • *Department of Biological Sciences, St. John's University, Queens, NY, USA*

OLIVIA HU • *Department of Biological Sciences, St. John's University, Queens, NY, USA*

ZIJUN HUO • *Department of Integrative Biology and Pharmacology, McGovern Medical School, The University of Texas Health Science Center at Houston, Houston, TX, USA; Department of Endocrinology, The First Affiliated Hospital of Sun Yat-sen University, Guangzhou, People's Republic of China*

YANFANG JIANG • *Department of Central Laboratory, The First Bethune Hospital, Jilin University, Changchun, China*

ZHENYU JIANG • *Department of Rheumatology and Immunology, The First Bethune Hospital, Jilin University, Changchun, China*

TAKAAKI KAMATANI • *Department of Oral and Maxillofacial Surgery, Showa University School of Dentistry, Ota-City, Tokyo, Japan*

PRITPAL KAUR • *Department of Biological Sciences, St. John's University, Queens, NY, USA*

AHRYUN KIM • *Department of Biological Sciences, St. John's University, Queens, NY, USA*

HELENA KUPCOVA SKALNIKOVA • *Laboratory of Applied Proteome Analyses, Institute of Animal Physiology and Genetics of The Czech Academy of Sciences, Libechov, Czech Republic*

DUNG-FANG LEE • *Department of Integrative Biology and Pharmacology, McGovern Medical School, The University of Texas Health Science Center at Houston, Houston, TX, USA*

AIHUA LI • *Epitomics—An Abcam Company, Burlingame, CA, USA*

ALEJANDRA M. MARTINEZ • *Department of Biological Sciences, St. John's University, Queens, NY, USA*

JOVAN MIRKOVIC • *Department of Biological Sciences, St. John's University, Queens, NY, USA*

VERONIKA MISKOLCI • *Department of Medical Microbiology and Immunology, University of Wisconsin–Madison, Madison, WI, USA*

SHREYA NAGAR • *Department of Biological Sciences, St. John's University, Queens, NY, USA*

SHEYDA NAJAFI • *Department of Pharmaceutical Sciences, College of Pharmacy and Health Sciences, St. John's University, Queens, NY, USA*

BENOIT P. NICOLET • *Department of Hematopoiesis, Sanquin Research-Amsterdam UMC Landsteiner Laboratory and Oncode Institute, Amsterdam, The Netherlands*

SVETA PADMANABHAN • *Department of Biological Sciences, St. John's University, Queens, NY, USA*

RYAN L. PANGILINAN • *Department of Biological Sciences, St. John's University, Jamaica, NY, USA*

VLADIMIR POLTORATSKY • *Department of Pharmaceutical Sciences, St. John's University, Queens, NY, USA; Department of Biological Sciences, St. John's University, Queens, NY, USA*

CAROL PRIVES • *Department of Biological Sciences, Columbia University, New York, NY, USA*

ALESSANDRO PROVVIDO • *Department of Biological Sciences, St. John's University, Queens, NY, USA*

SUSUMU ROKUDAI • *Department of Molecular Pharmacology and Oncology, Gunma University Graduate School of Medicine, Maebashi, Gunma, Japan*

MATTEO RUGGIU • *Department of Biological Sciences, St. John's University, Queens, NY, USA*

SAMUEL SABZANOV • *Department of Biological Sciences, St. John's University, Queens, NY, USA*

JUAN C. SANTOS • *Department of Biological Sciences, College of Liberal Arts and Sciences, St. John's University, Queens, NY, USA*

JEFFREY E. SEGALL • *Department of Anatomy and Structural Biology, Albert Einstein College of Medicine, Bronx, NY, USA; Gruss-Lipper Biophotonics Center, Albert Einstein College of Medicine, Bronx, NY, USA*

PINGFANG SONG • *Division of Arthritis and Rheumatic Diseases, Oregon Health & Science University, Portland, OR, USA; Rheumatology Section, VA Portland Health Care System, Portland, OR, USA*

SHAO TAO • *Division of Arthritis and Rheumatic Diseases, Oregon Health & Science University, Portland, OR, USA; Rheumatology Section, VA Portland Health Care System, Portland, OR, USA; Division of Experimental Medicine, Faculty of Medicine, McGill University, Montreal, QC, Canada*

JIAN TU • *Department of Integrative Biology and Pharmacology, McGovern Medical School, The University of Texas Health Science Center at Houston, Houston, TX, USA; Department of Musculoskeletal Oncology, The First Affiliated Hospital of Sun Yat-sen University, Guangzhou, People's Republic of China*

MOHAMMAD M. UDDIN • *Department of Biological Sciences, St. John's University, Queens, NY, USA*

ALES VANCURA • *Department of Biological Sciences, St. John's University, Queens, NY, USA*

IVANA VANCUROVA • *Department of Biological Sciences, St. John's University, Queens, NY, USA*

POLINA V. VERKHUSHA • *Department of Anatomy and Structural Biology, Albert Einstein College of Medicine, Bronx, NY, USA*

PETR VODICKA • *Laboratory of Applied Proteome Analyses, Institute of Animal Physiology and Genetics of The Czech Academy of Sciences, Libechov, Czech Republic*

KATERINA VODICKOVA KEPKOVA • *Laboratory of Applied Proteome Analyses, Institute of Animal Physiology and Genetics of The Czech Academy of Sciences, Libechov, Czech Republic*

HAICHAO WANG • *Laboratory of Emergency Medicine, The Feinstein Institute for Medical Research, Manhasset, NY, USA; Donald and Barbara Zucker School of Medicine at Hofstra/Northwell, Hempstead, NY, USA; The Feinstein Institute for Medical Research, Northwell Health System, Manhasset, NY, USA*

HERUI WANG • *Department of Biological Sciences, St. John's University, Jamaica, NY, USA*

RUIZHI WANG • *Department of Biological Sciences, St. John's University, Queens, NY, USA*

MONIKA C. WOLKERS • *Department of Hematopoiesis, Sanquin Research-Amsterdam UMC Landsteiner Laboratory and Oncode Institute, Amsterdam, The Netherlands*

WENJUN WU • *Department of Pharmaceutical Sciences, St. John's University, Queens, NY, USA*

ZHIHUI XIAO • *Department of Pharmaceutical Sciences, St. John's University, Queens, NY, USA*

CHONG XU • *Center for Cellular Immunotherapies, Perelman School of Medicine, University of Pennsylvania, Philadelphia, PA, USA; The Parker Institute for Cancer Immunotherapy, Perelman School of Medicine, University of Pennsylvania, Philadelphia, PA, USA; Department of Pathology and Laboratory Medicine, Perelman School of Medicine, University of Pennsylvania, Philadelphia, PA, USA; Department of Medicine, Perelman School of Medicine, University of Pennsylvania, Philadelphia, PA, USA*

DONG-HUA YANG • *Department of Pharmacology, College of Pharmacy and Health Sciences, St. John's University, Queens, NY, USA*

WAN SEOK YANG • *Department of Biological Sciences, St. John's University, Queens, NY, USA*

ZHUANG YE • *Department of Rheumatology and Immunology, The First Bethune Hospital, Jilin University, Changchun, China*

YIBO YIN • *Center for Cellular Immunotherapies, Perelman School of Medicine, University of Pennsylvania, Philadelphia, PA, USA; Department of Neurosurgery, Perelman School of Medicine, University of Pennsylvania, Philadelphia, PA, USA; The Fourth Section of Department of Neurosurgery, The First Affiliated Hospital of Harbin Medical University, Harbin, P.R. China*

ANDY QINGAN YUAN • *Department of Antibody Technology, EXCYTE LLC, Rockville, MD, USA*

XIAOWEI ZHANG • *Division of Arthritis and Rheumatic Diseases, Oregon Health & Science University, Portland, OR, USA; Rheumatology Section, VA Portland Health Care System, Portland, OR, USA*

LINGSHU ZHANG • *Division of Arthritis and Rheumatic Diseases, Oregon Health & Science University, Portland, OR, USA; Rheumatology Section, VA Portland Health Care System, Portland, OR, USA; Department of Rheumatology and Immunology, West China Hospital, Sichuan University, Chengdu, China*

LIN ZHAO • *Laboratory of Emergency Medicine, The Feinstein Institute for Medical Research, Manhasset, NY, USA*

LING ZHAO • *Department of Rheumatology and Immunology, The First Bethune Hospital, Jilin University, Changchun, China*

RUIYING ZHAO • *Department of Integrative Biology and Pharmacology, McGovern Medical School, The University of Texas Health Science Center at Houston, Houston, TX, USA*

YAN ZHU • *Department of Biological Sciences, St. John's University, Queens, NY, USA*

YUE ZOU • *Department of Biological Sciences, St. John's University, Queens, NY, USA*

Part I

Detection of Immune Mediators in Cancer Cells and Tissues

Chapter 1

A Useful Guide for Analysis of Immune Mediators in Cancer by Fluorochrome (Luminex) Technique

Maria Faresjö

Abstract

Immune cells and their mediators are key players in human cancer progression involving alternation in the number and function of immune cells, both peripheral and at the site of tumor. Through reliable predictive biomarkers, cancer can be predicted, and progression and response to therapy followed. Thereby immune biomarkers, e.g., cytokines and chemokines can serve as intermediate mediators of cancer diagnostics. Multiplex analysis of immune mediators in small blood volumes allows for rapid quantification of large number of circulating analytes. The fluorochrome (Luminex) technique is a bead-based sandwich immunoassay that combines the enzyme-linked immunosorbent assay (ELISA) with flow cytometry. The Luminex technique allows multiple immune mediators to be measured simultaneously in small volumes, and provides a convenient and sensitive tool for the detection of a large number of extracellular secreted cytokines and chemokines to be used in prediction and therapy prognosis of cancer.

The technique is based on so-called microspheres (beads) that serve as a solid phase for molecular detection. These individually dyed microbeads have monoclonal antibodies directed against the cyto- and chemokines of interest and allow a simultaneous detection of up to nearly 100 cyto- and chemokines in a dual-laser flow analyzer. Immune mediators can be detected in serum and plasma samples as well as in cell culture supernatants from in vitro stimulated peripheral blood mononuclear cells (PBMC). This chapter describes the Luminex technique for detection of immune mediators in cancer by using magnetic bead sandwich immunoassay, with focus on some important pre-analytic factors, e.g., cell separation and cryopreservation and thawing of PBMC that may affect the outcome of detection of immune mediators. The Luminex technique thus represents a very suitable method to identify immune mediators in cancer tissues in order to diagnose and improve clinical outcome of cancer.

Key words Luminex, Immune mediators, Cancer, Peripheral blood mononuclear cells, Cell separation and cryopreservation of PBMC

1 Introduction

Immune cells and their mediators are key players in human cancer progression. Alternation in the number and function of immune cells, both peripheral and at the site of tumor, has shown importance for both prediction and progression of disease. Circulating immune biomarkers, e.g., cytokine and chemokines, are parts of the

Ivana Vancurova and Yan Zhu (eds.), *Immune Mediators in Cancer: Methods and Protocols*, Methods in Molecular Biology, vol. 2108, https://doi.org/10.1007/978-1-0716-0247-8_1,

complex milieu of cancer, and thus they can serve as intermediate mediators of cancer diagnostics. Through reliable biomarkers progression of cancer can also be followed for cancer therapy. Taken together, immune mediators are of importance in the fight to improve clinical outcome of cancer.

The fluorochrome (Luminex) technique offers an opportunity for multiple analysis of a magnitude of biomarkers in a single assay. The fundament of the technique is a bead-based sandwich immunoassay [1]. The technique is based on so-called microspheres (beads) that serves as a solid phase for molecular detection. The microspheres are today available in one hundred different fluorescent color tones of red and infrared, each carrying its own detection reagent on the surface. As a result, the technique allows simultaneous detection of up to 100 parameters in a small single sample [2].

Each bead-set is coated with a capture antibody, specific to a particular bioassay, allowing the capture and detection of a specific analyte. In a secondary step, a biotinylated antibody together with streptavidin is captured to the bead complex and, finally, a phycoerytherin fluorescent reporter is coupled to the complex (Fig. 1).

In principle, the multiplex assay is performed directly in a microtiter plate. Each bead set, defined by an individual fluorescent color tone on its surface, is mixed to a multiplex bead mix and put into the wells on the plate. The sample (and standard) is, in a secondary step, mixed with the beads and thereafter the biotinylated antibody as well as streptavidin phycoerytherin (PE) are attached to the bead set of interest before readout of the plate (Fig. 2).

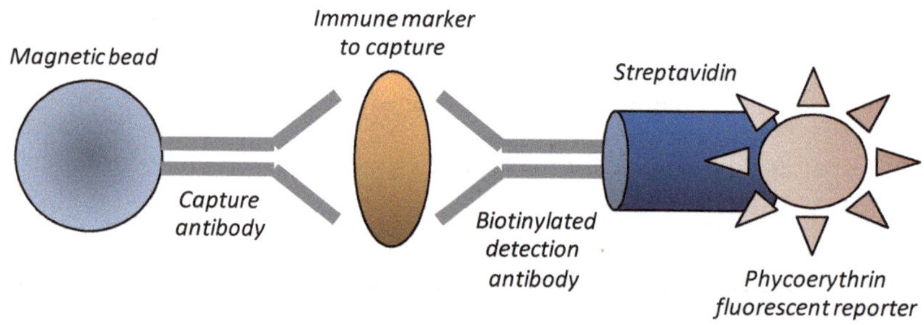

Fig. 1 Principle of magnetic bead sandwich immunoassay. Each magnetic bead-set is coated with a capture antibody for detection of each specific immune marker. In a secondary step, a biotinylated antibody together with streptavidin is captured to the bead complex and, finally, a phycoerytherin fluorescent reporter is coupled to the complex

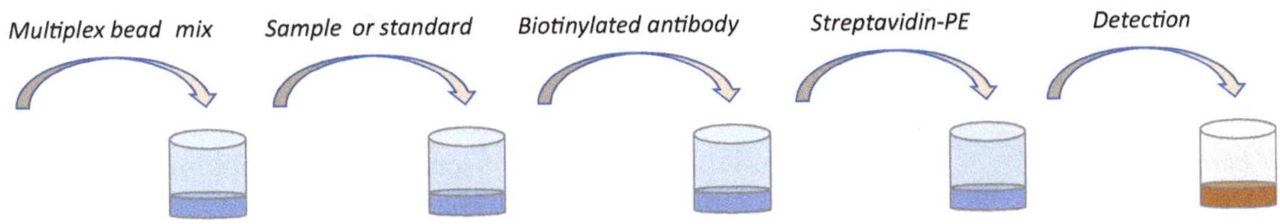

Fig. 2 Methodological principle of the Luminex technique. The multiplex assay is performed directly in a 96-well microtiter plate. Each bead set is mixed to a multiplex bead mix and put into the wells on the plate. The sample (and standard) is mixed with the beads and thereafter the biotinylated antibody and streptavidin phycoerytherin (PE) are attached to the bead set of interest and, finally, analyzed by reading each individual well on a dual-laser flow-based detector instrument

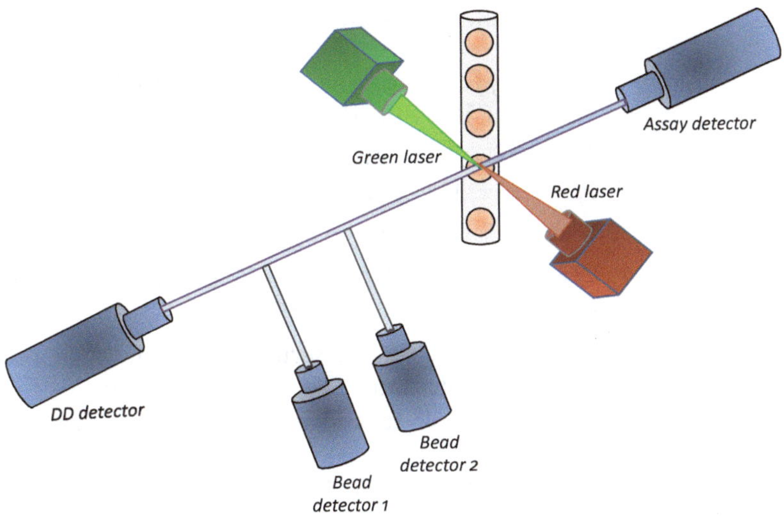

Fig. 3 Dual-laser flow-based detection. The beads are analyzed by a red laser (635 nm) that excites the internal dyes to identify each microsphere particle. The green laser (532 nm) excites the reporter dye (streptavidin-PE) to quantify the amount of bound immune marker on the beads

On a dual-laser flow-based detection instrument, the amount of bound analyte correlates directly with the fluorescent intensity, allowing the quantification of each specific analyte. During the readout of the plate the beads are analyzed by a red laser (635 nm) that excites the internal dyes to identify each microsphere particle. At the same time, a green laser (532 nm) excites the reporter dye (streptavidin-PE) in direct proportion of the fluorescence of the analyte, for quantification (Fig. 3).

The need for analyses of robust biomarkers to predict and follow therapy of cancer is obvious. The Luminex technique is one way of discovering immune mediators associated with cancer by analyzing, e.g., blood samples collected during pretreatment, treatment, and progression. This is in order to predict, prognose, and improve clinical outcome of cancer.

2 Materials

2.1 Isolation of Peripheral Blood Mononuclear Cells (PBMC)

1. Venous blood samples from cancer patients are drawn in tubes without supplement (for serum) or supplemented with K_2EDTA (for plasma and preparation of PBMC).
2. RPMI-1640 medium without glutamine.
3. Washing buffer: RPMI-1640 without glutamine, supplemented with 2% heat-inactivated fetal calf serum (FCS).
4. Separation reagent: Ficoll-Paque density gradient centrifugation.

2.2 Cell Number and Viability

1. Türk's solution.
2. Trypan Blue solution.

2.3 PBMC Cryopreservation and Stimulation

1. Freezing medium: 50% RPMI-1640 without glutamine, 40% FCS, and 10% dimethyl sulfoxide (Me_2SO).
2. Cryo 1 °C Freezing Container (Nalge Nunc International, Rochester, USA) containing isopropanol.
3. Vials appropriate for cryopreservation.
4. Washing buffer: RPMI-1640 without glutamine supplemented with 10% heat-inactivated FCS.
5. AIM V research-grade serum-free medium supplemented with 2 mM L-glutamine, 50 μg/L streptomycin sulfate, 10 μg/L gentamicin sulfate, and 2×10^{-5} M 2-mercaptoethanol.

2.4 Luminex

2.4.1 Luminex Kit

The Luminex kit includes the following reagents.

1. Standard for Luminex assay.
2. Luminex diluent for standard (standard diluent for serum and plasma or cell culture medium for cell culture supernatant).
3. Luminex sample diluent (for serum and plasma).
4. Luminex assay buffer.
5. Luminex wash buffer.
6. Coupled magnetic beads (10×).
7. Detection antibodies (10×).
8. Detection antibody diluent.
9. Streptavidin-PE (100×).
10. Flat-bottom plate (96-well).
11. Sealing tape.

2.4.2 Equipment

1. Wash station (for use with magnetic bead-based assays).
2. Microtiter plate shaker.
3. Dual-laser flow-based plate reader including software for data acquisition and analysis.

3 Methods

3.1 Isolation of PBMC

Separation of PBMC should be handled at room temperature in a ventilated hood (*see* **Notes 1** and **2**).

1. Centrifuge the blood samples at 2000 × *g* for 10 min and transfer the serum/plasma to sterile tubes.
2. Dilute venous heparinized blood in RPMI medium 1:1 (i.e., half volume blood, half volume RPMI).
3. To ensure a thorough mixing, invert the Ficoll-Paque bottle several times, and thereafter withdraw the required volume of Ficoll-Paque using aseptic technique; Ficoll:blood 3:5 (i.e., 12 mL of Ficoll:20 mL of diluted blood sample).
4. Transfer the required volume of Ficoll-Paque to a sterile centrifuge tube.
5. Carefully lay the diluted blood sample on the Ficoll layer to avoid mix between Ficoll and blood sample.
6. Centrifuge at 400 × *g* for 30 min, without brake, at 18–20 °C.
7. Carefully draw up the layer of PBMC using a clean Pasteur pipette and transfer PBMC to a sterile centrifuge tube.
8. Resuspend PBMC in 20 mL of washing buffer (RPMI-1640 supplemented with FCS).
9. Centrifuge at 400 × *g* for 10 min, with low brake, at 18–20 °C.
10. Remove the supernatant and wash PBMC by repeating **steps 8** and **9** once more.
11. Remove the supernatant.

3.2 Cell Number and Viability

1. Dissolve the PBMC pellet in 1 mL of washing medium.
2. For determination of number of PBMC, dilute 10 μL of PBMC suspension with 90 μL of Türk's solution (1:10).
3. Place 10 μL of PBMC suspension in a Bürker's chamber. Count the number of PBMC using a light microscope (*see* **Note 3**).
4. For determination of membrane integrity, dilute 10 μL of PBMC suspension with 10 μL of Trypan Blue solution (1:1).
5. Place 10 μL of PBMC suspension in a Bürker's chamber. Count 100 PBMC using a light microscopy (*see* **Note 4**).

3.3 Cryopreservation of PBMC (See Note 5)

1. Centrifuge the solution of PBMC at 400 × *g* for 10 min, at 18–20 °C.
2. Remove the supernatant.
3. Resuspend PBMC in freezing medium (4 °C) by adding freezing medium dropwise, while the tube is continuously agitated, to a concentration of 5–10 × 10^6 PBMC/mL.

4. Transfer 1 mL of PBMC solution to vials appropriate for cryopreservation.
5. Place the vials with PBMC in a precooled (4 °C) Cryo 1 °C Freezing Container containing isopropanol.
6. Place the container at −70 °C (the freezing rate is −1 °C/min).
7. Transfer the vials to liquid nitrogen (−196 °C) the following day.

3.4 Thawing of PBMC

1. Thaw PBMC, directly from −196 °C to +37 °C, in a water bath under continuous agitation.
2. Immediately thereafter, add washing buffer (RPMI 1640 supplemented with 10% FCS) dropwise to the cells until a total volume of 10 mL is reached.
3. Centrifuge the solution of PBMC at 400 × *g* for 10 min, at 18–20 °C.
4. Remove the supernatant.
5. Resuspend PBMC in 1 mL of AIM V research-grade serum-free medium with supplements.
6. Count the number and check the viability of PBMC (*see* Subheading 3.3).

3.5 Stimulation of PBMC and Collection of Cell Supernatant

1. Adjust the concentration of PBMC in AIM V, with supplements, to 1×10^6/mL.
2. Transfer 1 mL of PBMC to each tube for stimulation.
3. Add antigen or control to appropriate concentration.
4. Incubate PBMC between 24 and 96 h, at 37 °C with 5% CO_2.
5. After completed incubation of PBMC, centrifuge cells for 10 min at 400 × *g*.
6. Transfer aliquots of cell supernatants to sterile tubes.

3.6 Luminex

Standard, diluents, and cell culture medium should be at room temperature, while serum, plasma, or cell culture supernatants should be kept on ice before preparation.

3.6.1 Preparation of Standard and Blank

1. Reconstitute the vial of standard in 500 μL of diluent (standard diluent for serum and plasma or cell culture medium for cell culture supernatant), vortex, and incubate on ice for 30 min.
2. Prepare the 9-point standard dilution series and blank, by:
   (a) Mark tubes; S1–S9 and blank.
   (b) Add 72 μL of diluent (standard diluent for serum and plasma or cell culture medium for cell culture supernatant), into tube S1, and 150 μL diluent to S2–S9 and blank (Fig. 4).

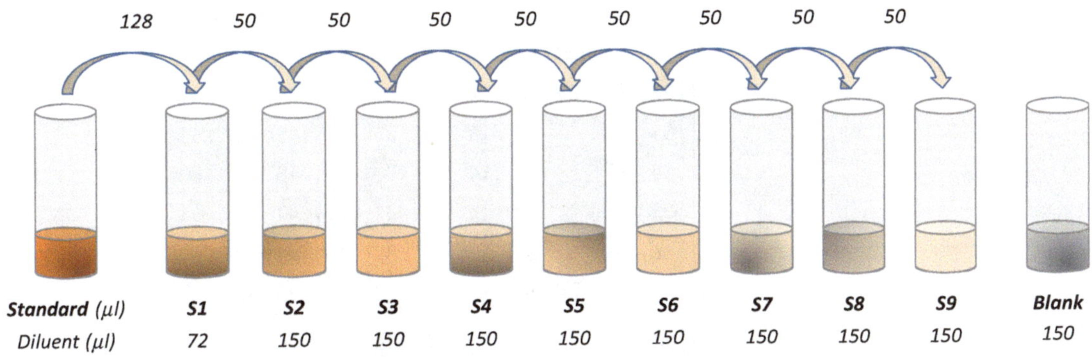

Fig. 4 Preparation of fourfold serious of standard. A 9-point standard dilution series is prepared by adding 72 μL of diluent to tube S1 (standard diluent for serum and plasma or cell culture medium for cell culture supernatant), and 150 μL of diluent to S2–S9. Reconstituted standard (128 μL) is transferred into S1, and thereafter serially diluted fourfold from S1 through S9 by transferring 50 mL between each tube. To the tube marked blank, exclusively 150 μL diluents (for serum samples) or cell culture medium (for cell culture supernatants) is transferred

3. Transfer 128 μL of reconstituted standard into S1.
4. Serially dilute fourfold from S1 through S9 by transferring 50 μL between each tube (vortex between each transfer).
5. To the tube marked blank, add 150 μL of diluent (for serum samples) or cell culture medium (for cell culture supernatants).

3.6.2 Preparation of Samples and Beads

1. Dilute serum samples in sample diluent (e.g., *1:4; 50 μL serum to 150 μL of sample diluent)*.
2. Dilute cell culture supernatants in cell culture medium (*if high concentration of immune markers is to be expected)*.
3. Dilute 575 μL of beads in 5175 μL of assay buffer (1:10).

3.6.3 Running the Assay

1. Add 50 μL/well of beads (diluted 1:10) to the assay plate.
2. Wash the plate by adding 100 μL/well of wash buffer and repeat this step once.
3. Add 50 μL of samples (serum or cell culture supernatants), standards (S1–S9), blank, and, if used, also control (Fig. 5).
4. Cover the plate with sealing tape and incubate for 30 min in the dark, at room temperature through continuous shaking at 300 rpm.
5. With 10 min remaining of the incubation step, prepare the detection antibody.

   Dilute 300 μL detection antibody in 2700 μL diluent (1:10).
6. Wash the plate by adding 100 μL/well of wash buffer and repeat this step twice.

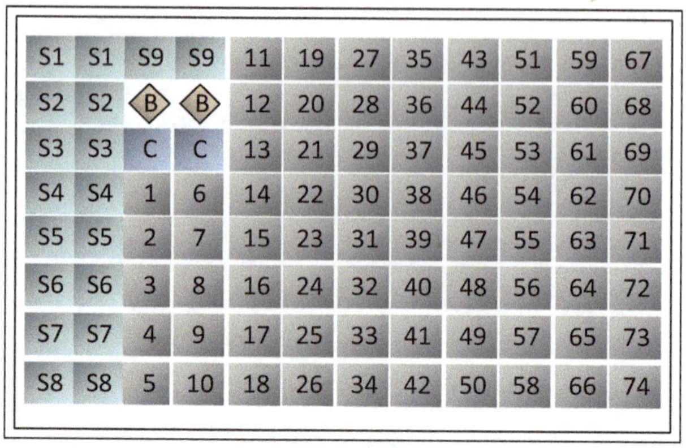

Fig. 5 Plate formation. An example of plate formation for standards (S1–S9), blank (B), control (C), and samples (serum or cell culture supernatants; position 1–74), for the wells on the plate

7. Add 25 μL/well of detection antibody (diluted 1:10) to the assay plate.
8. Cover the plate with sealing tape and incubate for 30 min in the dark, at room temperature through continuous shaking at 300 rpm.
9. Meanwhile, prepare software protocol, e.g., normalized standard (S1–S9) values.
10. With 10 min remaining of the incubation step, prepare 1× streptavidin-PE in assay buffer.

    Dilute 60 μL streptavidin-PE in 5940 μL assay buffer (1:100).
11. Wash the plate by adding 100 μL/well of wash buffer and repeat this step twice.
12. Add 50 μL/well of streptavidin-PE (diluted 1:100) to the assay plate.
13. Cover the plate with sealing tape and incubate for 10 min in the dark, at room temperature through continuous shaking at 300 rpm.
14. Wash the plate by adding 100 μL/well of wash buffer and repeat this step twice.
15. Resuspend beads in 125 mL assay buffer/well, cover the plate with sealing tape and shake at 1100 rpm for 30 s.
16. Remove the sealing tape and the plate cover and place the plate in the reader. Read the plate by choosing the running protocol (prepared in advance of the running and preparation of the plate). A minimum of 100 beads per region should be analyzed.

17. Raw data is thereafter analyzed with a suitable software to apply a standard curve, with a cutoff for minimum detectable concentration, for each individual immune marker.

4 Notes

1. Of great importance is the time period between blood sampling and processing of the sample. Our own research group has found that blood samples left at room temperature less than 24 h before separation of peripheral blood mononuclear cells (PBMC) will not change the percentages of $CD3^+$, $CD3^+CD8^+$, $CD19^+$, and $CD56^+CD16^+$ [3]. It has also been shown that PBMC handled and cryopreserved within 8 h from venipuncture has better viability, higher cell recovery, and higher concentration of, e.g., IFN-γ compared to PBMC handled after 8 h from blood sampling [4].
2. There are a number of different ways to enrich PBMC. The most frequently used techniques for isolation of PBMC are density gradient separation by Ficoll or Lymphoprep or separation by vacutainer CPT (cell preparation tube). Ficoll is routinely used to isolate mononuclear cells from bone marrow, peripheral blood, and umbilical cord blood. In principle, PBMC are enriched from whole blood that is layered onto a density gradient. Gentle centrifugation at room temperature results in a buffy coat of monocytes and lymphocytes under a layer of plasma, with the remaining white blood cells together with red blood cells passing through the interface and collecting at the bottom of the tube. The PBMC interface is collected and washed for several times in either phosphate-buffered saline (PBS) or cell culture medium (washing buffer) to remove any contaminating separation medium.

   The vacutainer CPT is a single tube system, supplemented with sodium citrate, for collection of whole blood and the separation of PBMC. In principle, blood is collected in the CPT tube, the tube is centrifuged, and the cell pellet is resuspended in PBS or cell culture medium, before subsequent assay or procedure.
3. In the most common design, the volume of each large square of a Bürker's chamber is 0.1 mm^3. The cells in four large squares are counted and cells over or touching the lines on top and on the left are counted, but cells over or touching the right or bottom lines are ignored. The concentration in cells per mL will be calculated as cells in four large squares/4 × 10,000.

4. Viability thresholds should be used in, e.g., clinical trials in order to obtain reliable results of functional assays. The most convenient way to check the viability of PBMC is to manually count PBMC by light microscopy after the cells have been pre-colored with, e.g., trypan blue. In a viable cell, trypan blue is not absorbed; however, it traverses the membrane of dead cells. Hence, dead cells are shown as distinctive blue color dots studied by light microscopy.

   In principle, the number of live (white) cells versus number of dead (blue) cells are counted. The number of white cells/100 PBMC gives the viability in percentage.

   A more reliable way to ensure the viability of cells is detection by flow cytometry. In principle, PBMC should be resuspended in a flow cytometry staining buffer and thereafter cell count and viability analysis is performed. However, this requires more cells and thus may not be possible in limited sample sizes.

5. The functional assays on cryopreserved PBMC are associated with viability of the cells. For practical reasons it can be an advantage to collect cells during a limited period of time and perform all analyses collectively, post cryopreservation, in order to overcome, e.g., inter-assay variation in the methodology analyzing cytokine secretion, e.g., by Luminex. Cryopreservation is a convenient way to handle PBMC. Actually, frozen cells are used in the great majority of all studies of cell-mediated immunity. We and others have been able to show that cryopreserved PBMC can be used, trustworthy after cryopreservation for detection of cytokines and chemokines [5], Treg-associated markers [6] and also that cryopreserved PBMC maintain a stable expression of the T-regulatory markers FOXP3 (% and MFI) in the $CD4^{+}CD25^{hi}$ cell population after cryopreservation [7]. Actually, subsets of $CD4^{+}$, $CD8^{+}$, and $CD25^{hi}$ lymphocytes are in general not influenced by isolation and long-term cryopreservation [3]. Collectively, these studies show that cryopreserved PBMC can be used and still give a trustworthy and useful information.

References

1. De Jager W, te Velthuis H, Prakken BJ et al (2003) Simultaneous detection of 15 human cytokines in a single sample of stimulated peripheral blood mononuclear cells. Clin Diagn Lab Immunol 10:133–139
2. Lagrelius M, Jones P, Franck K et al (2006) Cytokine detection by multiplex technology useful for assessing antigen specific cytokine profiles and kinetics in whole blood cultured up to seven days. Cytokine 33:156–165
3. Tompa A, Nilsson-Bowers A, Faresjö M (2018) Subsets of $CD4^{+}$, $CD8^{+}$, and $CD25^{hi}$ lymphocytes are in general not influenced by isolation and long-term cryopreservation. J Immunol 201:1799–1809
4. Bull M, Lee D, Stucky J et al (2007) Defining blood processing parameters for optimal detection of cryopreserved antigen-specific responses for HIV vaccine trials. J Immunol Methods 322:57–69

5. Axelsson S, Faresjö M, Hedman M et al (2008) Cryopreserved peripheral blood mononuclear cells are suitable for the assessment of immunological markers in type 1 diabetic children. Cryobiology 57:201–208
6. Kivling A, Nilsson L, Faresjö M (2009) How and when to pick up the best signal from markers associated with T-regulatory cells? J Immunol Methods 345:29–39
7. Rydén A, Faresjö M (2011) Efficient expansion of cryopreserved $CD^{4+}CD^{25+}CD^{127lo}/-$ cells in type 1 diabetes. Res Immunol 1:36–44

Chapter 2

Analysis of Circulating HMGB1 in Human Serum

Weiqiang Chen, Guoqiang Bao, Lin Zhao, and Haichao Wang

Abstract

As a ubiquitous nuclear protein, high-mobility group box 1 (HMGB1) is constitutively expressed and can be actively secreted by macrophages/monocytes, as well as passively released from damaged cells following pathological injuries. Studies indicate that HMGB1 functions as a mediator of infection- and injury-elicited inflammatory diseases. Although intracellular HMGB1 functions as a regulator of tumorigenesis, epigenetic anticancer agents or therapeutic γ-ray irradiation could also cause active secretion or passive release of HMGB1, enabling serum HMGB1 to serve as a biomarker for the diagnosis and therapy of various cancers. Here we describe a semiquantitative immune blotting method to measure HMGB1 in human serum, in comparison with a commercially available HMGB1 enzyme-linked immunosorbent assay (ELISA) technique.

Key words HMGB1, Western blotting, ELISA, Serum, Antibody

1 Introduction

The high-mobility group box 1 (HMGB1), a highly conserved 30 kDa DNA-binding protein, is expressed constitutively in most cells, and a large "pool" of preformed HMGB1 is stored in the nucleus due to the presence of two lysine-rich nuclear localization sequences [1, 2]. It contains two internal repeats of positively charged domains (known as "A box" and "B box") in the N-terminus, and a continuous stretch of negatively charged (aspartic and glutamic acid) acidic tail in the C-terminus. These HMG boxes enable HMGB1 to bind chromosomal DNA and fulfill its nuclear functions, such as maintaining the nucleosomal structure and stability and regulating gene expression [3]. In response to exogenous bacterial products (such as endotoxin or CpG-DNA) [1, 4] or endogenous inflammatory stimuli (e.g., TNF, IFN-γ, or hydrogen peroxide) [1, 5, 6], innate immune cells actively release HMGB1 in a dose- and time-dependent manner. In addition, HMGB1 can be released passively from damaged cells [7], and similarly triggers an inflammatory response [8]. The accumulated

Ivana Vancurova and Yan Zhu (eds.), *Immune Mediators in Cancer: Methods and Protocols*, Methods in Molecular Biology, vol. 2108, https://doi.org/10.1007/978-1-0716-0247-8_2, © Springer Science+Business Media, LLC, part of Springer Nature 2020

evidence has supported a pathogenic role for extracellular HMGB1 in infection- or injury-elicited inflammatory diseases [9–13]. In addition, HMGB1 is overly expressed in many types of tumor cells, and intracellular HMGB1 functions as a regulator of tumorigenesis [14, 15]. However, epigenetic anticancer agents [16], therapeutic γ-ray irradiation [17], or even harmful ultraviolet radiation [18] could cause active secretion of passive release of HMGB1. Consequently, serum HMGB1 has thus been proposed as a biomarker for the diagnosis and therapy of various types of cancers [19, 20]. Thus, it is important to measure plasma or serum HMGB1 levels in patients with various inflammatory diseases or cancers. In this chapter, two immunoassays, ELISA and western blotting, are described for measuring HMGB1 in human serum samples.

2 Materials

2.1 Sandwich ELISA

Several companies have developed HMGB1 Chemi-Luminescent ELISA kits based on standard sandwich enzyme-linked immunosorbent assay technology for the quantitative determination of HMGB1 levels in human plasma and serum. For instance, the IBL International HMGB1 ELISA kit contains the following components:

1. Microtiter Plate: 8-well strips coated with the capture antibody (polyclonal antibody generated against the peptide KPDAAKKGVVKAEK adjacent to the C-terminal acidic tail of HMGB1) (*see* **Notes 1** and **2**). One plate contains twelve 8-well strips.
2. Enzyme Conjugate (lyophilized): Peroxidase (POD)-conjugated anti-HMGB1 monoclonal antibody (lyophilized for making 12 mL solution).
3. HMGB1 Standard: contains pig HMGB1 protein.
4. Positive Control (lyophilized): contains pig HMGB1 protein.
5. Diluent Buffer: ready to use, contains buffer 0.01% NaN_3 '20 mL.
6. Enzyme Conjugate Diluent: ready to use, contains buffer in a total volume of 12 mL.
7. Color Reagent A: ready to use, contains 3,3′,5,5′-tetramethylbenzidine (TMB), 6 mL.
8. Color Reagent B: ready to use, contains buffer with 0.005 M hydrogen peroxide, 6 mL.
9. Color Stop Solution: ready to use, contains 0.35 M sulfuric acid, 12 mL.

10. 5× Washing buffer: contains phosphate buffer, <0.5% Tween 20, 200 mL.
11. Adhesive Foil: to seal the ELISA plate, 2 sheets.

2.2 Western Blotting

1. 10× Phosphate-Buffered Saline (10× PBS): 1.37 M NaCl, 27 mM KCl, 100 mM Na_2HPO_4, 18 mM KH_2PO_4, pH 7.4.
2. 10× Tris/Glycine/SDS Buffer: 0.025 M Tris, 0.192 M glycine, 0.1% SDS, pH 8.3.
3. 10× Tris/Glycine Buffer: 0.025 M Tris, 0.192 M glycine, pH 8.3.
4. SDS-PAGE gel: 4–20% Mini-PROTEAN® TGX™ Precast Gel.
5. PageRuler plus Prestained Protein Ladder 10–250 kDa molecular weight markers.
6. Immun-Blot PVDF Membrane.
7. CL-X Posure TM Film.
8. Amersham™ ECL™ western blotting Detection Reagents.
9. Anti-HMGB1 antibody (OncoImmune Inc., MI, USA, Cat# OI0001A-05).
10. ECL Rabbit IgG, HRP-linked whole antibody (from donkey).
11. Donkey anti-mouse IgG-HRP.
12. Laemmli 2× Buffer/Loading Buffer: 4% SDS, 10% 2-mercaptoethanol, 20% glycerol, 0.004% bromophenol blue, 0.125 M Tris–HCl, pH 6.8.
13. Running buffer (Tris/Glycine/SDS): 25 mM Tris base, 190 mM glycine, 0.1% SDS, pH 8.3.
14. Add 100 mL of 10× Tris/Glycine/SDS Buffer to 900 mL of ultrapure water, and mix thoroughly.
15. Transfer buffer: 25 mM Tris base, 190 mM glycine, 20% methanol, pH 8.0.
16. Add 100 mL of 10× Tris/Glycine Buffer to 200 mL of methanol and 700 mL of ultrapure water, and mix well. Chill buffer at 4 °C.
17. Washing buffer: Add 500 μL of Tween 20 to 1000 mL of 1× PBS, and mix thoroughly.
18. Blocking buffer: Add 5 g nonfat dry milk to 100 mL of washing buffer. Mix thoroughly, filter, and store at 4 °C. Failure to filter can lead to "spotting" tiny dark grains that will contaminate the blot during color development.

3 Methods

3.1 HMGB1 ELISA

Below is a brief protocol adapted from the IBL International HMGB1 ELISA kit for measuring HMGB1 in plasma or serum samples.

1. Prepare serum or plasma samples immediately after blood collection to prevent progressive HMGB1 leakage from blood cells (*see* **Note 3**). Samples containing concentrations higher than the highest standard have to be diluted with Diluent buffer.
2. Set each reagent in the ELISA kit at room temperature for at least 30 min before use.
3. Pipette 100 μL of Diluent buffer into the respective wells of the microtiter plate. Pipette 10 μL of Diluent buffer into the blank-well of the microtiter plate.
4. Pipette 10 μL of HMGB1 standard, positive control and each serum or plasma sample into the respective wells of the microtiter plate. Shake the plate briefly 30 s (*see* **Note 4**).
5. Cover plate with adhesive foil. Incubate for 20–24 h at 37 °C.
6. Remove adhesive foil. Discard incubation solution. Wash the plate five times with Wash Solution (400 μL/well) using microplate washer. Remove excess solution by tapping the inverted plate on a paper towel.
7. Pipette 100 μL of peroxidase-linked anti-HMGB1 MAb to each well. Cover plate with adhesive foil and incubate for 2 h at room temperature (25 °C).
8. Remove adhesive foil. Discard incubation solution. Wash the plate five times with Wash Solution (400 μL/well) using microplate washer. Remove excess solution by tapping the inverted plate on a paper towel.
9. For adding Color and Stop solutions, use an 8-channel micropipettor. Pipetting should be carried out in the same time intervals for both solutions. Pipette 100 μL of Color Solution (chromogen 3,3′,5,5′-tetra-methylbenzidine) to each well, and incubate for 30 min at room temperature.
10. Stop the color reaction by adding 100 μL of Stop Solution to each well in the same sequence and time intervals as the addition of Color solution. Briefly mix contents by gently shaking the plate.
11. Clean the back of the wells. Be careful not to scratch the wells as this may interfere with measurements.
12. Measure absorbance at 450 nm within 60 min after adding the Stop Solution (*See* **Notes 5–7**).

3.2 HMGB1 Western Blotting

Western blotting enables indirect detection of protein samples immobilized on a nitrocellulose or PVDF membrane, and serves as a useful tool to quantify HMGB1 in serum or plasma samples. Briefly, plasma or serum protein samples are first resolved by SDS-PAGE and then electrophoretically transferred to a membrane. Following a blocking step, the membrane is probed with a primary antibody raised against HMGB1. After subsequent washings, the membrane is incubated with an enzyme-conjugated secondary antibody that is reactive toward the primary antibody. The activity of the enzyme, such as alkaline phosphatase (AP) and horseradish peroxidase (HRP), is necessary for signal generation. Finally, the membrane is washed again and incubated with an appropriate enzyme substrate (e.g., chemiluminescent substrates for HRP), producing a recordable signal.

Carry out all procedures at room temperature unless otherwise specified.

3.2.1 Sample Preparation

1. Use a small volume (50 μL) of serum or plasma to determine the protein concentration.
2. Mix serum or plasma samples with an equal volume of 2× Laemmli Sample Buffer (*see* **Notes 8** and **9**). We recommend denaturing the sample using the following method unless nonreducing and nondenaturing conditions are required to investigate HMGB1/protein interactions (*see* **Note 10**).
3. To reduce and denature proteins, boil the sample mixtures at 100 °C for 5 min, and spin briefly to collect the condensed water from the tube cap immediately before loading to SDS-PAGE gel.

3.2.2 Protein Separation by Gel Electrophoresis

1. Mount the pre-casted SDS-PAGE gels onto the electrophoresis apparatus, and add running buffer to the top and bottom reservoirs. Remove any air bubbles.
2. Load equal amounts of serum or plasma proteins (20–30 μg) into the wells of the gel, along with molecular weight markers (*see* **Note 11**), as well as purified HMGB1 protein at several concentrations (e.g., 1, 5, 20 ng/well).
3. Attach the electrophoresis apparatus to a power supply; the positive electrode should be connected to the bottom buffer reservoir.
4. Run the gel for 1–2 h at 110 V. The time and voltage may require some optimization. We recommend following the manufacturer's instructions. A reducing gel should be used unless nonreducing conditions are required to investigate HMGB1/protein interactions (*see* **Note 10**).

5. Remove the plates from the electrophoresis apparatus and place them on a paper towel. Using a spatula, separate the plates apart.
6. Incubate the gels in Transfer Buffer for approximately 10 min to equilibrate them.

3.2.3 Protein Transfer to the Membrane

1. Cut the PVDF membrane to the dimensions of the gel, immerse it in 100% methanol for 5 min, and rinse with transfer buffer before preparing the transfer stack (*see* **Note 12**). Mark and/or clip one corner for orientation. Handle the membranes only with flat forceps.
2. Soak the member, filter paper, and fiber pads in transfer buffer for 10 min.
3. Prepare the transfer stack as shown below (*see* Fig. 1):
   (a) Place the cassette, with the gray side down, on a lean surface.
   (b) Place one pre-wetted sponge/fiber pad on the gray side of cassette.
   (c) Place a sheet of filter paper on the sponge pad.
   (d) Place the equilibrated gel on the filter paper.
   (e) Place the pre-wetted PVDF membrane on the gel.
   (f) Complete the sandwich by placing another piece of filter paper on the membrane.
   (g) Using a glass tube gently roll all air bubbles out.
   (h) Add the last sponge pad.
4. Close the cassette firmly and carefully to not move the gel and filter paper sandwich. Lock the cassette closed with the white latch, and place it in the electrophoresis module.
5. Add frozen Bio-Ice cooling unite into the tank, and completely fill the tank with buffer. Add standard stir bar to help maintain even buffer temperature and ion distribution in the tank.
6. Put on the lid, and plug the cable into the power supply.

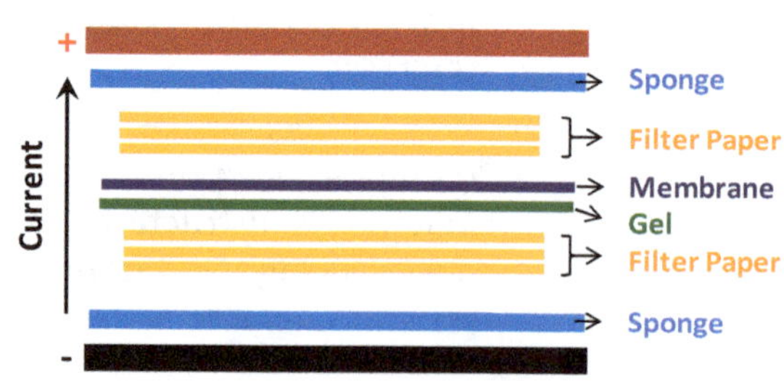

Fig. 1 Assembling the sandwich transfer stack

7. Transfer proteins at 200 mA for 60 min. The time and voltage may require some optimization. We recommend following the manufacturer's instructions. Transfer to the membrane can be checked using Ponceau Red staining before the blocking step.
8. After the transfer, unclamp the blot sandwich and remove the sheets of blotting paper, exposing the blot membrane.

3.2.4 Antibody Staining

1. Block the membrane for 2 h at room temperature, or overnight at 4 °C, using 5% nonfat milk blocking solution (*see* **Notes 13** and **14**).
2. Incubate membrane with appropriate dilutions of primary anti-HMGB1 antibody in 5% or 2% blocking solution overnight at 4 °C or for 2 h at room temperature (*see* **Notes 15, 16** and **17**).
3. Wash the membrane three times for 10 min each in Washing Buffer to remove unbound antibody.
4. Incubate the membrane with the recommended dilution of labeled secondary antibody in 5% Blocking Buffer at room temperature for 1 h.
5. Wash the membrane three times for 10 min each in washing buffer containing 0.05% Tween 20. Rinse the membrane with washing buffer without Tween 20 (*see* **Note 14**).
6. To prepare the substrate, proceed according to the kit manufacturer's recommendations. For instance, mix the black and white ECL solutions (1:1 ratio) of the Amersham ECL kit.
7. Aliquot sufficient volume of substrate solution to cover and wet the membrane, and incubate the blot with the substrate for 1 min (0.1 mL/cm^2) when using the Amersham ECL or 5 min when using the SuperSignal Substrates.
8. Remove excess reagent and cover the membrane in transparent plastic wrap. A plastic sheet protector works well, although plastic wrap also may be used. Remove all air bubbles between the blot and the surface of the membrane protector.
9. Acquire image using darkroom development techniques for chemiluminescence or normal image scanning methods for colorimetric detection.
10. The relative band intensity is quantified by using the NIH image 1.59 or other software to determine HMGB1 levels with reference to standard curves generated with purified HMGB1 at various dilutions (*see* **Notes 18–22**).

4 Notes

1. According to the manufacturer, the IBL international (manufactured under the license of Shino-Test Corporation), capture anti-HMGB1 antibodies are highly specific to HMGB1, but not to HMGB2. However, their cross-reactivity with other plasma or serum proteins is not yet known (*see* Table 1); it should be a subject of future investigations.
2. As a highly charged molecule, HMGB1 can interact with various plasma or serum proteins, such as immunoglobulins (IgGs) and thrombomodulin [21, 22]. It is not yet known how these and as-yet-unidentified HMGB1-binding molecules affect the detection of HMGB1 by using the Shino-Test or other HMGB1 ELISA kits [21].

Table 1
Commercially available anti-HMGB1 antibodies for western blotting analysis

Company	Sigma-Aldrich		Abcam		Cell signaling	OncoImmune Inc
Antibody type (Clone #)	M-MAb (Clone 2F6)	R-PAb	M-MAb	R-PAb	R-PAb	M-MAb (Clone 3B1 or 3E8)
Catalog No.	WH0003146M8	SAB2101049	ab77302	ab18256	3935	OI0001A or OI0001B
Species cross-reactivity	Human	Human, Mouse Rat Bovine Canine Chicken Pig	Human	Human Mouse Rat	Human, Mouse Rat Monkey	Human Mouse Rat Monkey Canine
Immunogen	Human HMGB1 residues 1–91	Human HMGB1, residue 1–91	Recombinant HMGB1, residue 1–216	Human HMGB1 residue 150–216	Synthetic peptide	Recombinant HMGB1 residue 1–216
Specificity to whole-cell lysate[a]	Hela	Hela	HMGB1-transfected 293 T cell	NIH/3T3 MEF1 e PC12	NIH/3T3 DLD-1 C6 COS	Mouse spleen cells
Cross-reactivity to serum proteins	Unknown	Unknown	Unknown	Unknown	Unknown	Unknown

M-MAb murine monoclonal antibodies, *R-PAb* rabbit polyclonal antibodies
[a]One specific band was detected in lysate of indicated cells

3. Prolonged storage of blood samples before centrifugation at room temperature often led to higher HMGB1 levels in sera [23], possibly due to leakage of HMGB1 from stressed/damaged blood cells. However, storage of serum samples after centrifugation for up to 7 days did not affect HMGB1 levels [23].
4. The minimal measurable HMGB1 concentrations are calculated by adding two standard deviations to the mean optical density value of several zero standard replicates. According to the Shino-Test Corporation, the limit of detection HMGB1 ELISA is approximately 0.3–1 ng/mL, making it suitable for measuring plasma or serum HMGB1 in patients with sepsis or other inflammatory diseases. If serum HMGB1 levels are relatively low, consider to use the recommended sensitive HMGB1 ELISA method by loading more serum samples and less HMGB1 standard on the ELISA plates (*see* Fig. 2a).
5. In agreement with previous report [24], the measurement of HMGB1 in healthy individuals showed low levels by using the Shino-Test Corporation HMGB1 ELISA kit (*see* Fig. 2a).
6. Research in Dr. Stoetzer's laboratory has shown that the measurement of HMGB1 in EDTA plasma samples yielded considerably lower values than in sera with a mean recovery <30% [23].
7. The ELISA method has been used by many investigators to measure HMGB1 levels in serum or plasma samples [23, 25–33].
8. Almost all serum or plasma proteins can be readily solubilized by sodium dodecyl sulfate (SDS), making SDS-PAGE the most widely used method for determining the molecular mass of serum or plasma proteins.
9. As an ionic detergent, SDS denatures proteins by wrapping around the polypeptide backbone at a fixed ratio (1.0 g of SDS: 0.7 g of polypeptide). Thus, more SDS can be added in the sampling buffer if excessive amount of plasma or serum proteins (up to 50–100 μg) are loaded onto SDS-PAGE gels in order to detect relatively lower HMGB1 levels.
10. To investigate the possibility whether HMGB1 interacts with itself (aggregation) or other proteins in plasma and serum samples, non-denaturing native conditions can be employed, where HMGB1 protein is electrophoresed in its native form based on charge-to-mass ratio.
11. When using different SDS-PAGE buffer systems (e.g., different pH), the charge and SDS-binding capacities of chemically modified proteins (e.g., pre-stained molecular weight standards) might be slightly affected. Consequently, there might

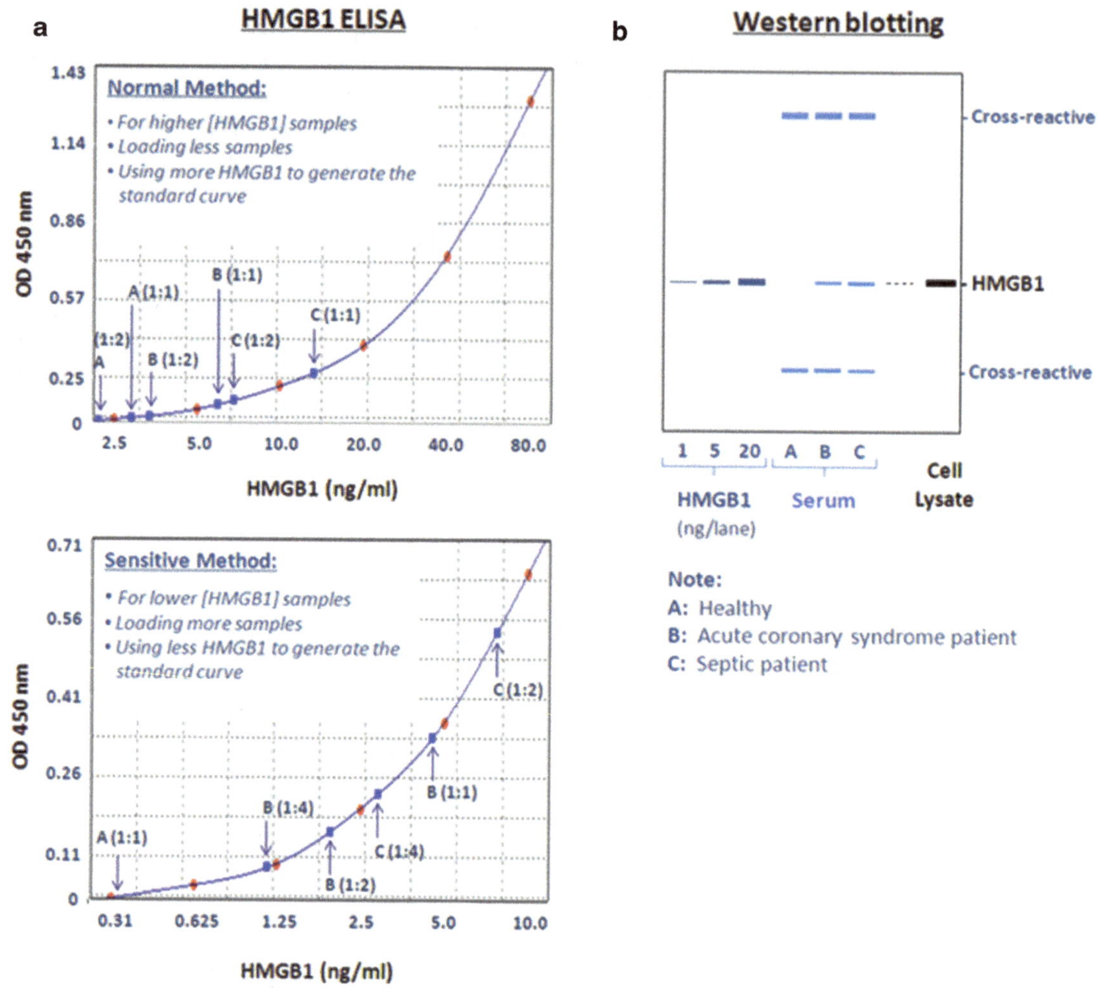

Fig. 2 Representative HMGB1 ELISA and western blotting results of human serum samples. (**a**) Measurement of human serum HMGB1 levels using the IBL International ELISA kit. As per the manufacturer's recommendation, two methods with different sensitivities were used to measure HMGB1 in human serum at various dilutions. (**b**) Measurement of human serum HMGB1 by western blotting analysis. Polyclonal antibodies were generated against recombinant HMGB1 in the authors' laboratory, and used in the western blotting analysis of human serum HMGB1 levels

be a slight deviation from the calculated molecular weight (based on the amino acid sequence). To confirm the identity of antibody-reactive band, whole-cell lysate can be used in parallel lanes as a reference size marker.

12. Several types of blotting membranes are commonly used, including nitrocellulose and PVDF membranes. Whereas nitrocellulose binds proteins better, and often gives better band signals, PVDF is more physically stronger and easy to handle. For best results, empirically determine which membrane type, manufacturer and lot is optimal for each western blotting system.

13. Many different blocking reagents are available for western blotting. Because milk contains variable amounts of endogenous biotin, it may produce higher background when using nonfat milk as a blocking reagent in the avidin/biotin systems.
14. Some systems may benefit from adding a surfactant, such as Tween® 20, to the blocking solution. Surfactants can minimize background by preventing the blocking reagent from nonspecifically binding to the target. Adding too much detergent, however, can prevent adequate blocking. Typically, a final concentration of 0.05% detergent is used; however, for best results, determine if detergents enhance a specific system and at what optimal concentrations. Always use a high-quality detergent that is low in contaminants.
15. As an alternative of the classical western blotting protocol using enzyme-conjugated secondary antibodies, direct detection using a labeled primary antibody can be tried. The direct detection takes less time and has less background signal (from the secondary antibody cross-reactivity) than a classical western blot. However, it is generally less sensitive than the indirect detection, because a labeled primary antibody cannot provide signal amplification, and occasionally loses immunoreactivity to the targeted antigen. One alternative option is biotinylating the primary antibody, which not only amplifies the signal but also eliminates the secondary antibody cross-reactivity.
16. HMGB1 is a highly conserved protein, making it difficult to generate highly reactive antibodies in many animal species. Currently, there are several commercial sources for HMGB1-reactive polyclonal or monoclonal antibodies. These antibodies normally recognize one single band on western blots of lysates of various types of cells (*see* Table 1), but their cross-reactivity with serum components remains largely unknown.
17. Based on our experience, most anti-HMGB1 antibodies tested cross-reacted with several other proteins in serum or plasma samples under denaturing conditions (*see* Fig. 2b).
18. Using highly reactive and specific polyclonal antibodies, we found that western blot often gave rise to higher values in serum HMGB1 levels as compared to commercially available HMGB1 ELISA (*see* Table 2). This observation was consistent with previous report by others that sandwich HMGB1 ELISA often gave false low or negative results as compared to western blots [21].
19. Although HMGB1 has been suggested as a feasible therapeutic target for experimental sepsis [3, 11, 34], its levels in un-fractionated crude serum of septic patients did not correlate well with their disease severity [35].

Table 2
Comparison of human serum HMGB1 levels measured by ELISA and western blotting analysis

	ELISA				
	Normal method		Sensitive method[a]		Western blotting[b]
Human serum	Dilution	[HMGB1] (ng/mL)	Dilution	[HMGB1] (ng/mL)	[HMGB1] (ng/mL)
A	1:1	ND	1:1	ND	ND
	1:2	ND	1:2	ND	
	1:4	ND	1:4	ND	
B	1:1	5.9	1:1	4.5	581
	1:2	5.7	1:2	3.3	
	1:4	8.8	1:4	4.5	
C	1:1	13.2	1:1	20.9	950
	1:2	13.5	1:2	15.3	
	1:4	13.4	1:4	11.5	

[a]The recommended sensitive method was achieved by increasing sample loading, and decreasing HMGB1 standard concentrations for the HMGB1 ELISA assay
[b]Using highly specific and reactive polyclonal antibodies generated in the authors' laboratory; ND: not detectable

20. Following ultrafiltration of serum proteins through membrane with 100 kDa cutoff, a 30 kDa HMGB1 band was detected by western blotting in both the filtrate (<100 kDa) and retentate (>100 kDa) fractions of some septic patients [1]. Interestingly, HMGB1 levels in the filtrate fraction correlated well with the outcome of sepsis [1]. It support the possibility that HMGB1 may interact with other serum components to form large (>100 kDa) complexes.
21. In addition, chemical modification may similarly affect the immuno-detection of HMGB1. For instance, a recent study indicated that reactive oxygen species (ROS) may oxidize HMGB1 to form intramolecular disulfide bond between thiol group of Cys^{106} and Cys^{23} or Cys^{45} [36]. It will be important to investigate whether oxidization affects the immuno-detection of HMGB1 in future studies.
22. We and others are still routinely using western blotting method to measure HMGB1 in serum samples [29, 37–48].

Acknowledgments

Work in the authors' laboratory was supported by grants from the National Institutes of Health (R01GM063075 and R01AT005076).

References

1. Wang H, Bloom O, Zhang M et al (1999) HMG-1 as a late mediator of endotoxin lethality in mice. Science 285:248–251
2. Bonaldi T, Talamo F, Scaffidi P et al (2003) Monocytic cells hyperacetylate chromatin protein HMGB1 to redirect it towards secretion. EMBO J 22:5551–5560
3. Lotze MT, Tracey KJ (2005) High-mobility group box 1 protein (HMGB1): nuclear weapon in the immune arsenal. Nat Rev Immunol 5:331–342
4. Ivanov S, Dragoi AM, Wang X et al (2007) A novel role for HMGB1 in TLR9-mediated inflammatory responses to CpG-DNA. Blood 110:1970–1981
5. Rendon-Mitchell B, Ochani M, Li J et al (2003) IFN-gamma induces high mobility group box 1 protein release partly through a TNF-dependent mechanism. J Immunol 170:3890–3897
6. Tang D, Shi Y, Kang R et al (2007) Hydrogen peroxide stimulates macrophages and monocytes to actively release HMGB1. J Leukoc Biol 81:741–747
7. Scaffidi P, Misteli T, Bianchi ME (2002) Release of chromatin protein HMGB1 by necrotic cells triggers inflammation. Nature 418:191–195
8. Wang H, Ward MF, Fan XG et al (2006) Potential role of high mobility group box 1 in viral infectious diseases. Viral Immunol 19:3–9
9. Zhu S, Li W, Ward MF et al (2010) High mobility group box 1 protein as a potential drug target for infection- and injury-elicited inflammation. Inflamm Allergy Drug Targets 9:60–72
10. Wang H, Ward MF, Sama AE (2009) Novel HMGB1-inhibiting therapeutic agents for experimental sepsis. Shock 32:348–357
11. Wang H, Yang H, Tracey KJ (2004) Extracellular role of HMGB1 in inflammation and sepsis. J Intern Med 255:320–331
12. Wang H, Li W, Goldstein R, Tracey KJ, Sama AE (2007) HMGB1 as a potential therapeutic target. Novartis Found Symp 280:73–85
13. Wang H, Zhu S, Zhou R et al (2008) Therapeutic potential of HMGB1-targeting agents in sepsis. Expert Rev Mol Med 10:e32
14. Kang R, Xie Y, Zhang Q et al (2017) Intracellular HMGB1 as a novel tumor suppressor of pancreatic cancer. Cell Res 27:916–932
15. Jiao Y, Wang HC, Fan SJ (2007) Growth suppression and radiosensitivity increase by HMGB1 in breast cancer. Acta Pharmacol Sin 28:1957–1967
16. Liu P, Zhao L, Loos F et al (2018) Epigenetic anticancer agents cause HMGB1 release in vivo. Oncoimmunology 7:e1431090
17. Wang L, He L, Bao G et al (2016) Ionizing radiation induces HMGB1 cytoplasmic translocation and extracellular release. Guo Ji Fang She Yi Xue He Yi Xue Za Zhi 40:91–99
18. Bald T, Quast T, Landsberg J et al (2014) Ultraviolet-radiation-induced inflammation promotes angiotropism and metastasis in melanoma. Nature 507:109–113
19. Kargi A, Demirpence O, Gunduz S et al (2016) Serum levels of HMGB1 have a diagnostic role in metastatic renal cell cancer. Cancer Biomark 17:17–20
20. Napolitano A, Antoine DJ, Pellegrini L et al (2016) HMGB1 and its hyperacetylated isoform are sensitive and specific serum biomarkers to detect asbestos exposure and to identify mesothelioma patients. Clin Cancer Res 22:3087–3096
21. Urbonaviciute V, Furnrohr BG, Weber C et al (2007) Factors masking HMGB1 in human serum and plasma. J Leukoc Biol 81:67–74
22. Sha Y, Zmijewski J, Xu Z, Abraham E (2008) HMGB1 develops enhanced proinflammatory activity by binding to cytokines. J Immunol 180:2531–2537
23. Lehner J, Wittwer C, Fersching D et al (2012) Methodological and preanalytical evaluation of an HMGB1 immunoassay. Anticancer Res 32:2059–2062
24. He RL, Zhou J, Hanson CZ et al (2009) Serum amyloid A induces G-CSF expression and neutrophilia via Toll-like receptor 2. Blood 113:429–437
25. Yasuda T, Ueda T, Takeyama Y et al (2006) Significant increase of serum high-mobility group box chromosomal protein 1 levels in patients with severe acute pancreatitis. Pancreas 33:359–363
26. Gaini S, Pedersen SS, Koldkjaer OG et al (2007) High mobility group box-1 protein in patients with suspected community-acquired infections and sepsis: a prospective study. Crit Care 11:R32
27. Okazaki K, Kondo M, Kato M et al (2008) Elevation of high-mobility group box 1 concentration in asphyxiated neonates. Neonatology 94:105–109
28. Karlsson S, Pettila V, Tenhunen J et al (2008) HMGB1 as a predictor of organ dysfunction

and outcome in patients with severe sepsis. Intensive Care Med 34(6):1046–1053

29. Rowe SM, Jackson PL, Liu G et al (2008) Potential role of high-mobility group box 1 in cystic fibrosis airway disease. Am J Respir Crit Care Med 178:822–831
30. Yoshizaki A, Komura K, Iwata Y et al (2009) Clinical significance of serum HMGB-1 and sRAGE levels in systemic sclerosis: association with disease severity. J Clin Immunol 29:180–189
31. Chung HW, Lee SG, Kim H et al (2009) Serum high mobility group box-1 (HMGB1) is closely associated with the clinical and pathologic features of gastric cancer. J Transl Med 7:38. https://doi.org/10.1186/1479-5876-7-38
32. Dupire G, Nicaise C, Gangji V, Soyfoo MS (2012) Increased serum levels of high-mobility group box 1 (HMGB1) in primary Sjogren's syndrome. Scand J Rheumatol 41:120–123
33. Lee H, Song M, Shin N et al (2012) Diagnostic significance of serum HMGB1 in colorectal carcinomas. PLoS One 7:e34318
34. Wang H, Yang H, Czura CJ, Sama AE, Tracey KJ (2001) HMGB1 as a late mediator of lethal systemic inflammation. Am J Respir Crit Care Med 164:1768–1773
35. Angus DC, Yang L, Kong L et al (2007) Circulating high-mobility group box 1 (HMGB1) concentrations are elevated in both uncomplicated pneumonia and pneumonia with severe sepsis. Crit Care Med 35:1061–1067
36. Kazama H, Ricci JE, Herndon JM et al (2008) Induction of immunological tolerance by apoptotic cells requires caspase-dependent oxidation of high-mobility group box-1 protein. Immunity 29:21–32
37. Park JS, Arcaroli J, Yum HK et al (2003) Activation of gene expression in human neutrophils by high mobility group box 1 protein. Am J Physiol Cell Physiol 284:C870–C879
38. Li W, Li J, Sama AE, Wang H (2013) Carbenoxolone blocks endotoxin-induced PKR activation and HMGB1 release. Mol Med 19:203–211
39. Li W, Li J, Ashok M et al (2007) A cardiovascular drug rescues mice from lethal sepsis by selectively attenuating a late-acting proinflammatory mediator, high mobility group box 1. J Immunol 178:3856–3864
40. Wang H, Liao H, Ochani M et al (2004) Cholinergic agonists inhibit HMGB1 release and improve survival in experimental sepsis. Nat Med 10:1216–1221
41. Li W, Zhu S, Li J et al (2011) A hepatic protein, fetuin-A, occupies a protective role in lethal systemic inflammation. PLoS One 6:e16945
42. Li W, Ashok M, Li J et al (2007) A major ingredient of green tea rescues mice from lethal sepsis partly by inhibiting HMGB1. PLoS One 2:e1153
43. Yang H, Ochani M, Li J et al (2004) Reversing established sepsis with antagonists of endogenous high-mobility group box 1. Proc Natl Acad Sci U S A 101:296–301
44. Manganelli V, Signore M, Pacini I et al (2010) Increased HMGB1 expression and release by mononuclear cells following surgical/anesthesia trauma. Crit Care 14:R197
45. Zhou Y, Xiong KL, Lin S et al (2010) Elevation of high-mobility group protein box-1 in serum correlates with severity of acute intracerebral hemorrhage. Mediat Inflamm 2010:142458. https://doi.org/10.1155/2010/142458. Epub 2010 Sep 29
46. Bruchfeld A, Wendt M, Bratt J et al (2011) High-mobility group box-1 protein (HMGB1) is increased in antineutrophilic cytoplasmatic antibody (ANCA)-associated vasculitis with renal manifestations. Mol Med 17:29–35
47. Shang GH, Jia CQ, Tian H et al (2009) Serum high mobility group box protein 1 as a clinical marker for non-small cell lung cancer. Respir Med 103:1949–1953
48. Goldstein RS, Gallowitsch-Puerta M, Yang L et al (2006) Elevated high-mobility group box 1 levels in patients with cerebral and myocardial ischemia. Shock 25:571–574

Chapter 3

Analysis of IL-22 and Th22 Cells by Flow Cytometry in Systemic Lupus Erythematosus

Zhuang Ye, Ling Zhao, Qi Gao, Yanfang Jiang, Zhenyu Jiang, and Cong-Qiu Chu

Abstract

Interleukin (IL)-22 belongs to the IL-10 family of cytokines. IL-22 exerts its biological effects via members of the cytokine receptor family class 2. CD4$^+$ T helper (Th) cells predominantly producing IL-22 have been designated as Th22 cells. IL-22/Th22 cells are functionally related to IL-17/Th17 cells, but are distinctly different. Both IL-22 and IL-17 are cytokines recruiting neutrophils in response to microbe invasion. In chronic inflammation, IL-22 mediates protective and regenerative processes, whereas IL-17 cytokines tend to induce inflammation. Studies found that increased IL-22 levels and Th22 cells in peripheral blood were associated with disease activity in patients with systemic lupus erythematosus (SLE), but decreased IL-22 and Th22 cells were also reported. Here we describe analysis of IL-22 and Th22 cells in peripheral blood quantified by flow cytometry, and correlate our findings with SLE disease activity.

Key words Interleukin-22, Th22 cells, Systemic lupus erythematosus, ELISA, Flow cytometry

1 Introduction

Interleukin (IL)-22 belongs to the IL-10 family of cytokines. Like all other members of the IL-10 family, IL-22 exerts its biological effects via members of the cytokine receptor family class 2. The cell surface IL-22 receptor (IL-22R) complex is a heterodimeric receptor consisting of IL-22R1 and IL-10R2 chains [1]. In addition to the cell surface-associated IL-22R complex, there is a secreted ("soluble"), single-chain, high-affinity IL-22-binding receptor named IL-22-binding protein (IL-22BP), which also demonstrates the features of the extracellular domain of the class 2 cytokine receptors [2–4]. IL-22BP functions as an IL-22 antagonist in vitro, while in vivo, it acts either as a cytokine carrier molecule or as a cytokine antagonist [2–4]. The primary physiological function of IL-22 is in host defense against microbes, and this function is related to IL-17 family of cytokines.

Ivana Vancurova and Yan Zhu (eds.), *Immune Mediators in Cancer: Methods and Protocols*, Methods in Molecular Biology, vol. 2108, https://doi.org/10.1007/978-1-0716-0247-8_3, © Springer Science+Business Media, LLC, part of Springer Nature 2020

In general, both IL-22 and IL-17 are known to be cytokines in the rapid response to microbe invasion by recruiting neutrophils and by inducing antimicrobial peptide production. Both IL-22 and IL-17 are produced by cells in epithelial tissues, and are thus important cytokines for host protection in mucosal membranes, such as intestinal and pulmonary defense. Like IL-17, IL-22 is produced by a variety of cell types from T cells to innate lymphoid cells [5, 6]. $CD4^+$ T helper (Th) cells producing IL-22 have been designated as Th22 cells [7, 8]. The activities mediated by IL-22 and Th22 cells have distinct features although they are often related to or overlapped with those of IL-17 and Th17 cells [5, 6]. In particular, in chronic inflammation, IL-22 appears largely protective and regenerative, whereas IL-17 cytokines are mainly involved in induction of inflammation [5, 6].

As a distinct subset of T helper cells, Th22 cells were first identified in 2009 [7, 8]. Th22 cells are characterized by abundant secretion of IL-22, but not IL-4, IL-17, or interferon (IFN)-γ [7, 8], and are important for skin homeostasis and pathology. Cytokines such as IL-13, fibroblast growth factor, and tumor necrosis factor (TNF) also can be secreted by Th22 cells, but in a very small amount [9, 10]. Th22 cells differentiate from naïve precursor $CD4^+$ T cells. TNF and IL-6 contribute to the generation of Th22 cells. Similar to Th17 cell differentiation, IL-23 is also required for Th22 cell differentiation [7, 8]. It was also demonstrated that resident Langerhans cells (LCs) and dermal dendritic cells (DCs) can induce the differentiation of Th22 cells in an IL-6- and TNF-independent way [11]. Th22 cells could be differentiated by stimulation of naïve $CD4^+$ T cells in the presence of conventional DCs and/or plasmacytoid DCs [8]. While aryl hydrocarbon receptor (AHR) was suggested as the main transcription factor of Th22 [7], basonucilin-2 (BNC-2) and FOXO4 were found to be expressed exclusively by Th22 cell clones [9], and thereby BNC-2 has been considered to be the distinct transcription factor driving Th22 cell differentiation. BNC-2 expression in combination with CD3 or CD4 expression have been used to identify Th22 cells in tissues [12, 13]. Once differentiated, the phenotype of Th22 cells remains stable over many weeks in culture and is not *skewable* into another phenotype [9]. This argues for Th22 cells being terminally differentiated effector cells. Th22 cells are characterized by the expression of chemokine receptor CCR6 and the skin-homing receptors CCR4 and CCR10 [7]. Besides the chemokine receptors mentioned above, as a subset of Th cells, Th22 cells express all typical markers of Th cells, such as CD3 and CD4 [9, 10]. Platelet-derived growth factor receptor (PDGFR) is also highly expressed on the surface of Th22 cells [9]. Chemokines that bind to CCR4, CCR6, and CCR10 are strongly expressed in the skin. This explains that numerous Th22 cells reside in tissues, but fewer circulate in the blood. Furthermore, due to the characteristic expression of these receptors, Th22 cells may be important in skin homeostasis and in the pathogenesis of skin diseases [7–9]. The frequency of Th22 cells among total IL-22-producing T cells ranges from 37% to 63%, whereas Th17 cells range from 10% to 18%, and the average frequency of Th1 cells is approximately 35% [7]. Of note, in addition to the distinct Th cell subsets, there seems to be a few "mixed" Th cells in the human blood that produce IL-17A, IFN-γ, and IL-22, and are $CCR6^+/CCR4^-/CXCR3^+$ [7, 8, 14, 15].

Systemic lupus erythematosus (SLE) is a chronic, multisystem, and multi-organ involved autoimmune disease. It usually occurs in women between adolescence and menopause age. The clinical manifestations are diverse and significantly heterogeneous. The etiology of SLE is not fully understood, but genetic and environmental factors are involved, leading to immune dysfunction at the levels of cytokines, T and B cells, DCs, and macrophages [16]. Our studies have focused on T cell responses in patients with SLE, in particular, on the activities of Th22 cells and levels of IL-22 in peripheral blood and in kidney of SLE patients with lupus nephritis. We found that the frequencies of Th22, $IL\text{-}22^+Th17$, and $IL\text{-}22^+Th1$ cells in the peripheral blood of SLE patients were significantly higher than those of healthy controls. In addition, the levels of plasma cytokines IL-22 and IL-17 were significantly increased in SLE patients. The frequencies of Th22 cells were positively correlated with the levels of plasma IL-22. Furthermore, the frequency of Th22 cells in SLE patients was positively correlated with SLE Disease Activity Index (SLEDAI) [17–19]. These results suggest that Th22 and IL-22 are involved in the pathogenesis of SLE. Data from another study suggests that Th22 cells are a better predictor of organ involvement in SLE patients compared with Th17 cells [20]. In SLE patients with skin involvement, the levels of IL-22 and Th22 cells were increased, and the proportion of Th22 cells was positively correlated with the level of plasma IL-22 [19, 20]. However, there were conflicting observations reported in earlier studies. For example, it was reported that IL-22 levels in peripheral blood of SLE patients were lower than those in normal controls [21–23], this is particularly more significant in new onset of patients with SLE [21]. Interestingly, a IL-22 gene polymorphism was found to be correlated with decreased levels of IL-22 in a Chinese population of SLE patients [23]. In contrast, a more recent study showed an increased serum IL-22 level in patients with lupus nephritis. In a murine lupus model, increased levels of IL-22 were detected in the kidney of MRL/lpr mice. Treatment with an anti-IL-22 monoclonal antibody significantly reduced proteinuria and reduced inflammatory cell infiltrate [24]. Moreover, impaired TGF-β signaling was observed in patients with active SLE and increased expression of IL-22 in the peripheral blood [25], suggesting that IL-22 is regulated by TGF-β in SLE. All these studies indicate the association of IL-22 and Th22 cells with SLE, but little is known what role of IL-22 and Th22 cells may contribute to the pathogenesis of SLE. The conflicting results may reflect the heterogeneity of SLE and/or the complex functional properties of IL-22. Furthermore, IL-22 signaling is also influenced by the presence of other cytokines, especially IL-17 and Th17 cells. Lessons learnt from host defense indicate an intimate interrelationship between IL-22/Th22 and IL-17/Th17 pathways [5, 6]. Given the fact that IL-22 and Th22 might be more involved in protection and regenerative process in host defense against infections, it is reasonable to speculate that similar effects of IL-22 and Th22 cells may also be in operation in SLE. There is no doubt that more mechanistic studies are required to provide insight for better understanding of the role of IL-22 and Th22 cells in the pathogenesis of SLE. Future studies will need to take into account the relationship of IL-22/Th22 with IL-17/Th17 in different stages of disease and disease activity. Here we share our experience in studies of IL-22 and Th22 cells in patients with SLE to assist future investigations in delineating the role of IL-22/Th22 pathways in the pathogenesis of SLE.

2 Materials

2.1 Collection of Human Plasma (See Note 1)

1. Blood collection tubes containing sodium heparin; store at room temperature.
2. Centrifuge 5180 R (Eppendorf).
3. Pipettes.

2.2 ELISA of Plasma IL-22

1. Human IL-22 Platinum ELISA kit; store at 2–8 °C.
2. 96 Test microwell plates coated with monoclonal antibody to human IL-22.
3. Biotin-conjugated monoclonal antibody to human IL-22.
4. Streptavidin-horseradish peroxidase (HRP).
5. Human IL-22 standard, lyophilized.
6. Sample diluent.
7. Assay buffer concentrate 20×: PBS with 1% Tween 20, 10% BSA.
8. Wash buffer concentrate 20×: PBS with 1% Tween 20.
9. Substrate solution: tetramethyl-benzidine.
10. Stop solution: 1 M phosphoric acid.
11. Adhesive films.

12. Pipettes.
13. Device for delivery of wash solution (multichannel wash bottle or automatic wash system).
14. Synergy HT Microplate reader (BIOTEK).

2.3 Peripheral Blood Mononuclear Cell (PBMC) Isolation

1. Blood collection tubes containing sodium heparin; store at room temperature.
2. Centrifuge 5180 R (Eppendorf).
3. Pipettes.
4. Ficoll-Paque; store at 4–30 °C.
5. Phosphate-buffered saline; store at 15–30 °C.
6. RPMI complete medium: RPMI-1640 supplemented with 10% fetal calf serum (FCS), 100 U/mL penicillin, and 100 U/mL streptomycin; store at 4 °C.
7. Hemocytometer.

2.4 Detection of Th22 Cells in PBMC by Flow Cytometry (FC)

All fluorescently labeled monoclonal antibodies are stored in dark at 4 °C.

1. FACS Aria II flow cytometer (Becton Dickinson).
2. Anti-human CD4-APC-H7 (Becton Dickinson).
3. Anti-human CD3-PerCP-Cy5.5 (Becton Dickinson).
4. Anti-human CCR4-BV510 (Becton Dickinson).
5. Anti-human CCR6-PE-Cy7 (Becton Dickinson).
6. Anti-human CXCR3-PE-CF594 (Becton Dickinson).
7. Anti-human CCR10-BB515 (Becton Dickinson).
8. Anti-human IFN-γ-FITC (Becton Dickinson).
9. Anti-human IL-17-Alexa-Flour (Becton Dickinson).
10. Anti-human IL-22-PE (R&D Systems).
11. Mouse IgG1-APC-H7 (Becton Dickinson).
12. Mouse IgG1-PerCP-Cy5.5 (Becton Dickinson).
13. Mouse IgG1-BV510 (Becton Dickinson).
14. Mouse-IgG1-PE-Cy7 (Becton Dickinson).
15. Mouse-IgG2a-BB515 (Becton Dickinson).
16. Mouse IgG1-PE-CF594 (Becton Dickinson).
17. FACS (fluorescence-activated cell sorting) buffer: PBS containing 1% BSA and 0.01% sodium azide; store at 4 °C.
18. Leukocyte Activation Cocktail with GolgiPlug (BD Pharmingen); store at −80 °C.

19. 2% Formaldehyde in PBS (*see* **Note 2**); store at 4 °C.
20. Permeabilization buffer: PBS containing 0.5% saponin and 1% BSA; store at 4 °C.

3 Methods

3.1 Quantification of IL-22 in Plasma

3.1.1 Collection of Plasma

1. Obtain blood samples by venipuncture in the morning after an overnight fasting period.
2. Store the blood samples in 10 mL sodium heparin tubes (*see* **Note 3**).
3. Centrifuge the anticoagulated blood at 513 × *g* for 5 min.
4. Collect the plasma on the top layer above the blood cells and store at −80 °C until use.

3.1.2 Preparation of Reagents

1. Wash buffer: Dilute wash buffer concentrate (20×) at a ratio of 1:20 with glass-distilled or deionized water and store at 2–25 °C for 30 days.
2. Assay buffer: Dilute assay buffer concentrate (20×) at a ratio of 1:20 with distilled water and store at 2–8 °C for 30 days.
3. Biotin-conjugated anti-human IL-22 monoclonal antibody: Make a 1:100 dilution of the concentrated biotin-conjugate solution with assay buffer (1×) in a clean plastic tube as needed (*see* **Note 4**).
4. Streptavidin-HRP: Make a 1:200 dilution of the concentrated streptavidin-HRP solution with assay buffer (1×) in a clean plastic tube as needed (*see* **Note 4**).
5. Preparation of human IL-22 standard:
   (a) Reconstitute human IL-22 standard with distilled water for 10–30 min (*see* **Note 5**).
   (b) Prepare 7 tubes.
   (c) Prepare 1:2 serial dilutions:
      - Pipette 225 μL of sample diluent into each tube.
      - Pipette 225 μL of reconstituted standard into the first tube, label as S1, and mix (concentration of standard 1 = 2000 pg/mL).
      - Pipette 225 μL of this dilution into the second tube, label S2, and mix thoroughly before the next transfer.
   (d) Repeat serial dilution five more times. The concentration of standard human IL-22 after dilution is 2000 pg/mL, 1000 pg/mL, 500 pg/mL, 250 pg/mL, 125 pg/mL, 62.50 pg/mL, 31.3 pg/mL (*see* **Note 5**).

3.1.3 ELISA Assay

1. Wash the microwell strips twice with approximately 400 μL of wash buffer per well. Leave wash buffer in wells for about 10–20 s each time. Empty wells and tap microwell strips on absorbent paper (*see* **Note 6**).
2. Add 100 μL of serial dilutions of human IL-22 into standard wells (*see* **Note 7**).
3. Add 100 μL of sample diluent in duplicate to the blank wells.
4. Add 50 μL of sample diluent and 50 μL of each sample to the sample wells (*see* **Note 7**).
5. Cover with an adhesive film, shake at 400 rpm, and incubate at room temperature for 2 h.
6. Remove adhesive film and empty wells. Wash microwell strips three times.
7. Add 100 μL of the diluted Biotin-conjugate to all wells. Cover with an adhesive film, shake at 400 rpm, and incubate at room temperature for 1 h.
8. Remove adhesive film and empty wells. Wash microwell strips three times.
9. Add 100 μL of diluted Streptavidin-HRP to all wells. Cover with an adhesive film, shake at 400 rpm, and incubate at room temperature for 1 h.
10. Remove adhesive film and empty wells. Wash microwell strips three times.
11. Pipette 100 μL of TMB Substrate solution to all wells. Incubate the microwell strips in the dark at room temperature for 10 min.
12. Add 100 μL of stop solution into each well to stop the enzyme reaction (*see* **Note 8**).
13. Read absorption wavelength at 450 nm and a reference wavelength at 570 nm; the calibrated optical density (OD) value is derived from the measured value at 450 nm minus the measured value at 570 nm.
14. Calculate IL-22 concentrations in the samples: Take the standard concentration as the ordinate, the calibrated OD value is the abscissa, and the sample concentration is calculated according to the standard curve (Fig. 1).

3.2 Detection of Th22 Cells in PBMC by FC

3.2.1 Isolation of PBMC

1. Add PBS to make up the volume of plasma, which was removed by centrifugation, and mix thoroughly.
2. Layer the whole blood over 4 mL of Ficoll-Paque in 15 mL conical polystyrene tubes (*see* **Note 9**).
3. Centrifuge tubes at 659 × *g* for 30 min with no brake at 20 °C.

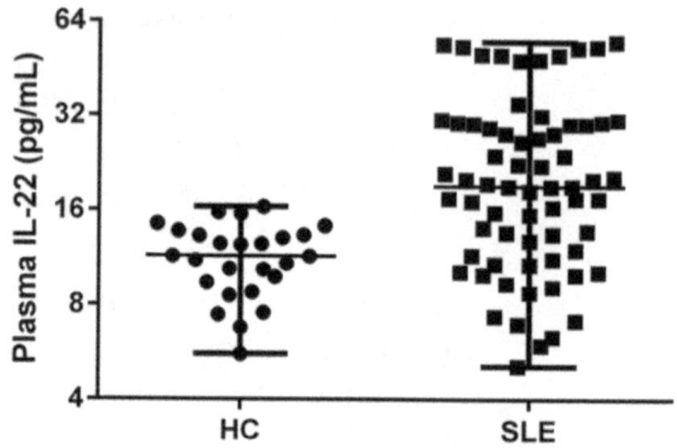

Fig. 1 Elevated IL-22 in plasma of patients with SLE. Levels of plasma IL-22 from healthy controls and patients with SLE were quantified by ELISA (modified with permission from Zhong et al., 2017, Fig. 3a [19]). *HC* healthy control, *SLE* systemic lupus erythematosus

4. Aspirate the milky white middle layer (containing PBMC) into a 15 mL tube.
5. Fill with PBS and centrifuge at 739 × *g* for 15 min to wash cells twice; discard the supernatant.
6. Resuspend the cell pellet in 400 μL of RPMI.
7. Pipette 2 μL of cell suspension into 198 μL of PBS.
8. Mix 10 μL of cell suspension in 90 μL of Trypan blue solution, and calculate cell viability using a hemocytometer.
9. Resuspend the cells at 1.0×10^7/mL for use.

3.2.2 FC Detection of Th22 Cells in PBMC

1. Pipette 200 μL of cell suspension and dispense into two wells of the incubation plate, 100 μL per well, labeled as control and detection well, respectively.
2. Add Leukocyte Activation Cocktail (including GolgiPlug) (*see* **Note 10**) to both wells, and incubate in an incubator at 37 °C in a 5% CO_2 humidified atmosphere for 4 h.
3. Aspirate the incubation plate wells as much as possible, and transfer to two tubes, labeled as a control tube and a detection tube, respectively. Mix cells with PBS, and centrifuge at 328 × *g* for 5 min; discard the supernatant.
4. Add 4 μL of antibodies (anti-CD4-APC-H7, anti-CCR6-PE-Cy7, anti-CXCR3-PE-CF594, anti- CCR4-BV510, anti-CCR10-BB515) to the detection tube, and add the corresponding isotype control antibodies to the control tube. Incubate for 30 min in the dark at 4 °C (*see* **Note 11**).
5. Wash cells by adding 500 μL of FACS buffer, resuspend the cells, and centrifuge at 228 × *g* for 5 min. Repeat once.
6. Fix cells by adding 500 μL of 2% paraformaldehyde, mix well, and incubate for at least 30 min at room temperature. Centrifuge at 513 × *g* for 5 min, and discard the supernatant.

7. Permeabilize cells by adding 500 μL of permeabilization buffer, resuspend, and incubate for at least 30 min at room temperature. Centrifuge at 513 × *g* for 5 min, and discard the supernatant.
8. Resuspend cells in 5 mL of permeabilization buffer, add 10 μL of normal mouse IgG at a final concentration of 10 μg/mL, and incubate for 10 min.
9. Add anti-IL-17A-Alexa Fluor, anti-IFN-γ-FITC, and anti-IL-22-PE, diluted in permeabilization buffer; isotope controls for each antibody to cytokines should be added in separate tubes; incubate for 30 min at room temperature.
10. Wash with 500 μL of permeabilization buffer for three times, and discard the supernatant.
11. Resuspend the cells in 300 μL of FASC buffer in a FACS tube for flow cytometry analysis (Fig. 2; *see* **Note 12**).

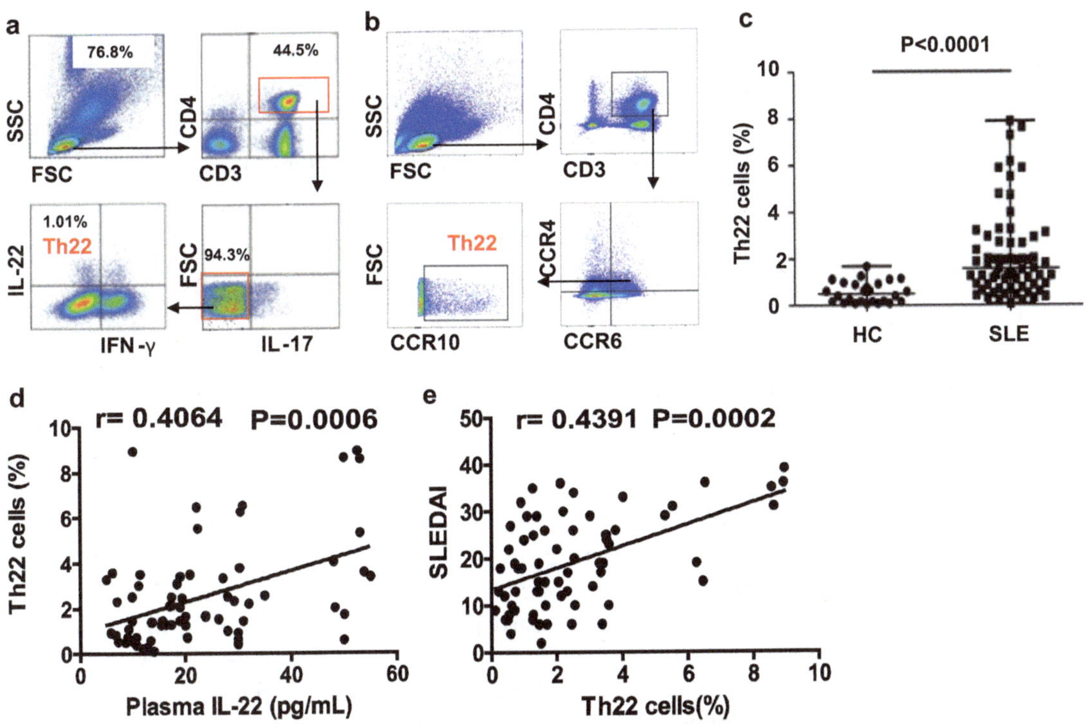

Fig. 2 Th22 cells in patients with SLE. Th22 cells in peripheral blood were identified (**a**) by intracellular staining of IL-22, and (**b**) by co-expression of CCR6, CCR4, and CCR10 (*see* **Note 11**). (**c**) An increased number of Th22 cells (identified by CCR6, CCR4, and CCR10 co-expression) is seen in SLE patients compared with that in healthy controls (modified with permission from Zhong et al., 2017, Fig. 2b [19]). (**d**) Correlation of Th22 cells with plasma IL-22 levels in patients with SLE (reproduced with permission from Zhong et al., 2017, Fig. 3e [19]; *see* **Note 13**). (**e**) Correlation of Th22 cells with SLE disease activity as measured by SLE disease activity index (SLEDAI) (reproduced with permission from Zhong et al., 2017, Fig. 4a [19]; *see* **Note 14**). *HC* healthy control, *SLE* systemic lupus erythematosus

4 Notes

1. This study was approved by the Human Ethics Committee of Jilin University.
2. Perform this procedure in a chemical fume hood. Preheat PBS to 80 °C and add paraformaldehyde slowly while PBS is being stirred. Keep stirring until paraformaldehyde is dissolved. Slowly cool solution down and store solution at 4 °C. Make fresh solution every 4–6 weeks.
3. Plasma should be separated as soon as possible the same day. The separated blood samples should be aliquoted into small aliquots as appropriate, and stored at −80 °C to avoid repeated freezing and thawing.
4. Please note that biotin-conjugate and streptavidin-HRP should be freshly prepared and used within 30 min after dilution.
5. Mix gently with the pipette to ensure complete solubilization of each diluted sample.
6. Microwell strips can be placed upside down on a wet absorbent paper for not longer than 15 min. Do not allow wells to dry.
7. Change pipette tips when you pipette 225 μL from S1 to S2. Change tips for each sample in the steps of adding samples.
8. It is recommended to add the stop solution when the highest concentration of standard has developed a dark blue color.
9. Add blood slowly along the wall of the tube. Avoid mixing the blood with the Ficoll. The interface of the blood and Ficoll is visible.
10. The Leukocyte Activation Cocktail, with BD GolgiPlug™ is a ready-to-use polyclonal cell activation mixture containing Phorbol 12-Myristate 13-Acetate (PMA), a calcium ionophore (ionomycin) and the protein transport inhibitor, brefeldin A (BD GolgiPlug™). The contents of each 100 μL vial is sufficient for treating up to 50 mL of cell cultures (at ~10^6 cells/mL); therefore one can stimulate $\geq 5 \times 10^7$ cells. This mixture represents a standard procedure for measuring cytokine production by intracellular staining. Otherwise, PMA at 50 ng/mL, ionomycin at 500 ng/mL, and brefeldin A at 10 μg/mL can be added to stimulate the cells for this purpose as described previously [26].
11. Expression of chemokines CCR6, CCR4, and CCR10 is correlated with IL-22 production by $CD4^+$ T cells and co-expression of CCR6, CCR4, and CCR10 has been used as a surrogate for Th22 cells [19].

12. The intracellular cytokine staining protocol is similar to that we described previously [26]. This can be done in combination with cell surface expression of chemokines as noted in **Note 11**.

13. IL-22 is produced by a variety of cells including Th22 cells [5, 6]. It is likely that plasma IL-22 in patients with SLE is contributed by other cell types although Th22 cells may contribute the most.

14. Systemic lupus erythematous disease activity index (SLEDAI) [27] has been developed and validated as a clinical index for the measurement of SLE disease activity, and has been used as a global measure of SLE disease activity since its introduction in 1985. It is valuable in both research and clinical settings. Here we show that the numbers of Th22 cells positively correlate with SLE disease activity as measured by SLEDAI (Fig. 2).

15. It is valuable to visualize and quantify IL-22-producing cells and Th22 cells at the site of diseased tissue. Here we show Th22 cells in kidney and skin biopsies from patients with SLE. The protocol of immunohistochemical staining is beyond the scope of this article and thereby not included, but a few points are provided. (a) The working dilutions of primary and secondary antibodies are determined by pilot experiments to optimize their concentrations. (b) After the tissue sections were fixed by formaldehyde and embedded in paraffin, some surface markers of Th22 cells, such as CCR6, could not be obtained due to technical limitations. (c) There are other methods for antigen retrieval described depending on tissues and antigens to be retrieved: https://www.rndsystems.com/resources/protocols/antigen-retrieval-methods. (d) It has been technically difficult to detect IL-22 in tissue sections. Since BNC2 is exclusively expressed by Th22 cells, but not by Th1, Th2, or Th17 cells [9], it has been used as a surrogate marker in combination with CD4 staining to identify Th22 cells in tissue sections [12, 13]. In this study, the expression of CD4 and BNC2 was used to identify Th22 cells in tissues (Figs. 3 and 4).

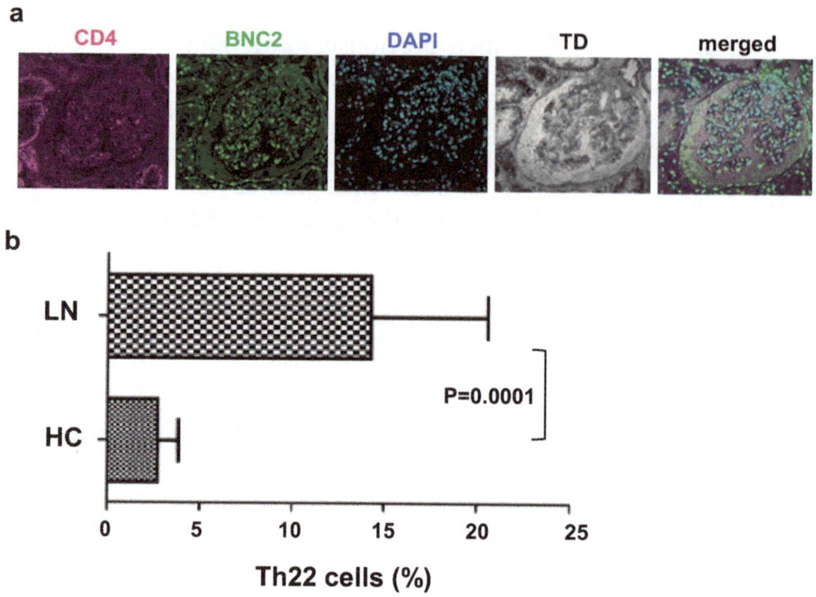

Fig. 3 Th22 cells in kidney of patients with lupus nephritis. Kidney biopsy samples from patients with lupus nephritis were stained with anti-CD4 and anti-BNC2 antibodies. (**a**) Th22 cells were identified as CD4 and BNC2 dual staining cells (*see* **Note 15**). (**b**) An increased number of Th22 cells in lupus nephritis compared with that in normal kidney. *HC* healthy control, *LN* lupus nephritis, *TD* transmitted light image

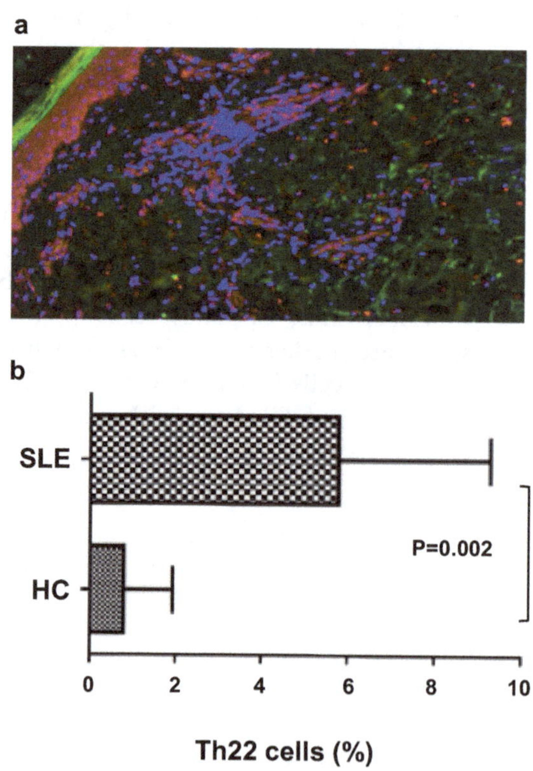

Fig. 4 Th22 cells in skin of patients with SLE. As in Fig. 3, (**a**) Th22 cells were identified as CD4 and BNC2 dual staining cells (*see* **Note 15**), and (**b**) an increased number of Th22 cells is seen in the skin of patients with SLE

Acknowledgments

This work was supported by grants from the National Natural Science Foundation of China (No. 81501343), Bethune Plan Project of Jilin University (2015410). CQC was supported by Rheumatology Research Foundation Innovative and Pilot grants.

References

1. Renauld JC (2003) Class II cytokine receptors and their ligands: key antiviral and inflammatory modulators. Nat Rev Immunol 3 (8):667–676
2. Dumoutier L, Lejeune D, Colau D, Renauld JC (2001) Cloning and characterization of IL-22 binding protein, a natural antagonist of IL-10-related T cell-derived inducible factor/ IL-22. J Immunol 166(12):7090–7095
3. Gruenberg BH, Schoenemeyer A, Weiss B, Toschi L, Kunz S, Wolk K, Asadullah K, Sabat R (2001) A novel, soluble homologue of the human IL-10 receptor with preferential expression in placenta. Genes Immun 2(6):329–334
4. Wei CC, Ho TW, Liang WG, Chen GY, Chang MS (2003) Cloning and characterization of mouse IL-22 binding protein. Genes Immun 4(3):204–211
5. Valeri M, Raffatellu M (2016) Cytokines IL-17 and IL-22 in the host response to infection. Pathog Dis 74(9):ftw111
6. McAleer JP, Kolls JK (2014) Directing traffic: IL-17 and IL-22 coordinate pulmonary immune defense. Immunol Rev 260 (1):129–144
7. Duhen T, Geiger R, Jarrossay D, Lanzavecchia A, Sallusto F (2009) Production of interleukin 22 but not interleukin 17 by a subset of human skin-homing memory T cells. Nat Immunol 10(8):857–863
8. Trifari S, Kaplan CD, Tran EH, Crellin NK, Spits H (2009) Identification of a human helper T cell population that has abundant production of interleukin 22 and is distinct from T(H)-17, T(H)1 and T(H)2 cells. Nat Immunol 10(8):864–871
9. Eyerich S, Eyerich K, Pennino D, Carbone T, Nasorri F, Pallotta S et al (2009) Th22 cells represent a distinct human T cell subset involved in epidermal immunity and remodeling. J Clin Invest 119(12):3573–3585
10. Eyerich K, Eyerich S (2015) Th22 cells in allergic disease. Allergo J Int 24(1):1–7
11. Fujita H, Nograles KE, Kikuchi T, Gonzalez J, Carucci JA, Krueger JG (2009) Human Langerhans cells induce distinct IL-22-producing CD4+ T cells lacking IL-17 production. Proc Natl Acad Sci U S A 106 (51):21795–21800
12. Moy AP, Murali M, Kroshinsky D, Duncan LM, Nazarian RM (2015) Immunologic overlap of helper T-cell subtypes 17 and 22 in erythrodermic psoriasis and atopic dermatitis. JAMA Dermatol 151(7):753–760
13. Moy AP, Murali M, Nazarian RM (2016) Identification of a Th2- and Th17-skewed immune phenotype in chronic urticaria with Th22 reduction dependent on autoimmunity and thyroid disease markers. J Cutan Pathol 43 (4):372–378
14. Volpe E, Servant N, Zollinger R, Bogiatzi SI, Hupe P, Barillot E, Soumelis V (2008) A critical function for transforming growth factor-beta, interleukin 23 and proinflammatory cytokines in driving and modulating human T(H)-17 responses. Nat Immunol 9(6):650–657
15. Acosta-Rodriguez EV, Rivino L, Geginat J, Jarrossay D, Gattorno M, Lanzavecchia A et al (2007) Surface phenotype and antigenic specificity of human interleukin 17-producing T helper memory cells. Nat Immunol 8 (6):639–646
16. Kaul A, Gordon C, Crow MK, Touma Z, Urowitz MB, van Vollenhoven R, Ruiz-Irastorza G, Hughes G (2016) Systemic lupus erythematosus. Nat Rev Dis Primers 22:16039
17. Zhao L, Jiang Z, Jiang Y, Ma N, Wang K, Zhang Y, Feng L (2013) IL-22+CD4+ T-cells in patients with active systemic lupus erythematosus. Exp Biol Med (Maywood) 238 (2):193–199
18. Zhao L, Ma H, Jiang Z, Jiang Y, Ma N (2014) Immunoregulation therapy changes the frequency of interleukin (IL)-22+ CD4+ T cells in systemic lupus erythematosus patients. Clin Exp Immunol 177(1):212–218
19. Zhong W, Jiang Y, Ma H, Wu J, Jiang Z, Zhao L (2017) Elevated levels of CCR6(+) T helper 22 cells correlate with skin and renal impairment in systemic lupus erythematosus. Sci Rep 7(1):12962

20. Yang XY, Wang HY, Zhao XY, Wang LJ, Lv QH, Wang QQ (2013) Th22, but not Th17 might be a good index to predict the tissue involvement of systemic lupus erythematosus. J Clin Immunol 33(4):767–774
21. Lin J, Yue LH, Chen WQ (2014) Decreased plasma IL-22 levels and correlations with IL-22-producing T helper cells in patients with new-onset systemic lupus erythematosus. Scand J Immunol 79(2):131–136
22. Pan HF, Zhao XF, Yuan H, Zhang WH, Li XP, Wang GH et al (2009) Decreased serum IL-22 levels in patients with systemic lupus erythematosus. Clin Chim Acta 401(1–2):179–180
23. Wang R, Zeng YL, Qin HM, Lu YL, Huang HT, Lei M et al (2018) Association of interleukin 22 gene polymorphisms and serum IL-22 level with risk of systemic lupus erythematosus in a Chinese population. Clin Exp Immunol 193(2):143–151
24. Yang X, Weng Q, Hu L, Yang L, Wang X, Xiang X, Hong B, Gong X, Wang Q (2019) Increased interleukin-22 levels in lupus nephritis and its associated with disease severity: a study in both patients and lupus-like mice model. Clin Exp Rheumatol 37(3):400–407
25. Rekik R, Smiti Khanfir M, Larbi T, Zamali I, Beldi-Ferchiou A, Kammoun O et al (2018) Impaired TGF-beta signaling in patients with active systemic lupus erythematosus is associated with an overexpression of IL-22. Cytokine 108:182–189
26. Zhao L, Chou Y, Jiang Y, Jiang Z, Chu CQ (2014) Analysis of IL-17 production by flow cytometry and ELISPOT assays. Methods Mol Biol 1172:243–256
27. Bombardier C, Gladman DD, Urowitz MB, Caron D, Chang CH (1992) Derivation of the SLEDAI. A disease activity index for lupus patients. The Committee on Prognosis Studies in SLE. Arthritis Rheum 35(6):630–640

Chapter 4

Application of Immunohistochemistry in Basic and Clinical Studies

Aihua Li and Dong-Hua Yang

Abstract

Immunohistochemistry (IHC), also known as immunohistochemical staining, is an immune morphological analysis. It is a process of selectively identifying antigens (proteins) by antibodies in cells or tissue sections. This chapter introduces the procedure and application of immunohistochemistry. Although immunohistochemistry has a vast application in basic and clinical studies, this chapter focuses on its application in biomarker study, particularly in biomarkers that related to cancer diagnosis, prognosis, and drug development. Detail protocol of immunohistochemistry in formalin-fixed and paraffin-embedded tissue sections is included.

Key words Immunohistochemistry, Immunofluorescence, Biomarkers, Diagnostics, Cancer treatment

1 Introduction

Immunohistochemistry (IHC), also known as immunohistochemical staining, is an immune morphological analysis. It is a process of selectively identifying antigens (proteins) in cells or tissue sections using antigen-antibody relationship. Immunohistochemical staining is generally known to start in 1941 [1]. However, histochemistry that utilize chemical methods for visualization of tissues or cells started much earlier when Dr. Paul Ehrlich, a German-Jewish physician scientist, published a paper about staining of animal tissue using aniline dye in 1878 [2]. Dr. Ehrlich also first used the term "antibody," in his article "Experimental Studies on Immunity," published in October 1891 [3]. The term Antikörper (the German word for antibody) appears in the conclusion of the article. Antigen and antibody binding can be traced back to 128 years ago, in doctor Emil von Behring's serum therapy of diphtheria in Marburg University, Germany, in 1890 [2]. Dr. Behring and Dr. Ehrlich worked together; they both received Nobel Prize in physiology or medicine in 1901 [4] and 1908 [5], respectively.

Ivana Vancurova and Yan Zhu (eds.), *Immune Mediators in Cancer: Methods and Protocols*, Methods in Molecular Biology, vol. 2108, https://doi.org/10.1007/978-1-0716-0247-8_4, © Springer Science+Business Media, LLC, part of Springer Nature 2020

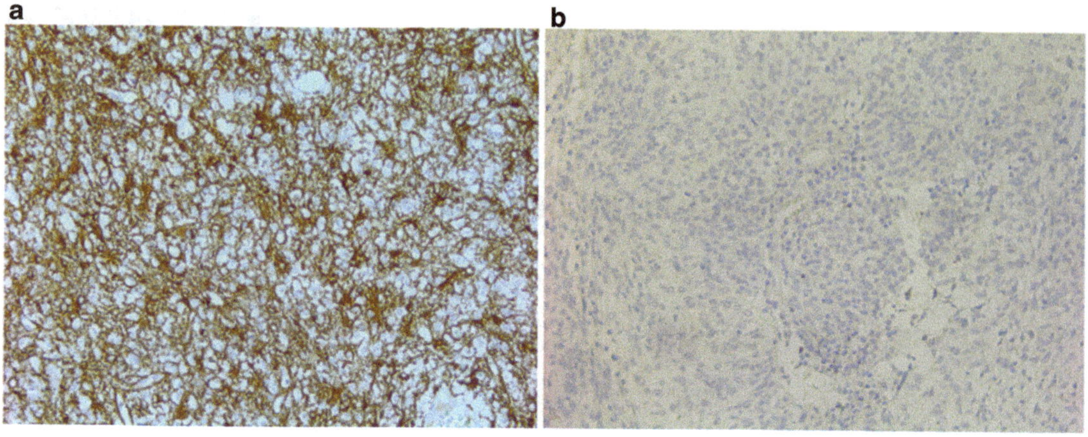

Fig. 1 Immunohistochemical staining on brain astrocytoma and non-small cell lung cancer. (**a**) GFAP positive staining in brain astrocytoma. (**b**) GFAP negative staining in lung cancer

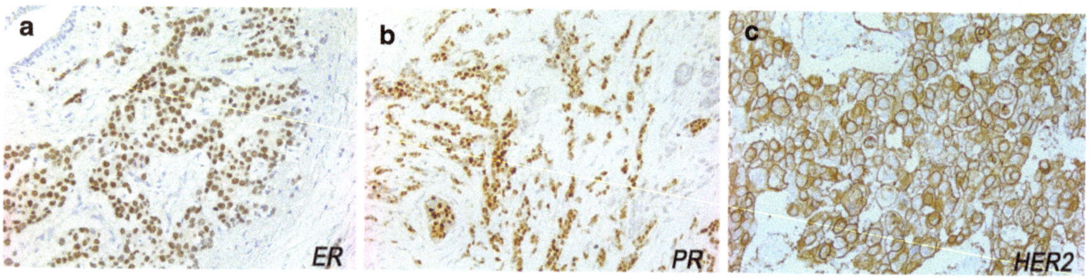

Fig. 2 Immunohistochemical staining on breast carcinoma. (**a**) Estrogen receptor positive staining in cell nucleus. (**b**) Progesterone receptor positive staining in cell nucleus. (**c**) Human epidermal growth factor receptor 2 staining in cell membrane

In the past decades, IHC has been an indispensable tool in various research, biomarker study, disease diagnostics, prognostics, theranostics, and drug development. IHC shows great benefit as a diagnostic adjunct in clinical pathology laboratories. It has been expended to become an essential component of histopathology practice especially for the diagnosis and management of cancers. From cytokeratins for diagnosis of epithelial tumors, Glial fibrillary acidic protein (GFAP) for identification of brain tumor (Fig. 1a, b), CD markers for differentiation of B-cell or T-cell lymphomas, cellular lineage biomarkers have been routinely used in clinical pathology for diagnosis, classification, and differential diagnosis of tumors. The testing of estrogen receptor (ER) alpha, progesterone receptor (PR), and human epidermal growth factor receptor 2 (HER2) using IHC (Fig. 2a–c) for guiding anticancer drug selection and prediction of treatment response, safety, and efficacy in breast cancer has brought IHC to a different level of application.

A biological marker or biomarker is defined as a substance with characteristics that can be objectively measured and evaluated as an indicator of normal biologic processes, pathogenic processes, or biological responses to a therapeutic intervention [6]. IHC is extremely helpful in biomarker studies. The unique feature that makes IHC stand out among many other protein detection methods is that it is performed with intact histologic architecture, the expression pattern of a protein molecule is visible, and thus the assessment of protein expression is possible in the context of microenvironment. Precise diagnosis and effective treatment are key to cancer management. Translational studies on discovery of biomarkers are important for prediction of the safety and effectiveness of new drugs [7–9].

In recent years, cancer diagnosis and treatment have gradually evolved into personalized medicine. Personalized medicine with targeted therapy offers great potential for cancer management. Targeted therapy is a treatment which targets the cancer's specific genes, proteins, or tissue environment that contributes to cancer growth and survival. The future of medicine is aimed at exploiting biomarkers to more precise diagnosis, prognosis, and prediction of the best strategy of cancer therapy.

IHC is a complex process. Antibody, tissue, and detection system may all cause variation in the reproducibility of immunohistochemical staining result. Pathologist and scientists have contributed much efforts in standardization of IHC from all aspects of IHC process [10–15]. College of American Pathologist recommend 10% neutral buffered formalin as fixative. Tissue must be received within 6 h after isolation and place in 10% neutral buffered formalin with a recommended fixation time of 6–72 h for ER alpha, PR, and HER2 IHC [16].

IHC has been used in basic and clinical research for more than 80 years. The application of IHC is extremely vast. We have applied IHC in our studies to elucidate the mechanism of embryogenesis [17], organ genesis and development [18–23], and tumorigenesis [24, 25]. We also used IHC to identify biomarkers in novel signaling pathways [26–35], clinical trials [36–38], and drug development [39].

The IHC detection method includes direct or indirect methods. In direct method, the primary antibody is conjugated with a label, such as fluorescein or HRP (horseradish peroxidase); in indirect method, an unconjugated primary antibody is used with a secondary antibody raised against the species of the primary antibody carries the label. The indirect method is a preferred method in IHC staining due to better signal amplification through labeled secondary antibody. Common detection labels for visualization include fluorescent labels which emit light, and enzymes which convert soluble substrates to chromogenic end products. Both chromogenic and fluorescent detection methods have unique advantages and disadvantages.

Table 1
IHC detection methods

	Advantages	Disadvantages
Enzymatic detection	• Good sensitivity—great signal amplification • Visualization by light microscope, easy review of cellular morphology and tissue structure, preferred by Pathologist • Resistant to photobleaching, can be stored for long time	• Limitation in multiplexing • Limitation in co-localization
Avidin-biotin complex (ABC)	• Good sensitivity	• Nonspecific (false positive) due to endogenous biotin activity
Labeled streptavidin biotin (LSAB)	• More sensitive than ABC method, popular in both diagnostic and research labs	• Nonspecific (false positive) due to endogenous biotin activity
Polymer	• Very sensitive • Avoid endogenous biotin background	
Tyramide signal enhancing (TSE)	• Very sensitive	• Nonspecific (false positive) due to endogenous biotin activity • Time-consuming due to more steps
Fluorescent detection	• Good for multiplexing • Good for co-localization • No substrate required for color development	• Low sensitivity • Photobleaching

Selection of detection/visualization may be based on the experimental need. Table 1 summarizes the advantages and disadvantages of various detection methods.

Immunofluorescence can be used on whole mount organs or tissues (Fig. 3a), tissue sections (Fig. 3b), or individual cultured cells (Fig. 3c), and may be used to analyze the distribution of proteins, glycans, and small biological and nonbiological molecules. Immunofluorescence can be used in combination with other, non-antibody methods of fluorescent staining, for example, use of DAPI to label DNA. The advantage of using immunofluorescence is multiplex and co-localization. More than one color can be stained in the same cells or tissues (Figs. 3 and 4).

2 Materials

1. Tissues: Formalin-fixed paraffin-embedded tissue or cells and frozen tissues or cells (*see* **Note 1**).
2. Xylene (or xylene substitute).

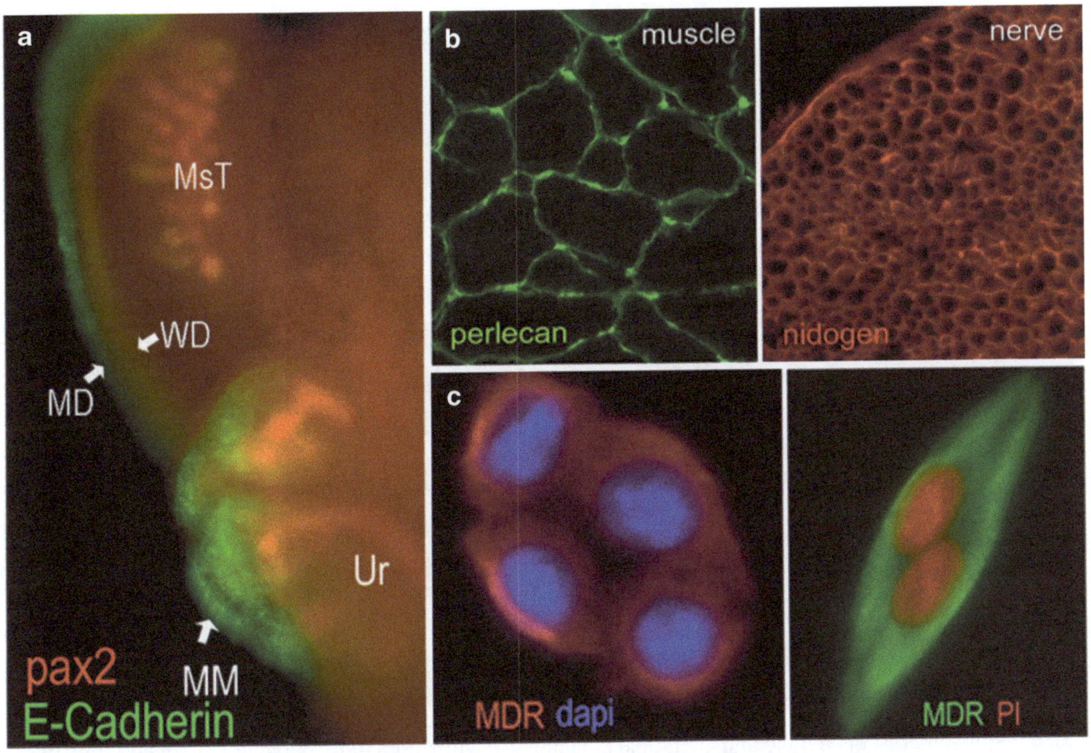

Fig. 3 Immunofluorescence single and double staining. (**a**) E-cadherin and Pax 2 staining double on developing mouse kidney. E-cadherin (red) stains the ureteric bub. Pax 2 (green) stains the mesonephrone mesenchyme. (**b**) Perlican staining (green) on muscle fibers and nidogen staining (red) on nerve fibers. (**c**) MDR staining (red or green) and DAPI (blue) or PI (red) nuclear staining on epidermoid cancer cells

3. 100%, 95%, 70%, and 50% ethanol.
4. 3% H_2O_2 solution in methanol.
5. Phosphate-buffered saline (PBS): 140 mM NaCl, 2.6 mM KCl, 2 mM Na_2HPO_4, 1.45 mM, pH 7.4.
6. Antigen retrieval buffers (*see* **Note 2**).
7. Primary antibodies (*see* **Note 3**).
8. Secondary antibodies (*see* **Note 4**).
9. Detection system: 0.05% 3,3′-Diaminobenzidine (DAB) with 0.015% H_2O_2 is used as an example (*see* **Note 5**).
10. Hematoxylin: There are various commercially available formula such as Harris Hematoxylin, Mayer's Hematoxylin, and Gill Hematoxylin.
11. Microscope (*see* **Note 6**).

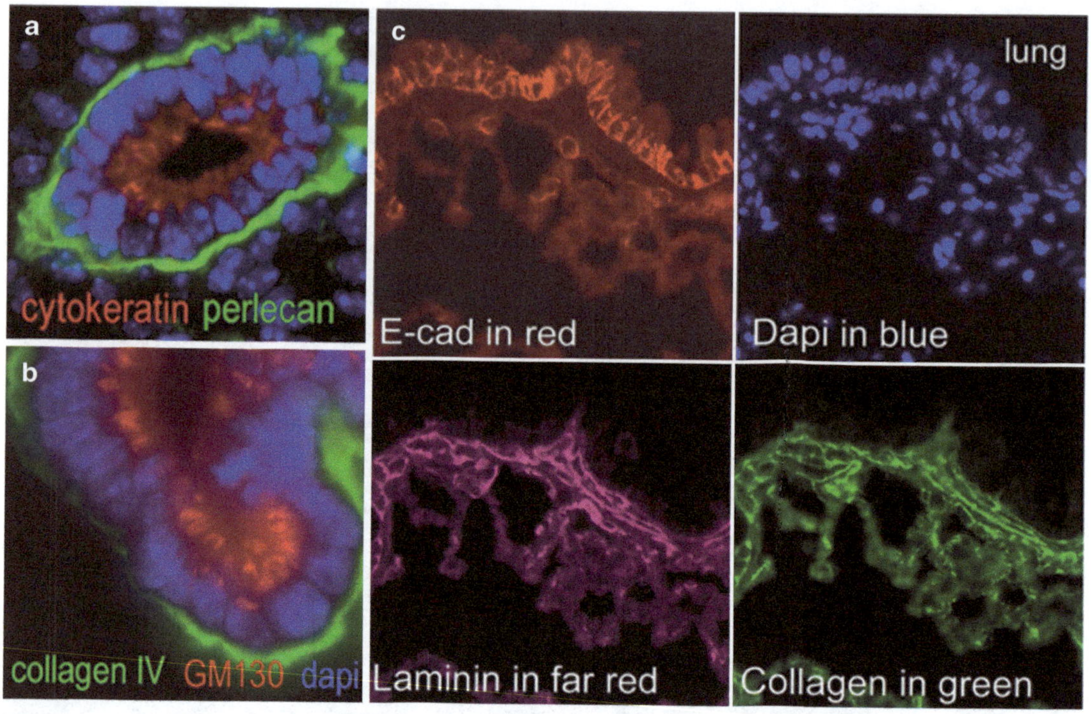

Fig. 4 Immunofluorescence triple and quadruple staining. (**a**) Cytokeratin (red), perlican (green) and DAPI (blue) staining on a kidney tubule. (**b**) GM130 (red), collagen (green) and DAPI (blue) staining on a kidney tubule. (**c**) E-cadherin (red), DAPI (blue), laminin (far red) and collagen (green) staining on a lung tissue with bronchial epithelium

3 Methods

The following steps describe a general IHC protocol using a formalin-fixed paraffin-embedded tissue section or cells. It can also apply to frozen tissues or cells.

1. Deparaffinize tissue slides in xylene (or xylene substitute) for three times, 5 min each (*see* **Note 1**).
2. Rehydrate through 100% ethanol for two times, 3 min each, then 95%, 70%, and 50% alcohols for 5 min each.
3. Rinse in distilled water.
4. Block endogenous peroxidase activity by incubation of tissue slide in 3% H_2O_2 solution in methanol for 10 min.
5. Rinse with PBS for two times, 5 min each.
6. Antigen retrieval by heating tissue slide at 92–100 °C in antigen retrieval buffer for 10–20 min or follow Manufacturer's instruction if using IHC pressure cooker. Cool the slide for 20 min at room temperature (*see* **Note 2**).
7. Rinse slides with PBS for two times, 5 min each.

8. Protein block by incubating tissue slide in 1% BSA or 5% normal serum. (This step is optional if using HRP polymer detection system).
9. Rinse slides with PBS for two times, 5 min each.
10. Dilute primary antibody in PBS with 1% BSA or blocking serum (*see* **Note 3**).
11. Apply 100 μL primary antibody on the slides and incubate in a humidified chamber (at room temperature for 1–2 h or 4 °C overnight).
12. Rinse slides with PBS for two times, 5 min each.
13. Apply 100 μL of secondary antibody on the slides and incubate in a humidified chamber at room temperature for 30 min (or follow Manufacturer's instruction).
14. Rinse slides with PBS for two times, 5 min each.
15. Apply 100 μL HRP conjugates on the slides and incubate in a humidified chamber at room temperature for 30 min (or follow Manufacturer's instruction).
16. Rinse slides with PBS for two times, 5 min each.
17. Prepare DAB substrate solution freshly with one part of 0.05% DAB and one part of 0.015% H_2O_2 (or follow Manufacturer's instruction).
18. Apply 100 μL DAB solution on slides and incubate for 1–10 min (*see* **Note 7**).
19. Rinse slides with water for two times, 5 min each.
20. Counterstain slides by immersing slides in hematoxylin for 1–2 min.
21. Rinse the slides in running tap water for 10 min.
22. Dehydrate with 70% and 95% ethanol for two times, 3 min each.
23. Dehydrate with 100% ethanol for two times, 3 min each.
24. Clear the tissue slides with xylene (or xylene substitute) for two times, 3 min each.
25. Mount slide with coverslip.
26. Visualize slide on microscope: IHC staining can be observed under a regular microscope. Fluorescent staining can be observed using a fluorescent microscope or confocal microscope.

4 Notes

1. It is recommended that fixation should be started as soon as possible, usually within 30 min of surgical removal of the tissue. Tissue fixation in 10% buffered formalin for at least 6–72 h. A 3–5 μm thickness is recommended for IHC staining of paraffin-embedded tissue, followed by tissue slide baking for 30 min at 60 °C or a few hours at 37–40 °C. Deparaffinization was generally performed by xylene in the past; it is highly recommended to use xylene substitutes like Histoclear for health and safety concerns.
2. Antigen retrieval is recommended for most antibodies [40]. The mechanism of antigen retrieval has been known to remove protein cross-links mediated by formalin fixation for better epitope exposure to antibody binding. There are two types of antigen retrieval methods, heat-induced with buffer solution at pH of 9 or 6, and enzymatic with trypsin, pepsin, or other protease. A manufacturer-recommended antibody retrieval buffer would work. Commonly used antibody retrieval buffers are as below.
   (a) Sodium Citrate Buffer (10 mM Sodium Citrate, 0.05% Tween 20, pH 6.0).
   Tri-sodium citrate (dihydrate) 2.94 g.

   Distilled water 1000 mL.

   Mix to dissolve. Adjust pH to 6.0 with 1 N HCl.

   Add 0.5 mL of Tween 20 and mix well. Store at 4 °C for long storage.

   (b) Tris-EDTA Buffer (10 mM Tris Base, 1 mM EDTA Solution, 0.05% Tween 20, pH 9.0).
   Tris 1.21 g.

   EDTA 0.37 g.

   Distilled water 1000 mL (100 mL to make 10×, 50 mL to make 20×).

   Mix to dissolve. pH is usually at 9.0.

   Add 0.5 mL of Tween 20 and mix well. Store at 4 °C for long storage.

   (c) Trypsin Stock Solution (0.5% in distilled water).
   Trypsin 50 mg.

   Distilled water 10 mL.

   Mix to dissolve. Store at −20 °C.

   • Calcium Chloride Stock Solution (1%).
   Calcium chloride 0.1 g.

Distilled water 10 mL.
Mix well and store at 4 °C.

- Trypsin Working Solution (0.05%).

Trypsin stock solution (0.5%) 1 mL.
Calcium chloride stock solution 1% 1 mL.
Distilled water 8 mL.

Adjust pH to 7.8 with 1 N NaOH. Store at 4 °C for 1 month or −20 °C for long-term storage.

Heat-induced epitope retrieval may be performed using a pressure cooker, microwave, steamer, or a water bath. The heating temperature of steamer, water bath, and microwave should be in the 92–100 °C range for a heating time of 10–20 min. Pressure cookers are capable of generating temperatures of 110–120 °C, the heating time may be 3 min depending on the manufacturer's recommended setting. The differences in temperature achieved by these devices may be compensated for by adjusting the duration of the heating period. The lower the temperature, the longer the heat time required to reach an equivalent intensity of staining observed with a higher temperature. When a microwave is used, large volume of retrieval buffer and pause of heating are recommended to avoid buffer evaporation and overheating. Cautions should be taken on higher temperature that may damage the tissue or cells and lead to loss of morphology. Due to the complexity of the IHC process, care should be taken on tissue fixation and processing. Staining process standardization and protocol optimization are highly recommended [10, 41, 42].

3. Primary antibody selection is a key to a successful experiment. Depending on experiment purpose, both monoclonal and polyclonal antibodies may be used for study. Monoclonal antibody offers the advantage of a specific epitope recognition. It is well known that rabbit monoclonal antibodies are the choice of IHC application, but some mouse monoclonal antibodies are also excellent for IHC staining. It is important to use antibody specific to target without cross reactivity. There are usually different commercially available antibodies for detection of the same protein. The first step is to look at the manufacturer's recommended application, an antibody with IHC application may be suitable. Antibody data provided by manufacturer and literature study using the same antibody (clone) gives good information on the quality of the antibody. Next, it is better to test two to three dilutions of an antibody for protocol optimization. High concentration of antibody may cause background staining or false positive result. The primary antibody raised in a species should be different from the tissue being

Table 2
Comparison of enzymatic detection and color development

Enzyme	Substrate	Color	Advantage	Disadvantage
Horseradish peroxidase (HRP)	3,3′-Diaminobenzidine (DAB)	Brown	Intense color, commonly used	• Endogenous peroxidase activity may cause nonspecific (false positive)
	3-Amino-9-ethyl carbazole (AEC)	Red	Good for co-localization/ double staining	• Endogenous peroxidase activity may cause nonspecific (false positive) • Alcohol soluble and incompatible with organic mounting media
Alkaline phosphatase (AP)	5-bromo-4-chloro-3-indoyl phosphate; Nitroblue tetrazolium (BCIP/NBT)	Blue	Good for co-localization/ double staining	Endogenous alkaline phosphatase activity may cause nonspecific (false positive)
Glucose oxidase	Nitroblue tetrazolium (NBT)	Blue	No endogenous enzyme activity	Low staining intensity

Table 3
Trouble shooting

Problem	Solution
No staining	Use positive and negative tissue control Titrate primary antibody at different dilutions Make sure to use matched second antibody (detection system)
Weak staining	Use positive and negative tissue control Titrate primary antibody at different dilutions Make sure to use matched second antibody (detection system)
Nonspecific staining	Use positive and negative tissue control Titrate primary antibody at different dilutions Contact antibody manufacturer
Background staining	Block endogenous enzyme activities using 3% hydrogen peroxide (block peroxidase) Block endogenous biotin activity using the avidin/biotin blocking reagent if use biotinylated second antibody Protein block if use biotinylated second antibody Change to use polymer based detection Keep tissue section wet without dry during staining

stained. For example, a primary antibody raised in rabbit is suitable for staining on mouse tissue, while both rabbit and mouse antibodies are suitable for staining on human tissue.

4. Commonly used dyes for detection are the following (Table 2): 3,3′-Diaminobenzidine (DAB), brown color

   3-Amino-9-ethyl carbazole (AEC), red color

5-bromo-4-chloro-3-indoyl phosphate; Nitroblue tetrazolium (BCIP/NBT), blue color

Nitroblue tetrazolium (NBT), blue color

Fluorescence (FITC, Texas Red, Alexa Flour et al.).

5. It is better to set the time of staining by observing the color change under a microscope.
6. The time of staining might vary depending on which brand of hematoxylin is used. The hematoxylin staining usually takes 1–5 min.
7. Troubleshooting for problems in IHC staining detection are summarized in Table 3.

References

1. Coons AH, Creech HJ, Jones RN (1941) Immunological properties of an antibody containing a fluorescent group. Proc Soc Exp Biol Med 47:200–202
2. Childs GV (2014) History of immunohistochemistry. In: McManus LM, Mitchell RN (eds) Pathobiology of human disease. Elsevier, San Diego, pp 3775–3796
3. Lindenmann J (1984) Origin of the terms "antibody" and "antigen". Scand J Immunol 19(4):281–285
4. The Nobel Prize in Physiology or Medicine (1901) nobelprize.org. https://www.nobelprize.org/prizes/medicine/1901/summary/
5. The Nobel Prize in Physiology or Medicine (1908) nobelprize.org. https://www.nobelprize.org/prizes/medicine/1908/summary/
6. Biomarkers Definitions Working Group (2001) Biomarkers and surrogate endpoints: preferred definitions and conceptual framework. Clin Pharmacol Ther 69(3):89–95
7. Khleif SN, Doroshow JH, Hait WN, AACR-FDA-NCI Cancer Biomarkers Collaborative (2010) AACR-FDA-NCI. Cancer biomarkers collaborative consensus report: advancing the use of biomarkers in cancer drug development. Clin Cancer Res 16:3299–3318
8. Smith NR, Womack C (2014) A matrix approach to guide IHC-based tissue biomarker development in oncology drug discovery. J Pathol 232(2):190–198
9. Howat WJ, Lewis A, Jones P et al (2014) Antibody validation of immunohistochemistry for biomarker discovery: recommendations of a consortium of academic and pharmaceutical based histopathology researchers. Methods 70 (1):34–38
10. Shi SR, Liu C, Taylor CR (2007) Standardization of immunohistochemistry for formalin-fixed, paraffin-embedded tissue sections based on the antigen-retrieval technique: from experiments to hypothesis. J Histochem Cytochem 55(2):105–109
11. Zu W, Li A, Chen T (2015) Rabbit monoclonal antibody. In: Fan L, Jeffrey P (eds) Handbook of practical immunohistochemistry: frequently asked questions, 2nd edn. Springer, New York
12. Schacht V, Kern JS (2015) Basics of immunohistochemistry. J Invest Dermatol 135:e30
13. Werner M, Chott A, Fabiano A et al (2000) Effect of formalin tissue fixation and processing on immunohistochemistry. Am J Surg Pathol 24(7):1016–1019
14. Grizzle WE (2009) Models of fixation and tissue processing. Biotech Histochem 84 (5):185–193
15. Taylor CR, Shi SR et al (1996) Comparative study of antigen retrieval heating methods: microwave, microwave and pressure cooker, autoclave, and steamer. Biotech Histochem 71 (5):263–270
16. Lott R, Tunnicliffe J, Sheppard E et al (2015) Practical guide to specimen handling in surgical pathology. College of American Pathologist, Northfield, IL
17. Yang DH, Smith ER, Roland IH, Sheng Z, He J, Martin WD, Hamilton TC, Lambeth JD, Xu XX (2002) Disabled-2 is essential for endodermal cell positioning and structural formation during mouse embryogenesis. Dev Biol 251:27–44
18. Yang DH, Kasamo H, Miyauchi M, Tsuyama S, Murata F (1996) Ontogeny of sulfated glycoconjugate producing cells in the rat fundic gland. Histochem J 28:33–43

19. Yang DH, Tsuyama S, Ge Y-B, Ohmori J, Wakamatsu D, Murata F (1997) Proliferation and migration kinetics of stem cells in the rat fundic gland. Histol Histopathol 12:717–728
20. Yang DH, Tsuyama S, Ohmori J, Hotta K, Katsuyama T, Murata F (1999) Phenotypic immunostaining of mucus-secreting cells of foregut origin. Acta Histochem Cytochem 32 (2):135–140
21. Yang DH, Tsuyama S, Murata F (2001) The expression of gastric H-K-ATPase mRNA and protein in developing rat fundic gland. Histochem J 33:159–166
22. Yang DH, Tsuyama S, Hotta K, Katsuyama T, Murata F (2000) Expression of N-acetylglucosamine residues in developing rat fundic gland cells. Histochem J 32 (3):187–193
23. Yang DH, Moss EG (2003) Temporally regulated expression of Lin-28 in diverse tissue of the developing mouse. Gene Expr Patterns 3 (6):719–726
24. Yang DH, Smith ER, Cohen C, Patriotis C, Godwin AK, Hamilton TC, Xu XX (2002) Molecular events associated with dysplastic morphological transformation and initiation of ovarian tumorigenicity. Cancer 94:2380–2392
25. Yang DH, Fazili Z, Smith ER, Cai Q, Klein-Szanto A, Cohen C, Horowitz IR, Xu XX (2006) Disabled-2 heterozygous mice are predisposed to endometrial and ovarian tumorigenesis and exhibit sex-biased embryonic lethality in a p53 null background. Am J Pathol 169:258–267
26. Yang DH, Cai KQ, Roland IH, Smith ER, Xu XX (2007) Disabled-2 is an epithelial surface positioning gene. J Biol Chem 282 (17):13114–13122
27. Yang DH, Smith ER, Cai KQ, Xu XX (2009) c-fos elimination compensates for disabled-2-requirement in mouse extraembryonic endoderm development. Dev Dyn 238(3):514–523
28. Yang DH, McKee KK, Chen ZL, Mernaugh G, Strickland S, Zent R, Yurchenco PD (2011) Renal collecting system growth and function depend upon embryonic gamma1 laminin expression. Development 138(20):4535–4544
29. Khan SA, Yang DH, Zhu F, Dubyk C, Tejani M, Cohen SJ, Hoffman JP, Burtness BA (2012) Survivin expression with resected pancreatic adenocarcinoma. Cancer Res 72 (8):714–714
30. Keller LM, Galloway TJ, Holdbrook T, Ruth K, Yang DH, Dubyk C, Flieder D, Lango MN, Mehra R, Burtness B, Ridge JA (2013) p16 status, pathologic and clinical characteristics, biomolecular signature, and long term outcomes in unknown primary carcinomas of the head and neck. Head Neck 36 (12):1677–1684
31. Mekee KK, Yang DH, Patel R, Chen ZL, Strickland S, Takagi J, Sekiguchi K, Yurchenco PD (2012) Schwann cell myelination requires integration of laminin activities. J Cell Sci 125 (Pt 19):4609–4619. https://doi.org/10.1242/jcs.107995. #equal contribution 1st author
32. Sukhanova A, Gorin A, Serebriiskii IG, Gabitova L, Zheng H, Restifo D, Egleston BL, Cunningham D, Bagnyukova T, Liu H, Nikonova A, Adams GP, Zhou Y, Yang DH, Mehra R, Burtness B, Cai KQ, Klein-Szanto A, Kratz LE, Kelley RI, Weiner LM, Herman GE, Golemis EA, Astsaturov IA (2013) Targeting C4-demethylating genes in the cholesterol pathway sensitizes cancer cells to EGFR inhibitors via increased EGFR degradation. Cancer Discov 3(1):96–111. https://doi.org/10.1158/2159-8290.CD-12-0031.
33. Gabitova L, Restifo D, Gorin A, Manocha K, Handorf E, Yang DH, Cai K, Klein-Szanto AS, Cunningham D, Kratz L, Herman G, Golemis EA, Astsaturov I (2015) Endogenous sterol metabolites regulate growth of EGFR/KRAS-dependent tumors via LXR. Cell Rep 12 (11):1927–1938. https://doi.org/10.1016/j.celrep.2015.08.023
34. Kudinov A, Deneka A, Nikonova A, Beck T, Ahn Y, Liu X, Yang DH, Golemis E, Boumber Y (2016) Musashi-2 (MSI2) supports TGF-β signaling and inhibits claudins to promote non-small cell lung cancer (NSCLC) metastasis. Proc Natl Acad Sci U S A 113 (25):6955–6960. https://doi.org/10.1073/pnas.1513616113
35. Sodani K, Patel A, Anreddy N, Singh S, Yang DH, Kathawala RJ, Kumar P, Talele TT, Chen ZS (2014) Telatinib reverses chemotherapeutic multidrug resistance mediated by ABCG2 efflux transporter *in vitro* and *in vivo*. Biochem Pharmacol 89(1):52–61
36. Mehra R, Zhu F, Yang DH, Cai KQ, Weaver J, Singh MK, Nikonova A, Golemis EA, Flieder DB, Cooper H, Lango MN, Ridge JA, Burtness B (2013) Quantification of excision repair cross complementing group 1 (ERCC1) and survival in p16-negative squamous cell head and neck cancers. Clin Cancer Res 19 (23):6633–6643
37. Egloff AM, Lee JW, Langer C, Quon H, Vaezi A, Grandis JR, Seethala RR, Wang L, Shin DM, Argiris A, Yang DH, Mehra R, Ridge JA, Patel UA, Burtness B, Forastiere AA (2014) Phase II study of cetuximab in

combination with cisplatin and radiation in unresectable, locally advanced head and neck squamous cell carcinoma: Eastern Cooperative Oncology Group trial E3303. Clin Cancer Res 20(19):5041–5051

38. Lee JW, Parameswaran J, Sandoval-Schaefer T, Eoh KJ, Yang DH, Zhu F, Mehra R, Sharma R, Gaffney SG, Perry EB, Townsend JP, Serebriiskii IG, Golemis EA, Issaeva N, Yarbrough WG, Koo JS, Burtness BA (2019) Combined Aurora kinase A (AURKA) and WEE1 inhibition demonstrates synergistic antitumor effect in squamous cell carcinoma of the head and neck. Clin Cancer Res 25(11):3430–3442
39. Xu S, Yao H, Luo S, Zhang YK, Yang DH, Li D, Wang G, Hu M, Yao H*, Wu X, Chen ZS, Xu J. (2017) A potent anticancer optimized from natural oridonin scaffold induces apoptosis and cell cycle arrest through the mitochondrial pathway, J Med Chem, 60 (4):1449-1468. doi: https://doi.org/10.1021/acs.jmedchem.6b01652
40. Pileri SA, Roncador G et al (1997) Antigen retrieval techniques in immunohistochemistry: a comparison of different methods. J Pathol 183(1):116–123
41. O'Leary TJ (2001) Standardization in immunohistochemistry. Appl Immunohistochem Mol Morphol 9(1):3–8
42. Lin F, Chen Z (2014) Standardization of diagnostic immunohistochemistry: literature review and geisinger experience. Arch Pathol Lab Med 138(12):1564–1577

Chapter 5

Interleukin-1 (IL-1) Immunohistochemistry Assay in Oral Squamous Cell Carcinoma

Takaaki Kamatani

Abstract

This section describes an immunohistochemistry method to analyze interleukin-1 (IL-1) in oral squamous cell carcinoma. The described protocol has been optimized for IL-1 detection in formalin-fixed, paraffin-embedded oral tissue sections by light microscopy. A few common pitfalls and problems associated with immunohistochemical staining are discussed.

Key words Immunohistochemistry, Interleukin-1, Oral squamous cell carcinoma, Formalin fixation, Paraffin embedding

1 Introduction

The interleukin-1 (IL-1) family comprises 11 cytokines, which play an important role in the regulation of immune and inflammatory responses [1]. The IL-1 family has a conserved beta-trefoil structure [2] that binds to the receptors belonging to the IL-1 receptor family [3]. The discovery of the cytokines began with studies on the pathogenesis of fever [4]. The basis of the term interleukin was to categorize the growing number of biological properties attributed to the soluble factors released from macrophages and lymphocytes. The cells of oral squamous cell carcinoma also express the IL-1 [5]. IL-1-alpha and IL-1-beta have been the focus of many studies [6], because they were the first to be discovered. IL-1-alpha and IL-1-beta bind to the same receptor molecule, which is called the type I IL-1 receptor [3].

Immunohistochemistry (IHC) is an immunoassay that is used to determine the localization of antigens in tissue sections using labeled antibodies as specific reagents for interaction with antigens; this reaction is visualized using markers, such as fluorescent dyes, enzymes, radioactive elements, or colloidal gold [7]. This assay was first developed in the year 1941 [8]. With the expansion and

Ivana Vancurova and Yan Zhu (eds.), *Immune Mediators in Cancer: Methods and Protocols*, Methods in Molecular Biology, vol. 2108, https://doi.org/10.1007/978-1-0716-0247-8_5, © Springer Science+Business Media, LLC, part of Springer Nature 2020

development of the immunohistochemistry technique, enzyme labels have been introduced, such as peroxidase and alkaline phosphatase [9]. The diaminobenzidine (DAB) molecule has been also developed for IHC during the same period [10]. Since immunohistochemistry involves a specific antigen-antibody reaction, it has an apparent advantage over the traditionally used enzyme-staining techniques, which identify only a limited number of proteins, enzymes, and tissue structures [11]. This is especially useful for assessing the progression and treatment of diseases. In basic research, this technique is also used for determining the localization and distribution of biomarkers within tissues. The selection of a suitable method from among the numerous immunohistochemistry methods that are available for determining antigen localization should be based on parameters, such as the type of specimen under investigation and the degree of sensitivity required.

2 Materials

1. 10% Neutral-Buffered Formalin (NBF): Add 6.5 g anhydrous di-sodium hydrogen phosphate (Na_2HPO_4), 4.0 g sodium di-hydrogen phosphate, monohydrate ($NaH_2PO_4{\cdot}H_2O$), and 100 mL of 37% formaldehyde solution to 900 mL of double distilled water. Adjust pH to 7.0 with 1 N NaOH or 1 M HCl. Adjust volume to 1000 mL. Store at 4 °C (*see* **Note 1**).
2. 10× Tris-Buffered Saline (10× TBS): Add 24.2 g Trizma base and 80 g NaCl to 900 mL of double distilled water. Adjust pH to 7.6 with concentrated HCl. Adjust volume to 1000 mL.
3. TBS with 0.05% Tween 20 (TBST): Add 100 mL of 10× TBS and 0.5 mL of Tween 20 to 900 mL of double distilled water. Adjust volume to 1000 mL.
4. Phosphate-Buffered Saline (PBS): Add 8 g NaCl, 0.2 g KCl, 1.44 g anhydrous disodium hydrogen phosphate (Na_2HPO_4), and 0.24 g potassium phosphate monobasic anhydrous (KH_2PO_4) to 900 mL of double distilled water. Adjust volume to 1000 mL.
5. Sodium Citrate Buffer: Add 2.9 g trisodium citrate dehydrate to 900 mL of double distilled water. Adjust pH to 6.0 with 1 M HCl. Add 0.5 mL of Tween 20. Adjust volume to 1000 mL. Store at room temperature, or at 4 °C for storing longer than 3 months.
6. 3% Hydrogen Peroxide: Add 10 mL of 30% H_2O_2 to 90 mL of double distilled water.
7. 1% DAB: Add 0.1 g of DAB to 10 mL of double distilled water. Add three to five drops (1 drop = 50 μL) of 10 N HCl; the solution turns light brown color. Shake for 10 min to dissolve DAB. Aliquot and store at −20 °C.

8. 0.3% H_2O_2: Add 1 mL of 30% H_2O_2 to 99 mL of double distilled water. Mix well. Store at 4 °C, or aliquot and store at −20 °C.
9. DAB Working Solution: Add 250 μL of 1% DAB to 5 mL of PBS, pH 7.2, and mix well. Add 250 μL of 0.3% H_2O_2 and mix well. Use the solution within 30 min after preparation (*see* **Note 2**).
10. Ethanol: anhydrous denatured, histological grade (100%, 95%, 80%, and 70%).
11. Xylene.

3 Methods

3.1 Tissue Fixation and Preparation

To ensure the preservation of tissue architecture and cell morphology, prompt and adequate fixation is essential. Inappropriate or prolonged fixation may significantly diminish the antibody binding capability (*see* **Note 3**). There is no one universal fixation that is ideal for the demonstration of all antigens. However, in general, many antigens can be successfully demonstrated in formalin-fixed, paraffin-embedded tissue sections with the use of antigen retrieval techniques (*see* **Note 4**). Tissues should be fixed by adding directly to the 10% NBF for at least 24 h. NBF has a very slow diffusion coefficient, so the tissue needs to be no more than 1 cm thick (*see* **Note 5**) (Fig. 1).

1. Prepare 3–5 μm sections using the microtome and place on clean, positively charged microscope slides (*see* **Note 6**).
2. Heat the slides on tissue drying oven at 60 °C overnight. Paraffin wax is the most widely used embedding medium for diagnostic histopathology in routine histological laboratories. This procedure makes the tissue to adhere better to the slides.

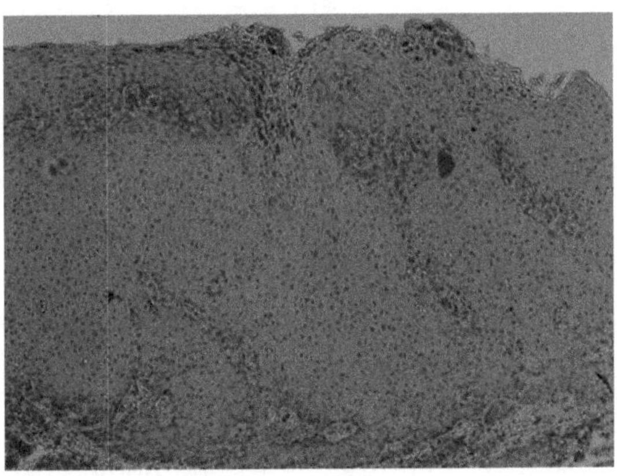

Fig. 1 Immunohistochemical staining of IL-1β in paraffin-embedded early-stage squamous cell carcinoma of the tongue tissue sections

3. For deparaffinization, incubate slides three times in xylene for 3 min each, followed by 3 min incubation in 100% ethanol, 3 min incubation in 95% ethanol, 3 min incubation in 80% ethanol, and 3 min incubation in 50% ethanol (*see* **Note 7**).
4. Wash slides two times in PBS for 5 min each.
5. Keep the slides in PBS until ready to perform antigen retrieval (*see* **Note 8**).

3.2 Antigen Retrieval

The demonstration of many antigens can be significantly improved by a pretreatment with antigen retrieval reagent that breaks the protein cross-links formed by formalin fixation, and thereby uncovers hidden antigenic sites. There are several methods of antigen retrieval. The techniques involved the application of heat for varying lengths of time to formalin-fixed, paraffin-embedded tissue sections in an aqueous solution. The most common method is the heat-mediated retrieval in sodium citrate buffer using microwave; we use this method for IL-1 IHC assay in oral squamous cell carcinoma.

1. Add 10 mM sodium citrate buffer to the microwaveable vessel, and place inside the microwave.
2. Heat slides in 10 mM sodium citrate buffer, pH 6.0 at 95–100 °C for 20 min.
3. Remove the slides from the microwave, and let stand at room temperature in buffer for 20 min.
4. Rinse in TBST for 1 min.
5. If using a domestic microwave, set to full power (*see* **Note 9**).

3.3 Blocking

Background staining may be specific or nonspecific. The main cause of nonspecific background staining is non-immunological binding of the specific immune sera by hydrophobic and electrostatic forces to certain sites within tissue sections. This form of background staining is usually uniform and can be reduced by blocking those sites with normal serum. Endogenous peroxidase activity is found in many tissues, and can be detected by reacting fixed tissue sections with DAB substrate. The solution for eliminating endogenous peroxidase activity is by the pretreatment of the tissue section with hydrogen peroxide prior to incubation with primary antibody (*see* **Note 10**).

1. Wash slides in 3% hydrogen peroxide in methanol for 10 min.
2. Wash sections twice in PBS for 5 min each.

3.4 Immunohistochemical Staining

Special controls must be run in order to validate the specificity of the antibody used. A positive tissue control is recommended to ensure that the antibody is performing as expected. It may also be useful to include a negative tissue control in which the protein of interest is absent.

1. Apply 100 μL of primary IL-1 antibody at recommended concentration diluted in TBS per slide. Incubate 60 min at room temperature or overnight at 4 °C (*see* **Notes 11–15**).
2. Wash slides in TBST four times for 5 min each.
3. Apply 100 μL of conjugated secondary antibody diluted in TBST per slide. Incubate for 30 min at room temperature in a moisture chamber.
4. Wash slides in TBST four times for 5 min each.
5. Apply DAB substrate solution. Incubate sections for 1–3 min at room temperature. Adjust the reaction time by microscopic observation.
6. Wash slides with distilled water at room temperature for 5 min.
7. Apply color development (i.e., hematoxylin) for 10 s.
8. Wash slides in distilled water for 1 min.

3.5 Mounting Slides

1. Wash slides two times in 80% ethanol for 1 min each.
2. Wash slides two times in 95% ethanol for 1 min each.
3. Wash slides three times in 100% ethanol for 1 min each.
4. Wash slides three times in xylene for 1 min each.
5. Apply coverslip with sealants.

4 Notes

1. Formaldehyde, a gas highly soluble in water, is typically sold as a saturated aqueous solution of 37% by mass. This is also referred to as "100% formalin." 10% Neutral-buffered formalin is the tenfold dilution of this solution, giving a final 3.7% concentration of formaldehyde.
2. The pH value is important; pH < 7.0 will reduce staining intensity, while pH >7.6 will cause background staining.
3. Inadequate or delayed fixation may give rise to false positive results due to the passive uptake of serum protein and diffusion of the antigen. Such false positives are common in the center of large tissue blocks or throughout tissues when fixation was delayed.
4. Certain cell antigens do not survive routine fixation and paraffin embedding. Thus, the use of frozen sections still remains essential for the demonstration of many antigens. However, the disadvantage of frozen section includes poor morphology, poor resolution at higher magnifications, special storage needs, limited retrospective studies, and cutting difficulty. IL-1 can be successfully detected in formalin-fixed paraffin-embedded oral tissue sections.

5. Delayed or inadequate fixation can cause no staining because antigen is denatured or masked during fixing process. Use less-potent fixative and decrease the fixing time.
6. Tissue sections are best mounted on positively charged- or APES (amino-propyl-tri-ethoxy-silane)-coated slides. Otherwise, tissue sections may come off from the slides.
7. Incomplete removal of paraffin can cause poor staining of the section. Remove paraffin thoroughly from the section.
8. Do not allow tissues to dry at any time during the staining procedure. Drying out will cause nonspecific antibody binding and therefore a high background staining.
9. Twenty minutes is only a suggested antigen retrieval time. Less than 20 min may leave the antigens under-retrieved, leading to a weak staining. More than 20 min may leave antigens over-retrieved, leading to a nonspecific background staining, and also increasing the chance of sections dissociating from the slides.
10. Endogenous biotin contained in some cells or tissues is a common cause of excessive background staining.
11. Antibodies, especially polyclonal antibodies, are sometimes contaminated with other antibodies due to impure antigen used to immunize the host animal.
12. Dilutions of the primary and secondary antibody are listed on the datasheets or are determined by testing a range. Adjust dilutions appropriately from the testing results obtained.
13. Inadequate incubation with antibody may cause no staining or only weak staining results. Provide sufficient time for reaction with antibody. In particular, primary antibodies should be applied for longer times.
14. A high room temperature can cause nonspecific staining due to accelerated enzyme reactions. Keep room temperature at 15–25 °C.
15. A shallow, plastic box with a sealed lid and a wet tissue paper at the bottom is an adequate chamber.

References

1. Jensen LE (2010) Targeting the IL-1 family members in skin inflammation. Curr Opin Investig Drugs 11:1211–1220
2. Murzin AG, Lesk AM, Chothia C (1992) beta-Trefoil fold. Patterns of structure and sequence in the Kunitz inhibitors interleukins-1 beta and 1 alpha and fibroblast growth factors. J Mol Biol 223:531–543
3. Sims JE, Gayle MA, Slack JL et al (1993) Interleukin 1 signaling occurs exclusively via the type I receptor. Proc Natl Acad Sci U S A 90:6155–6159
4. Dinarello CA (1994) The interleukin-1 family: 10 years of discovery. FASEB J 8:1314–1325
5. Kamatani T, Shiogama S, Yoshihama Y et al (2013) Interleukin-1 beta in unstimulated whole saliva is a potential biomarker for oral

squamous cell carcinoma. Cytokine 64:497–502

6. March CJ, Mosley B, Larsen A et al (1985) Cloning, sequence and expression of two distinct human interleukin-1 complementary DNAs. Nature 315:641–647
7. Matos LL, Trufelli DC, de Matos MG et al (2010) Immunohistochemistry as an important tool in biomarkers detection and clinical practice. Biomark Insights 5:9–20
8. Coons AH, Creech HJ, Jones RN (1941) Immunological properties of an antibody containing a fluorescent group. Exp Biol Med 47:200–202
9. Mason DY, Sammons R (1978) Alkaline phosphatase and peroxidase for double immunoenzymatic labeling of cellular constituents. J Clin Pathol 31:454–460
10. Vacca LL, Hewett D, Woodson G (1978) A comparison of methods using diaminobenzidine (DAB) to localize peroxidases in erythrocytes, neutrophils, and peroxidase-antiperoxidase complex. Stain Technol 53:331–336
11. Leong AS, Wright J (1987) The contribution of immunohistochemical staining in tumour diagnosis. Histopathology 11:1295–1305

Chapter 6

Luminex xMAP Assay to Quantify Cytokines in Cancer Patient Serum

Helena Kupcova Skalnikova, Katerina Vodickova Kepkova, and Petr Vodicka

Abstract

Cytokines, chemokines, and growth factors are key mediators of cell proliferation, migration, and immune response, and in tumor microenvironment, such factors contribute to regulation of tumor growth, immune cell recruitment, angiogenesis, and metastasis. In body fluids, levels of inflammatory mediators reflect the patient immune response to the disease and may predict the effects of targeted therapies. Significant improvements in cytokine detection techniques have been made during last 10 years leading to sensitive quantification of such potent molecules present in low pg/mL levels. Among the techniques, Luminex xMAP® multiplex assays allow for simultaneous quantification of up to 100 analytes with high sensitivity, broad dynamic range of quantification, high throughput, and minimal sample requirements. In this chapter we describe a detailed protocol for the application of xMAP assays using Luminex® 200™ analyzer with xPonent® acquisition software to quantify cytokines, chemokines, and growth factors secreted to blood serum and plasma of cancer patients. We also discuss how sample preparation, instrument settings, and standard curve fitting algorithms can influence validity of obtained results. Special attention is paid to data analysis using open source R statistical environment and we provide an example dataset of cytokine levels measured in serum and corresponding R script for standard curve fitting and concentration estimates.

Key words Luminex 200, xPonent software, Multiplex xMAP assays, Serum, Plasma, Cytokine, Cancer, R Bioconductor, drLumi, nCal

1 Introduction

Cytokines, chemokines, and growth factors are key mediators of cell proliferation, migration, and immune response. In cancer, cytokine regulatory networks participate in all stages of tumor development, including initialization and promotion, recruitment of inflammatory cells, promotion of cancer-related inflammation, angiogenesis, malignant cell invasiveness, and metastasis formation

---

Electronic supplementary material: The online version of this chapter (https://doi.org/10.1007/978-1-0716-0247-8_6) contains supplementary material, which is available to authorized users.

Ivana Vancurova and Yan Zhu (eds.), *Immune Mediators in Cancer: Methods and Protocols*, Methods in Molecular Biology, vol. 2108, https://doi.org/10.1007/978-1-0716-0247-8_6, © Springer Science+Business Media, LLC, part of Springer Nature 2020

[1, 2]. Not only intrinsic transformed cells and tumor-infiltrating immune cells, but also cancer-associated fibroblasts (CAFs) and other cell types produce autocrine and paracrine mediators and such complex interactions in tumor microenvironment have a pivotal role in regulation of cancer progress [3, 4]. Beside the local paracrine effects, inflammatory molecules are transported via blood or lymph vessels, influencing the whole organism. Blood cytokine levels may reflect the patient immune response to the disease and facilitate prediction of the treatment response, particularly to recently developed targeted therapies.

Significant improvements in cytokine detection techniques have been made during last 10 years leading to sensitive quantification of such potent molecules present in low pg/mL levels [5]. Most of the methods are antibody based and represent advanced variations of basic sandwich ELISA principle, usually in planar array or microbead assay multiplexed format [6]. Among such techniques, electrochemiluminescence-based planar assays (Meso Scale Discovery) and microbead-based xMAP immunoassays with fluorescence detection (Bio-Rad, Thermo Fisher, Merck, etc.) are favorable due to high sensitivity, broad dynamic range of quantification, high throughput, and minimal requirements for sample amounts [7, 8]. While Meso Scale Discovery platform might have slight edge in total dynamic range and seems to be less affected by matrix (serum, plasma) interference [8], it provides limited multiplexing of maximum ten spots per well. This means that for biomarker discovery projects, where screening of large set of analytes is required, kits must be split into multiple plates (e.g., V-PLEX Human Biomarker 54-Plex Kit, #K15248D-1 consist of 7 96-well plates), resulting in higher sample amount demands.

Multiplex xMAP assays (Fig. 1) are based on incubation of sample with fluorescent microbeads coated by capture antibodies, where each distinct capture antibody is conjugated to beads with unique spectral address. Combination of precise doses of 2 fluorophores inside the beads allows theoretically multiplexing of up to 100 individual analytes in one assay. Up to 80 analyte multiplexed

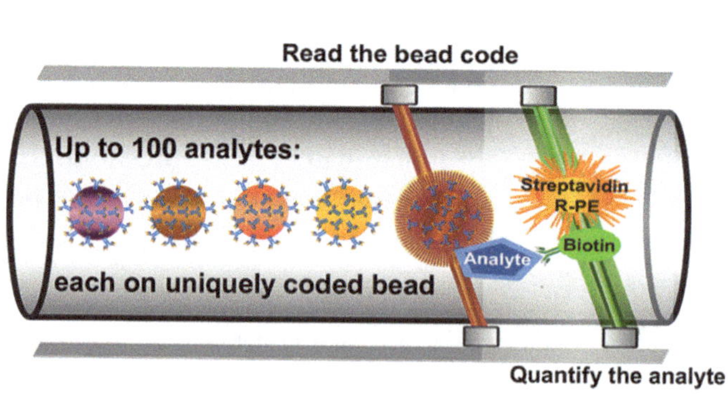

Fig. 1 Principle of xMAP assay

kits are commercially available (e.g., Immune Monitoring 65-Plex Human ProcartaPlex™ Panel, EPX650-10065-901). Moreover, up to 500 distinct bead spectral addresses may be distinguished by FlexMAP 3D Luminex platform incorporating three different fluorophores to the beads. All the beads with individual analytes are incubated in one well of 96-well plate with one aliquot of the sample. After washing out of the sample, biotinylated detection antibodies are added to the beads with captured analyte, followed by fluorescently labeled streptavidin (streptavidin-phycoerythrin conjugate). The beads with attached immunocomplexes are then read in Luminex analyzer, where fluorescent signal of the bead identifies an analyte and phycoerythrin fluorescence determines the quantity of the analyte. Both commercial multiplexed kits and in-house developed custom assays are possible to run on the Luminex platforms.

This chapter focuses on the application of Luminex xMAP assays using Luminex 200 analyzer with xPonent acquisition software to quantify cytokines, chemokines, and growth factors secreted to blood serum and plasma. We discuss how sample preparation, instruments settings, and standard curve fitting algorithms can influence validity of obtained results. Special attention is paid to data analysis using open source R statistical environment. We also provide example dataset of cytokine levels measured in serum of patients with malignant melanoma and corresponding R script for standard curve fitting and concentration estimates.

2 Materials

2.1 Luminex Analysis

1. Material for blood collection.
2. Analyzer Luminex® 200™.
3. Luminex 200 Calibration kit and Performance Verification kit.
4. Luminex Sheath Fluid.
5. Human cytokine multiplex magnetic kits containing assay diluent, beads with capture antibodies, biotinylated detection antibodies, streptavidin-phycoerythrin conjugate, cytokine standard mix, wash buffer, 96-well flat-bottom plate.
6. Refrigerated centrifuge with fixed angle rotor for microtubes, up to 16,000 × *g* at 4 °C.
7. Sonicating water bath.
8. Orbital 96-well plate shaker.
9. Handheld magnetic 96-well separator.
10. Calibrated adjustable 10 μL to 25 mL precision pipets with tips (200 μL multichannel pipet and electronic repetitive pipet is advantageous, e.g., Gilson Repetman).

2.2 Software

1. xPonent® software (description of procedures in protocol based on version 3.1) installed on acquisition computer connected to Luminex® 200™.
2. R interactive statistical programming environment [9].
3. Tidyverse set of packages (tidyverse) for data manipulation and graphing [10].
4. Cowplot package for publication ready graphical outputs from R [11].
5. Packages specific for reading multiplex data exported from xPonent—drLumi [12, 13] and standard curve fitting—drLumi [12, 13] and nCal [14, 15].
6. RStudio (RStudio)—not necessary, but useful, IDE (Integrated development environment) for R, provides syntax highlighting for R scripts, autocompletion and interactive R console as well as support for viewing and saving graphics and imported datasets [16].

3 Methods

3.1 Sample Collection and Processing (Fig. 2)

3.1.1 Preparation of Blood Serum

1. Collect 5–10 mL of blood and let to clot for 30 min at room temperature (*see* s **1** and **2**).
2. Centrifuge for 10 min at 1500 × g at 4 °C.
3. Transfer supernatant into a clean tube and centrifuge for an additional 10 min at 1500 × g and 4 °C.
4. Collect the supernatant into a new tube, aliquot (e.g., 250 μL aliquots) into polypropylene tubes, and store at −80 °C (*see* **Notes 3–5**).

3.1.2 Preparation of Blood Plasma

1. Collect 5–10 mL of blood with EDTA, citrate, or heparin used as an anticoagulant (*see* **Notes 1** and **2**).
2. Centrifuge for 10 min at 1500 × g at 4 °C.
3. Transfer supernatant into a clean tube and centrifuge for an additional 10 min at 1500 × g and 4 °C.
4. Collect the supernatant into a new tube, mix and aliquot (e.g., 250 μL aliquots) into polypropylene tubes and store at −80 °C (*see* **Notes 3–5**).

3.2 Preparation of Luminex System

1. Turn on the Luminex instrument, XY platform and sheath fluid delivery system. Allow the lasers warm up for 30 min (*see* **Note 6**).
2. Adjust needle height according to the plate type used. Wash the instrument with 70% ethanol or isopropanol to remove bubbles, followed by two water washes using commands in the Maintenance menu of the xPonent software (*see* **Note 7**).

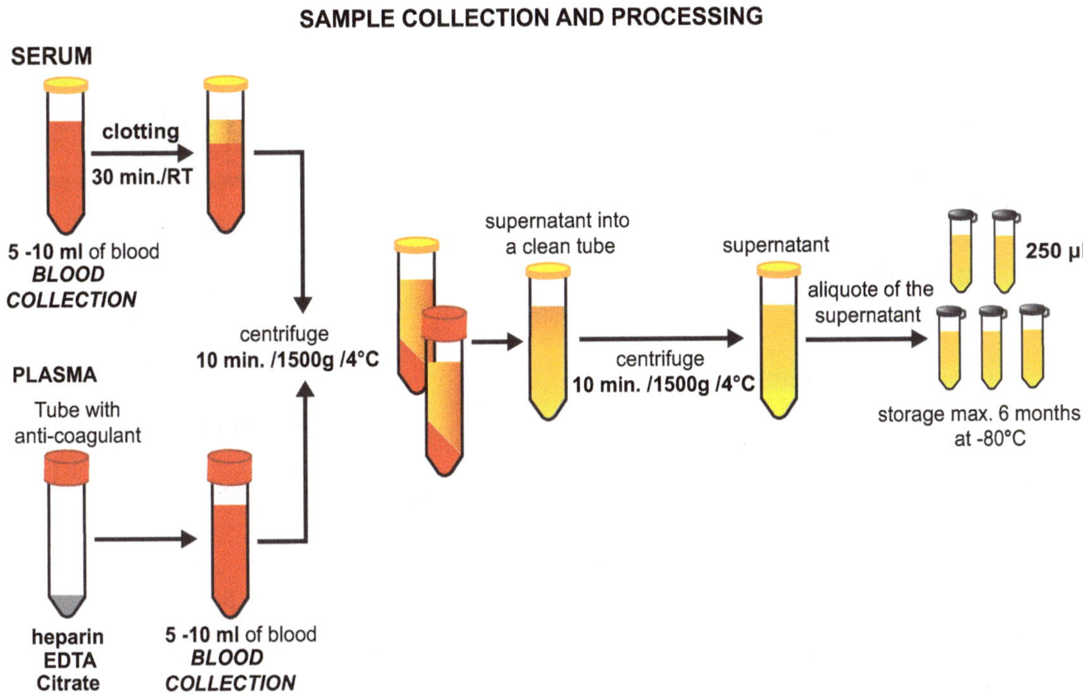

Fig. 2 Sample collection and processing

3. Calibrate the Luminex system according to the manufacturer's instructions using Luminex® 100/200 Calibration Kit and Luminex® 100/200 Performance Verification kit. Calibration is valid for maximum 1 week provided that the stable temperature (±2 °C) is guaranteed (*see* **Notes 8** and **9**).

3.3 Preparation of Assay Reagents (Fig. 3)

1. Determine the number of wells that will be used for background, standards, and samples and determine plate layout (*see* **Notes 10** and **11**).
2. Prepare wash buffer according to kit manual.
3. Thaw samples completely on ice, mix well (*see* **Note 12**), and clean samples by centrifugation at 16,000 × *g* for 10 min in prechilled centrifuge at 4 °C. Keep samples on ice.
4. Reconstitute lyophilized standards according to kit manual. Reconstituted standard should be used within 1 h of preparation (*see* **Notes 13–16**).
5. Prepare standard dilution according to kit manual or according to your own needs (*see* **Note 17** and Table 1).

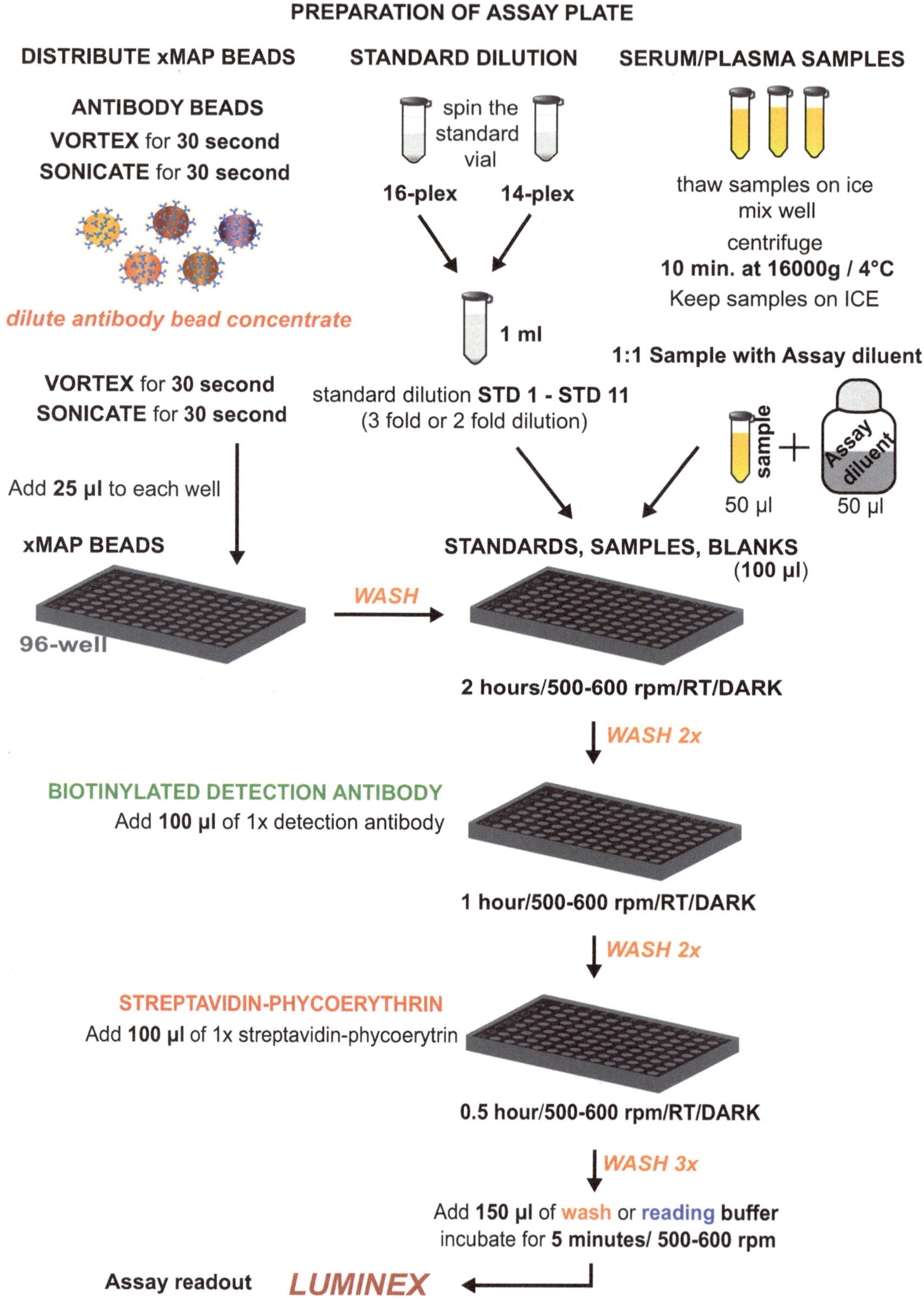

Fig. 3 Preparation of assay plate. Example standard preparation based on Invitrogen Cytokine 30-Plex Human Panel (# LHC6003M, Thermo Fisher), where two sets of standards must be mixed. This will vary based on kit/manufacturer

Table 1
Example of adjusted calibration standard preparation for more precise quantification of IL-6 in blood serum

	Recommended in kit		Adjusted			
	pg/mL	Dilution	pg/mL	Dilution	Assay diluent (μL)	Previous STD (μL)
STD 1	30,700.00		30,700.00			
STD 2	7675.00	4-fold	10,233.33	3-fold	400	200
STD 3	1918.75	4-fold	3411.11	3-fold	400	200
STD 4	479.69	4-fold	1137.04	3-fold	400	200
STD 5	119.92	4-fold	379.01	3-fold	400	200
STD 6	29.98	4-fold	126.34	3-fold	400	200
STD 7	7.50	4-fold	63.17	2-fold	250	250
STD 8			31.58	2-fold	250	250
STD 9			15.79	2-fold	250	250
STD 10			7.90	2-fold	250	250
STD 11			3.95	2-fold	250	250

3.4 Preparation of Assay Plate (Fig. 3)

3.4.1 Distribute xMAP Beads

1. Vortex antibody beads for 30 s, sonicate for 30 s. If provided as a concentrate, dilute the antibody bead concentrate according to the kit manual, followed by additional vortex and sonication, 30 s each.
2. Add 25 μL of antibody beads to each well of the 96-well plate using normal or electric repeated pipet (*see* **Notes 18–20**).

3.4.2 Plate Wash Step (Fig. 4)

1. Place the 96-well plate on magnetic plate separator and allow the beads to settle for 60 s. Hold securely together the plate and magnetic separator, turn them upside down to decant liquid, and blot excess fluid into a stack of paper towels (*see* **Note 21**). Turn the plate with magnetic separator back (plate wells facing up) and remove the plate from magnetic separator.
2. Add 200 μL of wash buffer to each well using multichannel pipette.
3. Repeat **step 1** of Subheading 3.4.2.

3.4.3 Plate Incubation Steps

1. Add 100 μL of each background (blank), standards, and samples to appropriate wells. Use reversed pipetting for accuracy and high reproducibility of replicates (*see* **Notes 22** and **23**). For serum and plasma samples, dilute them 1:1 in Assay Diluent (*see* **Notes 24** and **25**).

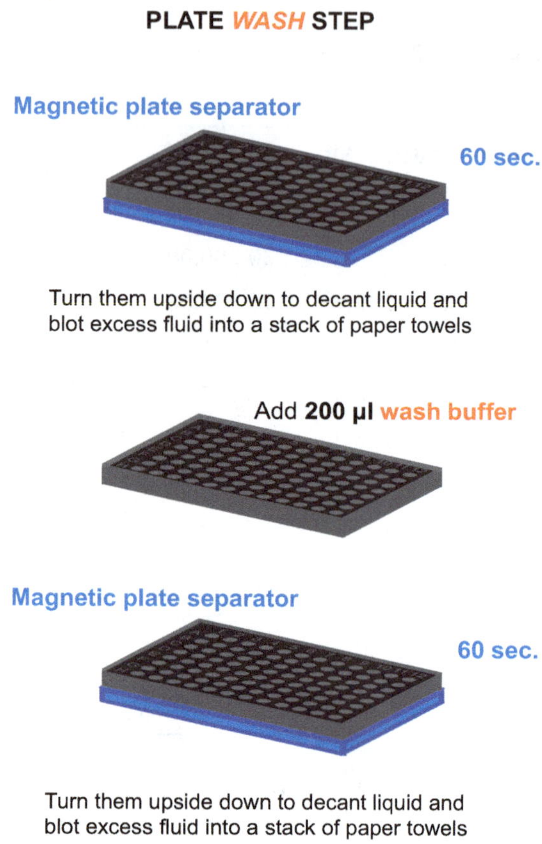

Fig. 4 Plate washing procedure

2. Seal the plate with plate sealer, cover with black lid, and incubate at room temperature on plate shaker for 2 h protected from light (*see* **Note 26**).
3. Prepare 1× biotinylated detection antibody (dilute the antibody concentrate according to kit manual). Place the plate on magnetic separator for 60 s, decant liquid, and perform two washing steps as described in Subheading 3.4.2, **step 2**. Completely blot the excess of fluid at the end of washing procedure. Add 100 µL of 1× detection antibody (or volume specified in kit manual) to each well. Seal the plate, cover, and incubate for 1 h at room temperature on orbital plate shaker protected from light.
4. Prepare 1× streptavidin-phycoerythrin (dilute according to kit manual). Place the plate on magnetic separator for 60 s and decant liquid and perform two washing steps as described in Subheading 3.4.2, **step 2**. Completely blot the excess fluid at the end of washing procedure. Add 100 µL of 1× streptavidin-phycoerythrin (or volume specified in kit manual) to each well. Seal the plate, cover, and incubate for 30 min at room temperature on orbital plate shaker protected from light.

5. Place the plate on magnetic separator for 60 s, decant liquid, and wash the plate three times as described in Subheading 3.4.2, **step 2**. Blot excess liquid after each wash step. Add 150 μL of wash buffer (or reading buffer—as specified in the kit manual) to each well and let the plate to shake for 5 additional minutes.

3.5 Assay Readout

1. During the incubation of plate with detection antibody, prepare Luminex system. If calibrated previous day, switch on the Luminex analyzer and let lasers to warm up for 30 min. Create protocol and batch in the xPonent software.
2. For Protocol, specify protocol name (version, description), manufacturer, and acquisition settings specified in the kit manual (e.g., bead type MagPlex, Volume 75 μL, Timeout 60 s, DD Gating and reporter gain using Default or High PMT) (*see* **Note 27** and Fig. 5).
3. Set xPonent software analysis settings to quantitative analysis using 5P Weighted Logistic curve fitting, define number of standards, and define analytes (analyte name, bead region, units, number of beads to analyze for each analyte) (*see* **Note 28**). Set plate layout and sample IDs (*see* **Notes 29** and **30**).
4. For Batch, specify batch name, protocol name, and kit (name, lot, expiration, manufacturer), assay standard information including name of standard, lot, expiration, manufacturer, concentrations of individual cytokines in individual standard dilutions (*see* **Note 31**), and plate layout (if not specified before in protocol), and proceed to Run Batch.
5. Uncover the 96-well plate and insert it into the XY platform of the Luminex instrument, retract the plate, and analyze samples (*see* **Note 32**).
6. At the end of the run, remove the 96-well plate and sanitize the analyzer using the System Shutdown command (sanitize with 10% bleach, followed by 2 water washes and soak in water) (*see* **Note 33**).
7. Export the resulting csv file for analysis in R (*see* **Notes 34–37**).

3.6 Data Processing and Analysis

For most downstream analysis, fluorescence intensities acquired during data readout are converted to analyte concentrations using standard curves fitted to appropriate standard dilutions. Although these dose-response curves are approximately linear over some limited range, at both low and high analyte concentration the response is highly nonlinear. Of the many nonlinear regression models used to fit dose-response curves, symmetric four-parameter (4PL) [eq. (1)] and asymmetric five-parameter logistic (5PL) [eq. (2)] functions describing sigmoidal curves are the most widely used today [17].

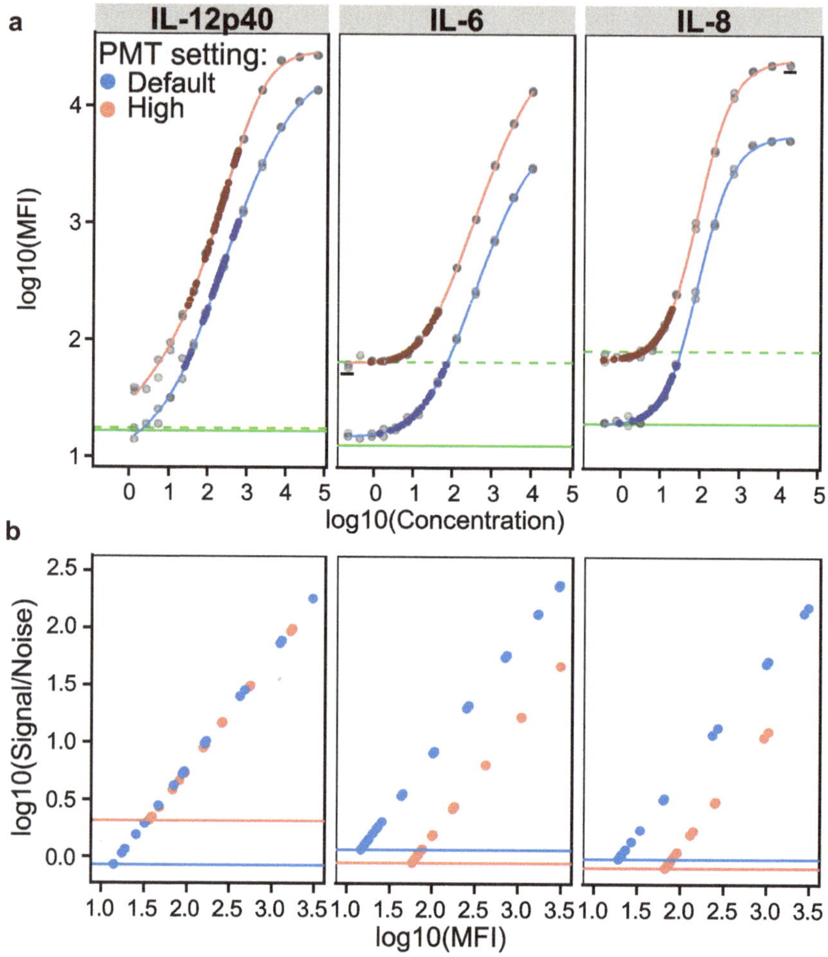

Fig. 5 Example of influence of Luminex 200 PMT sensitivity setting on assay sensitivity. Standard curves (**a**) and signal-to-noise ratio plots (**b**) for ProcartaPlex triplex kit measured at Default PMT (recommended by manufacturer) and High PMT settings are shown. (**a**) For IL-12p40 the standard curve shifts upward with High PMT setting, while background sample level (dashed green line) stays close to Default PMT background level (green line). This results in improved signal-to-noise ratio (*see* orange line higher than blue line in corresponding plot of panel) (**b**) and increased sensitivity of the assay. For the other two analytes, IL-6 and IL-8, background levels at High PMT setting rise comparatively higher than the shift in standard curve itself, leading to worse signal-to-noise ratio and loss of the assay sensitivity. Both IL-12p40 and IL-8 show curve flattening at high concentration range, leading to loss of dynamic range at High PMT setting

$$y = d + \frac{a - d}{1 + \left(\frac{x}{c}\right)^b} \tag{1}$$

where x is the independent variable (dose, unknown analyte concentration), y is the dependent variable (response, in xMAP assay fluorescence intensity), and four parameters to be estimated during curve fitting procedure represent the following:

a = the minimum value that can be observed (value at 0 dose, lower asymptote of the curve).

d = the maximum value that can be observed (at infinite dose, upper asymptote of the curve).

c = inflection point of the curve (EC50, dose corresponding to 50% response).

b = Hill's slope of the curve (steepness of the curve at point c, EC50).

As some assays show asymmetric dose-response relationship, asymmetric 5PL equation with additional parameter e is more appropriate.

$$y = d + \frac{a - d}{\left(1 + \left(\frac{x}{c}\right)^b\right)^e} \quad (2)$$

where e is an asymmetry factor. When $e = 1$, curve equation is identical to 4PL equation and represents symmetric sigmoidal curve (*see* **Note 38**).

As assay data are often heteroscedastic (variability of dependent variable is not constant across the range of independent variable), variance stabilizing data transformation (e.g., log transformation of either response variable—log 5PL or both dose and response variable log-log 5PL) [18] or data weighting (e.g., $1/y^2$ as implemented in xPonent analysis module) is often performed before curve fitting.

Default xPonent analysis setting uses 5P Weighted Logistic curve fitting on untransformed background corrected fluorescence data (net MFI—net median fluorescence intensity). This method leads to several problems:

1. Due to the matrix effects, background (blank) samples might have sometimes higher MFI values than legitimate analyte or standard readouts in actual sample matrix (e.g., serum or plasma), leading to negative fluorescence values after background correction.
2. $1/y^2$ weighting leads often to overcorrection and poor curve fit in the region of higher fluorescence intensities (*see* Fig. 6a, standard curve for EGF and RANTES).

For this reason, we recommend against using built-in xPonent analysis function and describe in following protocol curve fitting procedure and estimation of analyte concentrations implemented in two packages for open source R statistical environment, drLumi [12, 13] and nCal [14, 15]. Both packages use log-log 5PL and 4PL curve fitting and generally provide better curve fits (*see* Fig. 6b, resp. c).

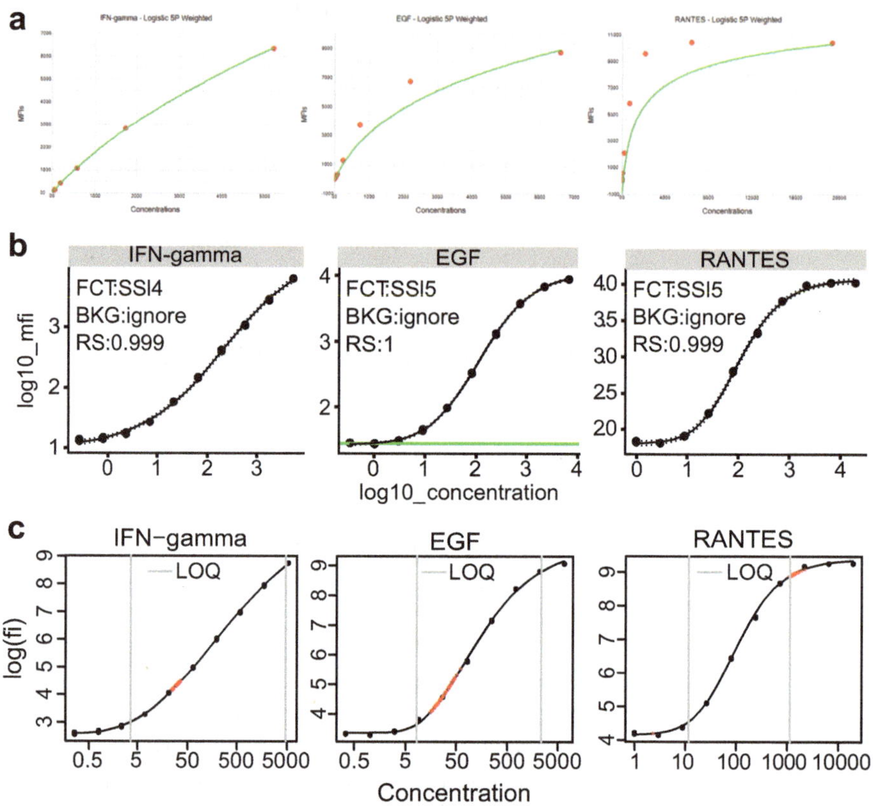

Fig. 6 Example calibration curves fitted using xPONENT (**a**), drLumi (**b**), and nCal (**c**). Standard curves were fitted to the provided sample dataset using (**a**) default settings in xPonent software (5PL weighted curve), (**b**) drLumi with log-log 5PL curve and ignored background, with 4PL curve as fallback option, and (**c**) Bayesian hierarchical log-log 5PL curve fitted by nCal package. Note the generally poor fit for EGF and RANTES generated by xPonent

More details are given for procedure implemented in drLumi package, as it can directly import csv data files acquired by xPonent, while nCal needs additional software (PERL) to import raw Luminex files. Commented scripts (30-plex_sample-script_drLumi.R, 30-plex_sample-script_nCal.R) are available as supplementary file of this chapter on the book's website and demonstrate analyte concentration estimation from provided sample dataset (Human30plex_sample-data.csv) acquired on serum samples using Invitrogen Cytokine 30-Plex Human Panel (# LHC6003M, Thermo Fisher). These scripts should be easily adaptable to user needs for different kit formats and samples, as long as recommended sample naming schemes are followed.

1. Prepare the directory structure: Create the master folder for each assay/set of assays to be analyzed together. Create subfolders in this master folder as follows—sources subfolder, where all the assay input files will be placed, plots subfolder,

where standard curve plots generated during analysis will be saved, and outputs subfolder, where estimated analyte concentrations will be saved. Place the provided R script into the master folder (*see* **Note 39**).

2. Copy csv file with acquired assay data (or sample data included as Supplementary File) into sources folder.
3. Start R session, preferably using R Studio IDE. Open provided example script (30-plex_sample-script_drLumi.R) or script adapted to your data. If using R Studio, set working directory to your master folder using menu Session > Set Working Directory > To Source File Location.
4. If running the script for the first time, install required R packages using the following command: `install.packages(c("drLumi", "nCal", "tidyverse", "cowplot"))` (*see* **Note 40**).
5. Load the required packages using set of `library()` commands. drLumi is the main package used for curve fitting and concentration estimation. Tidyverse is set of packages useful for data filtering and transformations. Cowplot is a package setting some ggplot2 graphical package parameters to defaults more in line with general journal requirements for publication ready figures.
6. Use `plate[i] <- lum_import("path/filename[i]")` command to import xPonent csv file (*see* **Note 41**).
7. Export only the data needed for downstream analysis using `exp.data[i] <- lum_export(plate[i])` command.
8. Filter out "Total Events" data rows, which are summary bead counts included together with individual analytes data and not needed for further analysis. Also remove non-needed columns, such as "`batch_well_analyte`" (the same data are in the dataset in the form of individual batch, well, and analyte columns) and "`net_mfi`" (background subtracted fluorescent intensities—not needed, as raw median fluorescent intensities and background levels are still present in the data). Store the resulting response variables (median fluorescent intensities) together with sample, plate, and analyte identifiers in `mfidata[i]` dataframe.
9. Prepare the `ecdata[i]` dataframe, which describes concentrations of your Standards.
10. Using `data_selection()` command, prepare the `datasets[i]` dataframe, combining raw fluorescence intensities from `mfidata[i]` with expected standard concentrations of `ecdata[i]`. At this step pay particular attention to describing your Sample, Blank, and Control naming scheme.

```
datasets1 <- data_selection(x = mfidata1,
                              ecfile = ecdata1,
                              byvar.ecfile =
c("sample","analyte"),
                              backname = "Background",
                              stanname="Standard",
posname = "Controls")
```

In given example, expected Background/Blank sample names in xPonent csv output is starting with "Background" (Background, Background0, BackgroundA would be all valid and recognized names), Standards (dilutions used for standard curve fitting) are expected to start with "Standard" (e.g., Standard1, Standard2), and positive control samples (optional) are expected to start with "Controls." These names should be adjusted as needed to fit names used during pre-acquisition batch setup. All the samples not specified as background, standard, or control above will be treated as "unknown" samples and their concentration will be estimated based on constructed standard curve in later steps.

11. Fit the standard curve using `scluminex()` command and assign resulting curve fits to `allanalytes[i]` object.

```
allanalytes1 <- scluminex(plateid = "Plate1",
                standard = datasets1$Plate1$standard,
                background =
datasets1$Plate1$background,
                bkg = "constraint", lfct =
c("SS15","SS14"),
                fmfi = "median", verbose = FALSE)
```

where Standards and Background samples are specified based on previously created `datasets[i]` dataframe, `bkg` specifies how to deal with assay background (*see* **Note 42**), `lfct` parameter specifies which curve fitting model to use (*see* **Note 43**), and `fmfi` specifies name of the column with response fluorescence values to use.

12. Plot fitted standard curves using `plot(allanalytes[i])` command and carefully check fitted curves for possible artifacts and outlier values. Curves can be saved in several image formats (png, pdf) from R Studio "Plots" panel or directly from provided script using `save_plot()` command. Saving to pdf format directly from script is recommended if publication use of plots is expected, as it provides resolution-independent vector format.

13. If some of the standard dilutions (which should be always run in duplicates or triplicates!) is obvious outlier, it can

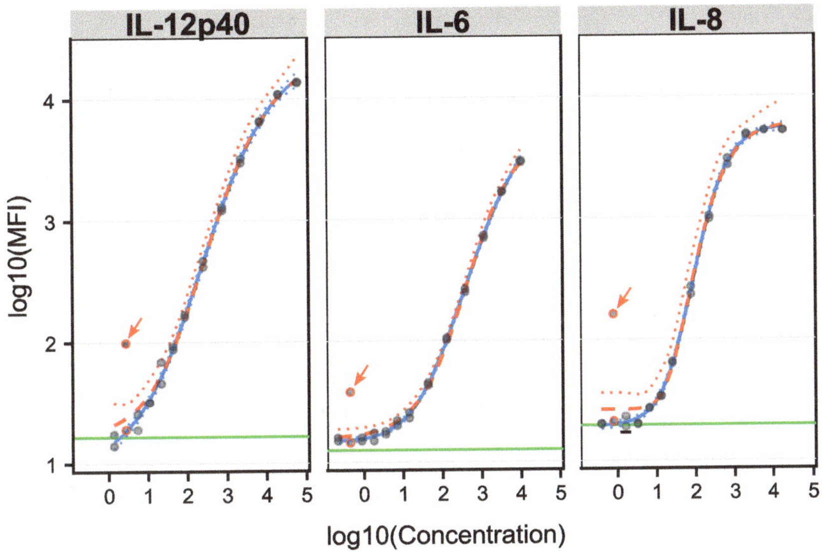

Fig. 7 Example of outlier influence on calibration curve fitting. Calibration curves generated from ProcartaPlex triplex kit data by drLumi package, with one outlier (highlighted in red and labeled by arrow) present out of two technical duplicates of one standard (second replicate only highlighted in red). Note how the presence of this outlier influences standard curve fit (dashed red line) and curve confidence interval (only upper confidence interval—dotted red line, is shown for standard curve including outlier). Other standards shown as gray circles, standard curve fitted after removing outlier shown as full blue line, with confidence intervals as dotted blue lines. Green indicated assay background level

significantly influence curve fit (*see* Fig. 7 for example). In such case it might be necessary to identify offending well, discard it from dataset, and repeat **steps 10–12** to fit corrected standard curves. Detailed example how to identify and filter potential outlier is provided in example script. Briefly, code below will remove all standard measurements in well B3:

```
datasets1$Plate1$standard <- datasets1$Plate1$standard
%>%
                                        filter(well != "P1_B3")
```

While following line will remove only standard measurements for IL-6 and IL-8 in well B3:

```
datasets1$Plate1$standard <- datasets1$Plate1$standard
%>%
    filter(!(analyte %in% c("IL-6", "IL-8") & well ==
"P1_B3"))
```

14. Estimate limits of quantification for individual analytes. Three methods are implemented for limits of quantification estimation in drLumi package. Interval method uses crossing of lower and upper asymptote of the model with the standard curve:

```
loq1 <- loq_interval(allanalytes[i], low.asymp=2,
high.asymp=3)
```

Derivative method uses the second-order derivative of the model and is the most conservative LOQ estimation method, which limits valid assay interval mostly to the linear part of the curve:

```
loq1 <- loq_derivatives(allanalytes[i])
```

Coefficient of variation method estimates CV of fitted concentrations and range of concentration values for which the CV will be held under provided limit. This is the most flexible method, leaving the decision what is acceptable variability in concentration estimates to the user (`set max.cv` parameter to your desired cutoff):

```
loq1 <- loq_cv(allanalytes[i], max.cv = 0.2)
```

15. Estimate concentration of your unknown samples using `est_conc()` function and store estimates in `estim[i]` object.

```
estim[i] <- subset(datasets[i]$Plate1$unknowns) %>%
est_conc(allanalytes[i], .,fmfi = "median", dilution =
2)
```

In example above, we select unknown samples stored in `datasets[i]` Plate1 unknowns section and estimate concentrations of these unknowns using standard curves stored in `allanalytes[i]` object. `Fmfi` again serves as an identifier of the response variable (here raw median fluorescence intensity). It is important to set correct dilution factors for your samples! The dilution is given relative to the standard concentration (e.g., If 100 μL of Standard 1 in Table 1 at 30700.00 pg/mL was added to the plate, while 50 μL of serum sample was mixed with 50 μL of Assay Diluent and added to the plate, resulting dilution factor is 2).

16. In similar way, estimate concentration of your standards from fitted curves (*see* **Note 44**).

```
estim_std[i] <- subset(datasets1$Plate1$standard) %>%
est_conc(allanalytes1, .,fmfi = "median", dilution =
1)
```

17. Comparing estimated with expected standard concentration allows calculating Recovery and CV of our standards. We first group data by individual sample (duplicated or triplicated

standard) and analyte using `group_by()` function, then calculate summary values for grouped data using `summarise()` with appropriate function. Here we calculate mean expected concentration (`Exp_conc`), mean estimated concentration (`Estim_conc`, individual estimates labeled as `dil.fitted.con` in dataframe), and finally calculate `Recovery` as ratio of estimated vs. expected concentration and `CV` as ratio of SD of estimated concentration to mean estimated concentration.

```
recovery[i] <- estim_std[i] %>% group_by(sample,
analyte) %>%
  summarise(Exp_conc = mean(ec, na.rm = TRUE),
            Estim_conc = mean(dil.fitted.conc, na.rm =
TRUE),
            Recovery = (Estim_conc/Exp_conc),
            CV = sd(dil.fitted.conc, na.rm =
TRUE)/Estim_conc)
```

18. Join estimated concentrations for your unknown samples and standards with `rbind()` command, add estimated limits of quantification with `left_join()` command, and save the concentration estimates and recovery data into outputs folder using `write.csv()` command.

```
all.data[i] <- rbind(estim[i], estim_std[i])
all.data[i] <- left_join(all.data[i], loq[i])
write.csv(all.data[i],
file = "./outputs/Concentrations_Plate[i].csv",
row.names = FALSE)
write.csv(recovery[i],
file = "./outputs/Recovery_and_CV_Plate[i].csv",
row.names = FALSE)
```

Package nCal provides two alternative ways for standard curve fitting, one based on drc package [19] and similar to drLumi default method, and second implementing a robust Bayesian hierarchical five-parameter logistic model. One advantage of Bayesian model is a possibility to borrow information across multiple assay runs for the given analyte and thus reduce standard curve variability and mitigate effect of outliers present in individual runs. Minimal script describing import of xPonent csv data using drLumi package, transformation into nCal compatible format and standard curve fitting and concentration estimation is provided as supplementary file (30-plex_-sample-script_nCal.R). Detailed description of all the nCal options is beyond the scope of this protocol and we direct reader to paper by Fong et al. [14] and to nCal package vignette and manual [15].

3.7 Downstream Data Analysis

We provided protocol for constructing standard curves based on measured responses of dilution series of standards with known concentration and for estimating concentrations of analytes in assayed unknown samples, as this is usually of biological interest. However, it is important to understand that the process of concentration estimation from standard curve adds uncertainty and can also be biased by systematic effects, such as matrix effect, where the same concentration of given analyte leads to different response in, e.g., serum vs. plasma vs. diluent used for standard preparation [8, 20]. For some applications, such as biomarker discovery projects, it might be advantageous to skip the step of concentration estimation entirely and rely on direct analysis of measured fluorescence values [21]. Advanced methods, employing analysis of the whole bead population for each analyte, instead of median fluorescence intensity reported by xPonent software are also available [22].

Detailed protocol for downstream data analysis is not provided, as it is highly dependent on study design and intended outputs. For simple designs, such as case (treatment)—control or pre–post measurement, common statistical test such as *t*-test, respective paired *t*-test might be usable, but should employ appropriate multiple testing correction in case of highly multiplexed assays. More complicated study designs, with more than two groups or repeated measures and time-course experiments, require complex approaches such as repeated measure ANOVA or mixed effect models [23]. Breen [24] recently described use of lme4 [25, 26] package for analysis of Luminex xMAP data using mixed-effect model approach.

As multiplexed immunoassay can provide high-dimensional data, with multiple analytes measured over multiple conditions, dimensionality reduction approaches for data visualization (e.g., Principle Component Analysis—PCA, [27] or t-distributed Stochastic Neighbor Embedding—tSNE, [28]) and data mining/machine learning approaches for data analysis and classification [29] can be employed.

4 Notes

1. Various factors influence cytokine levels, including chronobiology, mental stress, physical exercise, blood collection technique, sample storage, etc. [30], standardized procedure should be followed to minimize pre-analytical factors. Fasting is not required but avoid the use of lipemic or hemolytic samples. Do not use blood that has been stored for several hours as the cytokine levels are strongly influenced by cytokines released from blood cells and platelets [31], while other cytokines may undergo degradation.

2. Plasma and serum are not interchangeable, as plethora of factors are released from platelets during blood clotting. Similarly, the choice of anticoagulant influences total cytokine level as different pathways are activated by individual anticoagulants leading to cytokine release from cells [32, 33].
3. Aliquots are for single use, do not repeatedly freeze-thaw samples. Tubes should be resistant minimally to 20,000 × *g*.
4. Storage longer than 6 months is not recommended due to cytokine loss during long-term storage.
5. Tumor-originating cytokines may be highly diluted in blood. On the other hand, other cells and tissues participate in cytokine release to blood stream. Our preliminary results from MeLiM porcine melanoma model show up to 10–1000 times higher concentration of selected cytokines in tumor homogenates than in blood plasma. Tissue homogenate in both plain phosphate-buffered saline (isotonic PBS, pH 7.4) and nondenaturing detergent-containing buffers (e.g., Bio-Plex Cell Lysis Buffer, ProcartaPlex Cell Lysis Buffer) is compatible with xMAP assays.
6. If the system is idle for 4 h without acquiring data, the lasers will automatically turn off and additional 30-min laser warm-up is required.
7. Use the pre-set System Initialization procedure in xPonent software for alcohol and water washes, calibration and verification in one step.
8. Stable temperature is crucial for stable laser intensities.
9. If unused for longer time, calibrate the Luminex instrument in 1-month intervals to ensure proper function, prevent bubble formation and clogging. If low bead numbers per second are recorded or abnormal scatterplot populations appear, consider sample probe flush or sonication.
10. Each background, standard, and serum samples should be analyzed in duplicates. It is recommended to include in-house controls in every assay.
11. The assay is designed for 96-well plate. If less samples are to be run, the leftover of the kit can be used next time (using a new tube with lyophilized standard). Leftovers from kits with the same Lot number can be combined together. Never combine different Lots or kits from various manufacturers! Do not substitute reagents from different kits and Lots.
12. Mix samples using a pipette. Vortex is not sufficiently effective in mixing viscous plasma/serum samples and vigorous vortexing may lead to cytokine loss.

13. Spin the standard vial briefly before opening and open the vial carefully as the lyophilized powder tends to fly away. Use the appropriate diluent for standard reconstitution; e.g., for serum and plasma samples use the Assay Diluent (cytokine-free serum substitute) provided in the kit to ensure the most identical matrix for samples and standards.
14. Do not vortex the reconstituted standard to avoid foaming.
15. Do not reuse or store resuspended standards.
16. Always carefully read the Lot specific Certificate of Analysis and kit manual before preparation of standards. Some assays come with standards separated into two distinct tubes, e.g., Human Cytokine Magnetic 30-plex Panel (# LHC6003M) requires mixing of 16-Plex and 14-Plex standards into the final volume of 1 mL. On the other hand, standards in the ProcartaPlex simplex assays contain premixed set of several cytokines and imprudent combination of several simplex kit standards into one multiplex assay may lead to redundant cytokine standards.
17. For precise quantification of a broad dynamic range of cytokine concentrations, we recommend threefold or even twofold dilution of calibration standards, leading to a higher number of calibration standards. Example of adjusted standard dilution to cover broad dynamic range as well as low cytokine concentration is given in Table 1. For higher accuracy and good reproducibility, perform all pipetting steps using reversed pipetting.
18. As the magnetic beads tend to settle to the bottom of the tube, briefly vortex the tube with beads approximately every 30 s to ensure even bead distribution in wells.
19. Beads are fluorescently labeled, minimize exposure of the beads and plate to the light (keep the plate covered by black lid whenever possible). Additional cover of the plate (e.g., by aluminum foil) might be necessary during incubation steps.
20. When running two plates at the same day, assure the same incubation times for both plates (e.g., start processing of the second plate with 1-h delay to have time to prepare second plate and samples).
21. Blotting of the excess of fluid is crucial in each wash step to avoid cross contamination.
22. See recommended volumes in kit manual.
23. Use the Assay Diluent as background (blank) for serum and plasma samples.
24. For serum and plasma samples, it is recommended to dilute the samples 1:1 in Assay Diluent to decrease sample viscosity, reduce matrix effects, and increase availability of epitopes to the antibodies. For 1:1 dilution, add to each well designed for

samples 50 μL of Assay Diluent followed by 50 μL of each sample (100 μL in total, samples are twofold diluted, which needs to be considered during data analysis).

25. In some kits, additional 50 μL of Incubation Buffer are added to each well (background, standard, sample) resulting in 150 μL total volume.
26. Orbital shaker with a 3-mm orbital radius at a speed 500–600 rpm is recommended. Set appropriate rpm to avoid splashing of the liquid onto the lid (sealer).
27. For magnetic beads, Doublet Discriminator Gating is usually set between 7500 and 20,000 and removes doublets or larger clusters of multiple beads from fluorescence intensity counting. Correct PMT setting is usually specified in manufacturer's instructions for given kit and should be followed unless specifically optimized by user on different setting. While high PMT might provide higher sensitivity for some analytes, it might also rise assay background and lead to loss of total assay dynamic range by saturating detectors (Fig. 5).
28. 100 beads per analyte are recommended in most kits. However, measurements on min. of 30 beads could be considered valid [34].
29. For analysis in R software, keep the labeling Background, Standard#, and Unknown# in the beginning of sample name. Sample IDs can be imported as a text file (.txt).
30. Plate layout can be set later in Batch settings.
31. Cytokine concentrations can be copied from excel file.
32. The analysis of 96-well plate may take over 1 h, depending on the number of samples and analytes simultaneously quantified.
33. System sanitization is crucial for successful calibration and to prevent clogging.
34. CSV files can be found under Results/Saved Batches.
35. Make sure the acquisition computer is set to English locale and language settings, as this influences delimiters used in csv files (e.g., colon is used as decimal point delimiter and semicolon as field delimiter in some locales, which prevents data import into R session).
36. If a mistake in sample labeling or order is noted at the end of analysis, the analysis can be replayed from the previously recorded raw bead data files using new settings of Batch or Protocol. The Replay function can be found under Results/Saved Batches option in xPonent software.
37. Result reports generated by built-in xPonent analysis module can be generated as pdf files under Results/Reports option in the xPonent software. These data include information about %

recovery of standards and % CV of Replicates. Standards with % recovery over 130 or below 70 should be discarded from analysis. In most kits, % CV of replicates up to 30 is acceptable. If you plan to analyze data in R, do not use this information and rely on CV and recovery calculated there.

38. For 5PL curve parameter c is not equal to EC50.
39. Within provided example script, all paths for saving plots and data are listed relative to the master folder where script should be placed. The recommended folder structure should keep data organized and clearly distinguish input and output data, but experienced users can adapt it to their needs.
40. This step needs to be performed just once! Do not run this command on subsequent script runs.
41. Standard R assignment operator `<-` is used throughout protocol to denote storing R objects such as data-frames in variable of given name. Tidyverse `%>%` operator forwards output of given operation to subsequent command, allowing natural command chaining, instead of using nesting. `[i]` represents plate number, in provided scripts `plate1` notation is used for analysis of one assay plate.
42. Procedures for dealing with assay background are provided in drLumi package. Setting bkg parameter to "ignore" simply ignores background information altogether and uses raw MFI values of standards vs. expected concentrations, "constraint" fixes background MFI level as a lower asymptote of 4PL or 5PL model (parameter *a* of Eqs. (1) and (2)), "subtract" subtracts mean background MFI from all samples and standards, and "include" includes background as additional "Standard" with 1/2 concentration of lowest present standard in curve fitting model. Based on our experience, "ignore" and "constraint" bkg options provide reasonable curve fits in most assays.
43. Option set to `c("SS15", "SS14")` as shown in example code directs drLumi to fit 5PL model as a first option, with 4PL model fitted in case 5PL model didn't converge.
44. Dilution for standards will always be 1, as we estimate the same concentration that was used for curve fitting in the first place.

Acknowledgements

This study was supported by Ministry of Education, Youth and Sports of the Czech Republic under National Sustainability Program I (project LO1609) and under Operational Programme Research, Development and Education (project CZ.02.1.01/0.0/0.0/16_019/0000785).

References

1. Molinaro R, Corbo C, Livingston M et al (2018) Inflammation and cancer: in medio stat nano. Curr Med Chem 25:4208–4223
2. Nakamura K, Smyth MJ (2017) Targeting cancer-related inflammation in the era of immunotherapy. Immunol Cell Biol 95:325–332
3. Lacina L, Plzak J, Kodet O et al (2015) Cancer microenvironment: what can we learn from the stem cell niche. Int J Mol Sci 16:24094–24110
4. Dvořánková B, Szabo P, Kodet O et al (2017) Intercellular crosstalk in human malignant melanoma. Protoplasma 254:1143–1150
5. Kupcova Skalnikova H, Cizkova J, Cervenka J et al (2017) Advances in proteomic techniques for cytokine analysis: focus on melanoma research. Int J Mol Sci 18:2697
6. Valekova I, Skalnikova HK, Jarkovska K et al (2015) Multiplex immunoassays for quantification of cytokines, growth factors, and other proteins in stem cell communication. Methods Mol Biol 1212:39–63
7. Fu Q, Zhu J, Eyk JEV (2010) Comparison of multiplex immunoassay platforms. Clin Chem 56:314–318
8. Rosenberg-Hasson Y, Hansmann L, Liedtke M et al (2014) Effects of serum and plasma matrices on multiplex immunoassays. Immunol Res 58:224–233
9. R Core Team (2018) R: a language and environment for statistical computing. R Foundation for Statistical Computing, Vienna
10. Wickham H, RStudio (2017) tidyverse: easily install and load the "tidyverse". https://CRAN.R-project.org/package=tidyverse
11. Introduction to cowplot. https://cran.r-project.org/web/packages/cowplot/vignettes/introduction.html
12. Sanz H, Aponte JJ, Harezlak J et al (2017) drLumi: an open-source package to manage data, calibrate, and conduct quality control of multiplex bead-based immunoassays data analysis. PLoS One 12:e0187901
13. Sanz, H, Aponte JJ, Harezlak J et al (2015) drLumi: Multiplex Immunoassays Data Analysis. https://CRAN.R-project.org/package=drLumi
14. Fong Y, Sebestyen K, Yu X et al (2013) nCal: an R package for non-linear calibration. Bioinformatics 29:2653–2654
15. Fong Y, Sebestyen K, Yu X (2018) nCal: Nonlinear Calibration. https://CRAN.R-project.org/package=nCal
16. RStudio Team (2018) RStudio: integrated development environment for R. RStudio, Inc., Boston, MA
17. Findlay JWA, Dillard RF (2007) Appropriate calibration curve fitting in ligand binding assays. AAPS J 9:E260–E267
18. Fong Y, Yu X (2016) Transformation model choice in nonlinear regression analysis of fluorescence-based serial dilution assays. Stat Biopharm Res 8:1–11
19. Ritz C, Streibig JC (2005) Bioassay analysis using R. J Stat Softw 12:1–22
20. Chaturvedi AK, Kemp TJ, Pfeiffer RM et al (2011) Evaluation of multiplexed cytokine and inflammation marker measurements: a methodologic study. Cancer Epidemiol Biomark Prev 20:1902–1911
21. Breen EJ, Tan W, Khan A (2016) The statistical value of raw fluorescence signal in Luminex xMAP based multiplex immunoassays. Sci Rep 6:26996
22. Won J-H, Goldberger O, Shen-Orr SS et al (2012) Significance analysis of xMap cytokine bead arrays. Proc Natl Acad Sci U S A 109:2848–2853
23. Clarke DC, Morris MK, Lauffenburger DA (2013) Normalization and statistical analysis of multiplexed bead-based immunoassay data using mixed-effects modeling. Mol Cell Proteomics 12:245–262
24. Breen EJ (2017) Protein multiplexed immunoassay analysis with R. In: Greening DW, Simpson RJ (eds) Serum/plasma proteomics: methods and protocols. Springer New York, New York, NY, pp 495–537
25. Bates D, Mächler M, Bolker B et al (2015) Fitting linear mixed-effects models using lme4. J Stat Softw 1406:67
26. Bates D, Mächler M, Bolker B, et al (2018) lme4: Linear Mixed-Effects Models using "Eigen" and S4. https://CRAN.R-project.org/package=lme4
27. Ringnér M (2008) What is principal component analysis? Nat Biotechnol 26:303–304
28. van der Maaten L, Hinton G (2008) Visualizing data using t-SNE. J Mach Learn Res 9:2579–2605
29. Mani A, Ravindran R, Mannepalli S et al (2015) Data mining strategies to improve multiplex microbead immunoassay tolerance in a mouse model of infectious diseases. PLoS One 10:e0116262
30. Dugué B, Leppänen E, Gräsbeck R (1996) Preanalytical factors and the measurement of

cytokines in human subjects. Int J Clin Lab Res 26:99–105

31. Lee J-E, Kim J-W, Han B-G et al (2016) Impact of whole-blood processing conditions on plasma and serum concentrations of cytokines. Biopreserv Biobank 14:51–55
32. Brøndum L, Sørensen BS, Eriksen JG et al (2016) An evaluation of multiplex bead-based analysis of cytokines and soluble proteins in archived lithium heparin plasma, EDTA plasma and serum samples. Scand J Clin Lab Invest 76:601–611
33. Scholman RC, Giovannone B, Hiddingh S et al (2018) Effect of anticoagulants on 162 circulating immune related proteins in healthy subjects. Cytokine 106:114–124
34. Moncunill G, Campo JJ, Dobaño C (2014) Quantification of multiple cytokines and chemokines using cytometric bead arrays. Methods Mol Biol 1172:65–86

Chapter 7

Detection of Cytokine Receptors Using Tyramide Signal Amplification for Immunofluorescence

Herui Wang, Ryan L. Pangilinan, and Yan Zhu

Abstract

Tyramide signal amplification (TSA) is an enzyme-mediated method to enhance the immunohistochemical detection of protein, nucleic acid, or other molecules in situ.

Here we describe immunofluorescent detection of a low-abundance cytokine receptor, interleukin-17 receptor B (IL17RB) in U2OS cells, using tyramide signal amplification. In addition, we present a tyramide signal amplification compatible double-color immunostaining protocol using primary antibodies from the same host species. Those applications allow detection of cellular proteins with enhanced sensitivity and add flexibility on primary antibody selection in double- or multicolor immunofluorescence staining assays.

Key words Tyramide signal amplification, Immunofluorescence, Double-color immunostaining, Interleukin-17 receptor B

1 Introduction

Tyramide signal amplification (TSA) utilizes the catalytic activity of horseradish peroxidase (HRP) to deposit of a labeled (e.g., fluorophore, biotin, or other labeling moieties) tyramide onto target proteins that are previously blotted with primary antibody or nucleic acid sequences in situ [1–3]. In TSA-based immunohistochemical (IHC) or immunofluorescence (IF) detection, activated tyramide forms covalent bonds with tyrosine residues on the target protein, resulting in permanent high-density labeling. The signals can then be detected by standard chromogenic or fluorescent techniques [4, 5]. As this technique is based on detection via indirect immunostaining involving primary and secondary antibodies, TSA promotes enhanced sensitivity and high specificity for target protein detection, especially for those low-abundance proteins [6].

Double- or multicolor immunofluorescence staining is useful to examine the distribution of two (or more) different antigens in the same sample of cells. It requires unlabeled primary antibodies

Ivana Vancurova and Yan Zhu (eds.), *Immune Mediators in Cancer: Methods and Protocols*, Methods in Molecular Biology, vol. 2108, https://doi.org/10.1007/978-1-0716-0247-8_7, © Springer Science+Business Media, LLC, part of Springer Nature 2020

from different hosts or different fluorescently labeled primary antibodies for different antigens. The availability of primary antibodies restricts the usage of the application. TSA-based covalently linked labeling can preserve antigen-associated signal even after serial stripping of the primary/secondary antibody pairs, making this process amenable to multiple rounds of staining in a sequential fashion [1–3]. Most importantly, immunostaining with tyramide signal amplification allows double- or multicolor immunofluorescence staining being performed using unlabeled primary antibodies from the same hosts without the concern for crosstalk. This will add flexibility to the primary antibody selection and facilitate multiplex staining design.

Il17RB is a cytokine receptor that binds to interleukin 17 (IL-17) cytokine family members IL-17B and IL-17E (IL-25) [4]. It has been detected in kidney, pancreas, liver, brain, and intestine [5]. Amplification of IL-17B/RB signaling has been linked to tumorigenesis in breast [6], gastric [7], pancreatic [8], and thyroid [9] cancers. We have observed low levels of IL17RB expression in U2OS cells by western blot analysis. Here, we present the detection of IL17RB in U2OS cells using tyramide signal amplification for immunofluorescence (Fig. 1). In addition, we describe a tyramide signal amplification compatible double-color immunostaining protocol using primary antibodies against IL17RB and p53, a tumor suppressor, from the same host species (Fig. 2).

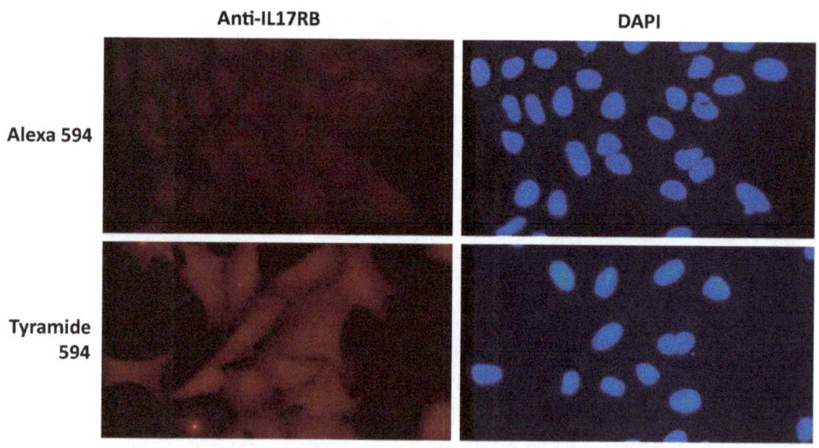

Fig. 1 Detection of low-abundance cytokine receptor IL17RB with tyramide signal amplification. Immunofluorescence staining of IL17RB in U2OS cells with goat anti-rabbit IgG (H + L) Alexa Fluor™ 594 secondary antibody or Alexa Fluor™ 594 Tyramide SuperBoost™ Kit, goat anti-rabbit IgG

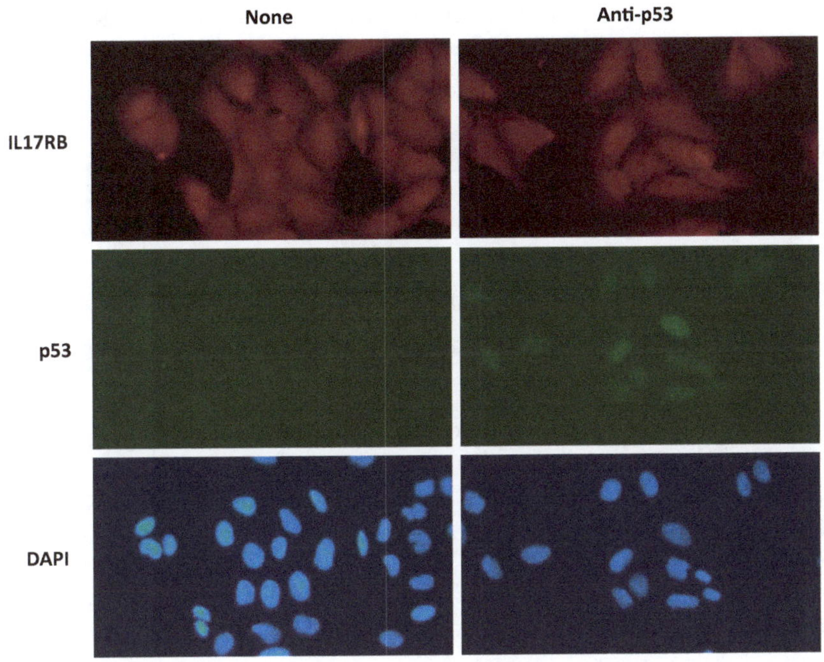

Fig. 2 Double-color immunostaining of IL17RB and p53 using primary antibodies from the same host species with tyramide signal amplification. IL17RB in U2OS cells was stained with Alexa Fluor™ 594 Tyramide SuperBoost™ Kit, goat anti-rabbit IgG as in Fig. 1. Then the cells were stained with or without anti-p53 antibody followed by immunostaining of goat anti-rabbit IgG (H + L) Alexa Fluor™ 488 secondary antibody. Primary antibodies against IL17RB and p53 are both rabbit polyclonal antibodies

2 Materials

All reagents and solutions are stored according to the manufacturer's instructions.

2.1 Cell Culture

1. Human osteosarcoma U2OS cells.
2. DMEM complete medium: Dulbecco's modified Eagle medium supplemented with 10% fetal bovine serum and 100 μg/mL penicillin/streptomycin.
3. 1× Phosphate-buffered saline (PBS, pH 7.2): 140 mM NaCl, 2.6 mM KCl, 2 mM Na_2HPO_4, 1.45 mM KH_2PO_4.
4. 4% Paraformaldehyde in 1× PBS (*see* **Note 1**).
5. Alexa Fluor™ 594 Tyramide SuperBoost™ Kit, goat anti-rabbit IgG (*see* **Note 2**).
6. Antibodies: anti-p53 (FL393; Santa Cruz); anti-IL17RB (NBP2-43767; Novus); goat anti-rabbit IgG (H + L) Alexa Fluor™ 594 secondary antibody; goat anti-rabbit IgG (H + L) Alexa Fluor™ 488 secondary antibody.
7. Blocking buffer: 0.5% BSA in 1× PBS.

8. Permeabilization buffer: 0.5% Triton X-100 in 1× PBS.
9. 10 mM sodium citrate (pH 6.0): fleshly made from 1 M sodium citrate (pH 6.0) stock.
10. 5 mg/mL DAPI in DMSO.
11. Fluorescence microscope (Nikon Eclipse Ti2).
12. Cell culture dishes: diameter 35 mm.
13. Cover slides: 22 × 22 mm.
14. Microscope slides: 75 × 25 mm.
15. Microwave-safe container: about 76 × 150 mm (*see* **Note 3**).
16. Microwave.
17. CO_2 incubator: set to 5% CO_2 and 37 °C.

3 Method

3.1 Immunofluorescent Staining with Tyramide Signal Amplification

1. Perform cell culture procedures in biosafety cabinets using sterile equipment and pre-warmed (37 °C) reagents.
2. The day before immunostaining, place sterile glass coverslips in each 35 mm cell culture dish using sterile forceps.
3. Seed 6 × 105 U2OS cells into each 35 mm dish with glass coverslips.
4. Incubate the cells with 2 mL DMEM in a 37 °C CO_2 incubator.
5. On the second day, aspirate the DMEM medium from the dish and wash the cells twice with 1 mL 1× PBS at room temperature.
6. Fix cells with 1 mL 4% paraformaldehyde in 1× PBS, at room temperature for 20 min.
7. Wash the cells with 1× PBS.
8. Permeabilize the cells with permeabilization buffer at room temperature for 90 s.
9. Wash the cells with 1× PBS.
10. Block the cells with blocking buffer at room temperature for 20–30 min.
11. Incubate the cells with the 100 μL anti-IL17RB antibody (1:500 dilution in blocking buffer) at room temperature for 1 h (*see* **Note 4**).
12. Wash the cells three times with 1× PBS.
13. Incubate the cells with the anti-rabbit second antibody with HRP at room temperature for 2 h (*see* **Note 5**).
14. Wash the cells three times with 1× PBS.

15. Prepare the following solutions during washing (*see* **Note 6**):
    (a) 100× H_2O_2: one drop (50 μL) of stock (3%) to 1 mL distilled water.
    (b) 1× Reaction Buffer (RB): one drop of stock to 1 mL distilled water.
    (c) Stop solution: 1:11 dilution in 1× PBS (10 μL stock in 100 μL 1× PBS).
16. Prepare the tyramide solution by mixing 100 μL of 1× RB + 1 μL of 100× H_2O_2 + 1 μL of Tyramide stock (*see* **Note 7**). Mix the solution by briefly vortexing.
17. Add the tyramide solution to the cells on and incubate them in the dark for 5 min (*see* **Note 8**).
18. Add the 100 μL stop solution to the cells and wash them using 1× PBS.
19. Counterstain cells with 0.5 μg/mL DAPI (freshly diluted in 1× PBS) for 1 min.
20. Wash the cells three times using 1× PBS.
21. Mount the cover slip onto a frosted microscope slide preloaded with 9 μL cold 50% glycerol.
22. Seal the cover slips with nail polish (fix the corners first and then spread it to all the edges).
23. Incubate for 15 min at room temperature in the dark to allow the nail polish to dry.
24. Store the cover slips in a dark place at 4 °C in a slide box.

3.2 Double-Color Immunofluorescent Staining with Tyramide Signal Amplification

1. Perform procedures as in Subheading 3.1, **steps 1–17**, to immunostain IL17RB with tyramide signal amplification.
2. Wash the cells three times using 1× PBS.
3. Aliquot 40 mL sodium citrate into a microwave-safe container and microwave at Hi power for 1 min with cap on (*see* **Note 9**).
4. Take out the cover glass from 35 mm dish with thin-tipped forceps, place it (the cell side up) in the heated sodium citrate solution, and microwave at Hi power for 30 s (*see* **Note 10**).
5. Take out the cover glass from the container and put it back into 35 mm dish with 1× PBS.
6. Wash the cells three times with 1× PBS.
7. Block the cells with blocking buffer at room temperature for 20–30 min.
8. Incubate the cells with the 100 μL anti-p53 antibody (1:500 dilution in blocking buffer) at room temperature for 1 h in the dark.
9. Wash the cells three times with 1× PBS.

10. Incubate the cells with the100 μL goat anti-rabbit IgG (H + L) Alexa Fluor™ 488 secondary antibody (1:200 dilution in blocking buffer) at room temperature for 1 h in the dark.
11. Wash the cells three times with 1× PBS.
12. Counterstain them with 0.5 μg/mL DAPI (freshly diluted in 1× PBS) for 1 min.
13. Wash the cells three times using 1× PBS.
14. Mount the cover slip onto a frosted microscope slide preloaded with 9 μL cold 50% glycerol (*see* **Note 11**).
15. Seal the cover slips with nail polish (fix the corners first and then spread it to all the edges).
16. Incubate for 15 min at room temperature in the dark to allow the nail polish to dry.
17. Store the cover slips in a dark place at 4 °C in a slide box.

3.3 Fluorescence Microscopy

1. Place the microscope slides containing coverslips (with the coverslips facing down) on the Nikon Eclipse Ti2 fluorescence microscope.
2. Obtain all images with a 50× fluorescent oil objective using 470 (green), 590 (red), and DAPI (blue) channels.
3. Adjust the exposure time and light intensity to obtain an optimum contrast between the signal and the background fluorescence. Use the same setting to take images for all the slides (*see* **Note 12**).

4 Notes

1. Paraformaldehyde is toxic and hard to dissolve. To make 4% paraformaldehyde in 50 mL 1× PBS:
   (a) Add 2 g of paraformaldehyde to 40 mL 65 °C ddH_2O.
   (b) Add 150 μL of 1 M NaOH (or 30 μL of 5 M NaOH) to help paraformaldehyde dissolve faster. Mix the solution until it is clear and all the paraformaldehyde has dissolved.
   (c) Add 5 mL of 10× PBS.
   (d) Adjust the pH of solution using 1 M HCl to 7.2.
   (e) Add ddH_2O to bring the volume to 50 mL.
   (f) Filter the solution using 45 μm filter.

   The solution can be stored at 4 °C for up to 3 days. For long-term storage, an aliquot of the solution should be kept at −20 °C.

2. There are tyramide signal amplification kits from different vendors. SuperBoost kit is used in the present protocol because it has two to ten times greater sensitivity than regular tyramide amplification techniques. Depending on the availability of antibodies and the choice of Alex Fluor dyes, different kits can be used. In SuperBoost kit it contains 1× blocking buffer, 1× poly-HRP-conjugated secondary antibody, Alexa Fluor tyramide reagent, stabilized 3% hydrogen peroxide solution, 20× reaction buffer, reaction stop solution, and dimethylsulfoxide (DMSO). Please see manufacturer's brochure for details.
3. Any microwave-safe container can be used. Based on the size of the container, the volume of sodium citrate and microwave time need to be adjusted to make sure that the sodium citrate buffer is boiled and the cover glass is immersed in the buffer all the time.
4. Depending on the primary antibody used, 1 h room temperature or 4 °C overnight primary antibody incubation can be performed. For overnight incubation, a humidified chamber such as a covered box with damp paper towel is needed to avoid sample dry out.
5. Anti-rabbit secondary antibody with poly-HRP from the SuperBoost kit is used here. In this system, several HRP enzymes are conjugated with short polymers to enhance the signal over the regular HRP system. The optimal incubation time is 2 h but it can be adjusted to achieve the best specific signal/background signal ratio.
6. 100× H_2O_2, 1× Reaction buffer, and Stop solution need to be prepared fresh. The reaction stop reagent stock solution is prepared according to manufactures' instruction and stored at −20 °C.
7. 100× Tyramide stock solution: the Alexa Fluor tyramide reagent is dissolved in DMSO according to manufactures' instruction and stored at 4 °C in dark. Depending on the choice of Alex Fluor dyes, a SuperBoost kit with a specific Alexa Fluor tyramide reagent is needed.
8. Incubation time can be adjusted to achieve the best specific signal/background signal ratio. Five minutes incubation works for most of the applications in our hand.
9. For a microwave safe container with size about 76 × 150 mm, 40 mL sodium citrate is optimal for the application. Based on the container used, the volume of sodium citrate need to be adjusted. In addition, since different microwave oven models have different power setting, the microwaving time need to be adjusted accordingly. The sodium citrate buffer needs to be boiled before putting in the coverslip. The coverslip needs to be immersed in the buffer all the time during the microwaving.

10. The microwaving time need to be adjusted depending on different microwave oven models to keep the buffer in boil but not dry. For tissue samples, it has been suggested to place the sample in citrate buffer and heat with 100% power until boiling and then reduce the power to 20% and keep microwaving for additional 15 min.
11. A mountant with antifade properties is preferred but cold 50% glycerol is OK for normal use.
12. Depending on the signal observed from fluorescence microscopy, adjustment can be made for immunostaining steps. If there is low signal, primary antibody dilution and incubation time can be optimized. Also, the incubation time with tyramide reagent for Subheading 3.1, **step 17**, can be lengthened. If there is excess signal, primary antibody dilution and incubation time can be optimized. In addition, the incubation time with tyramide reagent for Subheading 3.1, **step 17**, can be

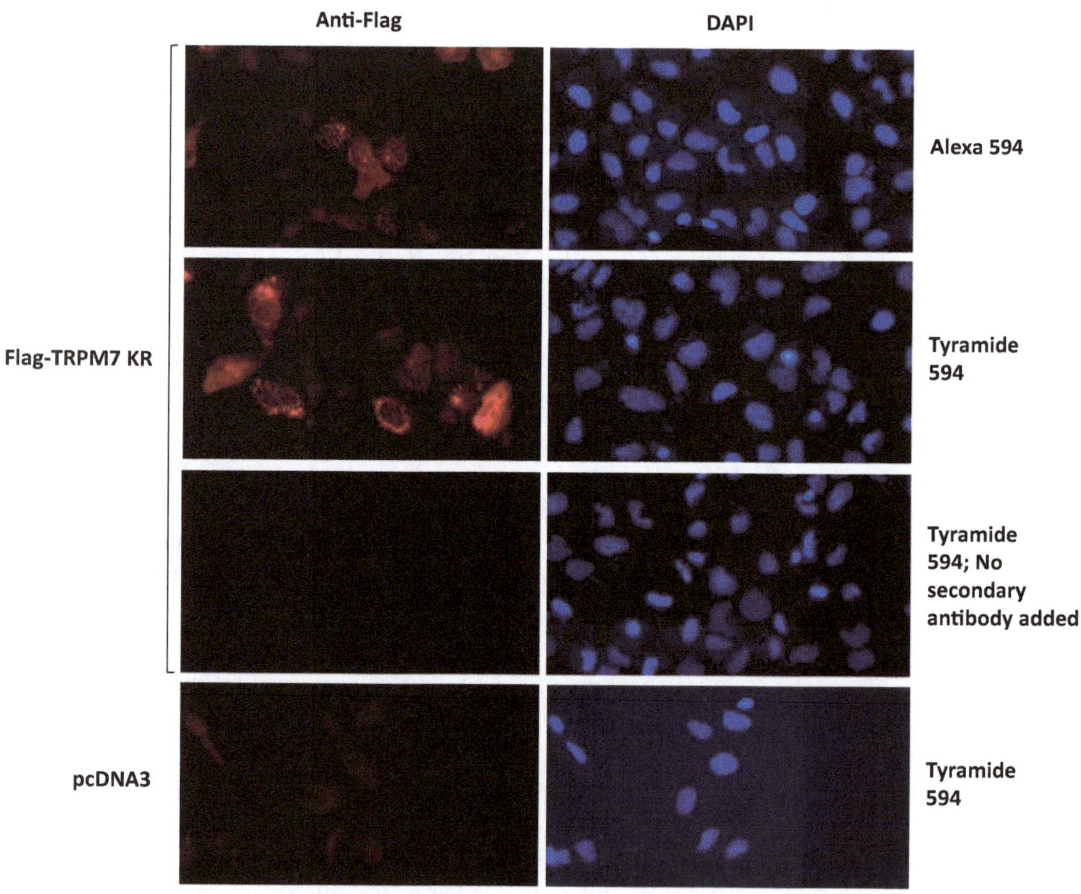

Fig. 3 Optimizing staining condition for tyramide signal amplification using a transfected protein. U2OS cells were transfected with Flag-TRPM7-KR or empty vector pcDNA3 and then subjected to immunostaining using anti-Flag antibody with goat anti-rabbit IgG (H + L) Alexa Fluor™ 594 secondary antibody or Alexa Fluor™ 594 Tyramide SuperBoost™ Kit, goat anti-rabbit IgG

shortened and the working concentration of tyramide reagent can be decreased. If there is high background, primary antibody dilution and incubation time can be optimized. Also, the concentration of secondary antibody can be decreased and incubation time with tyramide reagent for Subheading 3.1, **step 17**, can be shortened. Include a primary antibody only and a second antibody only staining control can help on which action is needed to optimize the staining condition (Fig. 3). Here, staining of a transfected protein (Flag-TRPM7-KR) is carried out with staining controls to optimize the condition. This protein is normally weakly stained with standard immunostaining procedure using Alexa Fluor™ 594 secondary antibody.

Acknowledgements

This work was supported by St. John's University and NIH grant CA213426 to Yan Zhu.

References

1. Parra ER, Uraoka N, Jiang M, Cook P, Gibbons D, Forget MA, Bernatchez C, Haymaker C, Wistuba II, Rodriguez-Canales J (2017) Validation of multiplex immunofluorescence panels using multispectral microscopy for immune-profiling of formalin-fixed and paraffin-embedded human tumor tissues. Sci Rep 7 (1):13380. https://doi.org/10.1038/s41598-017-13942-8
2. Stack EC, Wang C, Roman KA, Hoyt CC (2014) Multiplexed immunohistochemistry, imaging, and quantitation: a review, with an assessment of Tyramide signal amplification, multispectral imaging and multiplex analysis. Methods 70(1):46–58. https://doi.org/10.1016/j.ymeth.2014.08.016
3. Hunyady B, Krempels K, Harta G, Mezey E (1996) Immunohistochemical signal amplification by catalyzed reporter deposition and its application in double immunostaining. J Histochem Cytochem 44(12):1353–1362
4. Monin L, Gaffen SL (2018) Interleukin 17 family cytokines: signaling mechanisms, biological activities, and therapeutic implications. Cold Spring Harb Perspect Biol 10(4):a028522. https://doi.org/10.1101/cshperspect.a028522
5. Kolls JK, Linden A (2004) Interleukin-17 family members and inflammation. Immunity 21 (4):467–476. https://doi.org/10.1016/j.immuni.2004.08.018
6. Alinejad V, Dolati S, Motallebnezhad M, Yousefi M (2017) The role of IL17B-IL17RB signaling pathway in breast cancer. Biomed Pharmacother 88:795–803. https://doi.org/10.1016/j.biopha.2017.01.120
7. Bie Q, Zhang B, Sun C, Ji X, Barnie PA, Qi C, Peng J, Zhang D, Zheng D, Su Z, Wang S, Xu H (2017) IL-17B activated mesenchymal stem cells enhance proliferation and migration of gastric cancer cells. Oncotarget 8 (12):18914–18923. https://doi.org/10.18632/oncotarget.14835
8. Wu HH, Hwang-Verslues WW, Lee WH, Huang CK, Wei PC, Chen CL, Shew JY, Lee EY, Jeng YM, Tien YW, Ma C, Lee WH (2015) Targeting IL-17B-IL-17RB signaling with an anti-IL-17RB antibody blocks pancreatic cancer metastasis by silencing multiple chemokines. J Exp Med 212(3):333–349. https://doi.org/10.1084/jem.20141702
9. Ren L, Xu Y, Liu C, Wang S, Qin G (2017) IL-17RB enhances thyroid cancer cell invasion and metastasis via ERK1/2 pathway-mediated MMP-9 expression. Mol Immunol 90:126–135. https://doi.org/10.1016/j.molimm.2017.06.034

Part II

Cytokine Bioassays

Chapter 8

Analysis of IFNγ-Induced Migration of Ovarian Cancer Cells

Bijaya Gaire, Mohammad M. Uddin, Yue Zou, and Ivana Vancurova

Abstract

IFNγ is a pleiotropic cytokine that has both antitumor functions and pro-tumorigenic effects. Recent studies have shown that IFNγ induces expression of the immune checkpoint PD-L1 in ovarian cancer (OC) cells, resulting in their increased proliferation and tumor growth. Here, we tested the hypothesis that IFNγ induces migration of OC cells. Using the scratch wound healing assay, our results demonstrate that IFNγ promotes OC cell migration, thus adding to the complexities of IFNγ pro-tumorigenic mechanisms. This chapter describes analysis of the IFNγ-induced migration of OC cells by the wound healing assay followed by quantification of the obtained images using ImageJ software.

Key words Cell migration, Cell proliferation, Interferon-γ, Ovarian cancer, Scratch assay, Wound healing assay

1 Introduction

IFNγ is a pleiotropic cytokine that can have, depending on the cellular and molecular context, both antitumor functions and pro-tumorigenic effects [1–6]. One of the principle mechanisms of the IFNγ immunomodulatory effects is its ability to induce expression of the immune checkpoint PD-L1 (CD274) on cancer cells [3]. By binding to its receptor PD-1 on T cells, PD-L1 induces T cell apoptosis and tolerance, thus inhibiting the antitumor immunity [7–10]. However, tumor PD-L1 has also tumor-intrinsic effects that include increased cancer cell survival, mTOR signaling, and proliferation [11–13]. These autocrine, tumor-intrinsic effects of PD-L1 likely contribute to the IFNγ pro-tumorigenic functions.

Recent studies have shown that IFNγ induces PD-L1 expression in ovarian cancer (OC) cells, resulting in their increased proliferation and tumor growth [14–16]. In this study, we tested hypothesis that IFNγ induces migration of OC cells. Using the scratch wound healing assay, our results demonstrate that IFNγ promotes migration of OC cells (Fig. 1), thus adding to the complexities of IFNγ pro-tumorigenic functions. The scratch wound

Ivana Vancurova and Yan Zhu (eds.), *Immune Mediators in Cancer: Methods and Protocols*, Methods in Molecular Biology, vol. 2108, https://doi.org/10.1007/978-1-0716-0247-8_8, © Springer Science+Business Media, LLC, part of Springer Nature 2020

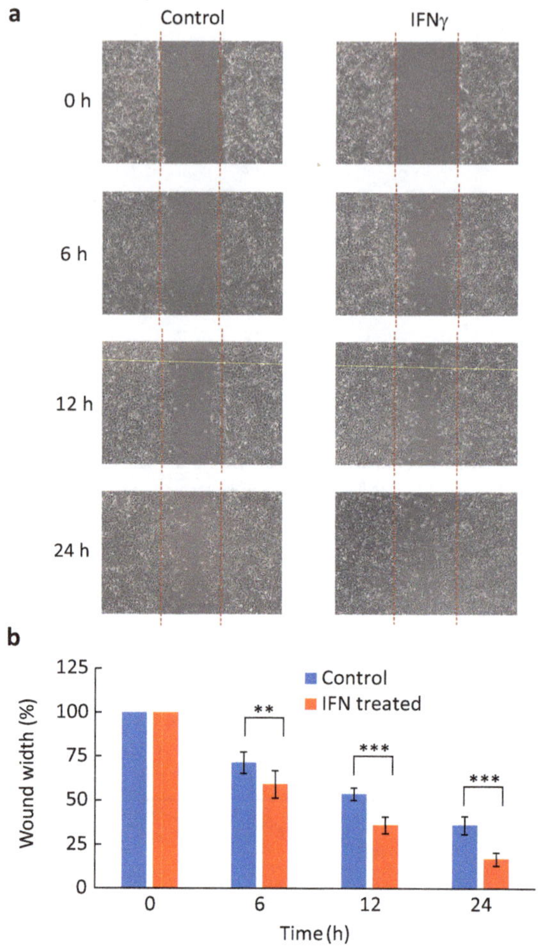

Fig. 1 IFNγ induces migration of OC cells. (**a**) Wound healing assay of SKOV3 cells incubated with 50 ng/mL IFNγ. Representative photographs at the indicated times from three independent experiments performed in triplicates are shown. Magnification: 4×. (**b**) Images from panel (**a**) were quantified using ImageJ software, and the data were expressed as wound width at the indicated time compared to the corresponding wound width at 0 h. The samples were measured in triplicates and expressed as mean ± S.E. (Mann-Whitney U test)

healing assay is a simple and inexpensive method that has been successfully used by many laboratories to study the cell migration in vitro [17–19]. This method can be easily modified and adjusted to different cell types and conditions, and can be on average performed in 3 days.

2 Materials

2.1 Cell Culture

1. SKOV3 cells (American Type Culture Collection).
2. RPMI complete medium containing low serum: RPMI medium supplemented with 1% fetal bovine serum (FBS), 2 mM glutamine, 1 mM sodium pyruvate, 10 mM HEPES, and 1% penicillin-streptomycin solution.
3. 6-Well plates with clear flat bottom.

2.2 Wound Healing Assay

1. Sterile 200 μL pipette tip.
2. RPMI complete medium containing low serum: RPMI medium supplemented with 1% FBS, 2 mM glutamine, 1 mM sodium pyruvate, 10 mM HEPES, and 1% penicillin-streptomycin solution (*see* **Note 1**).
3. IFNγ stock solution: Dissolve IFNγ in sterile deionized H_2O to a final concentration of 50 μg/mL. Store at −80 °C (*see* **Note 2**).
4. Phosphate-buffered saline (PBS) solution, pH 7.4.
5. Phase-contrast microscope with camera.
6. ImageJ software.

3 Methods

In this section, we describe the protocol for analysis of IFN-γ-induced migration of ovarian cancer cells by using the scratch wound healing assay. The scratch wound healing assay is a simple and inexpensive method to study cell migration in vitro; the method can be easily modified for different conditions and purposes. The principle of the assay is that upon creating a "scratch" in a cell monolayer, cells will migrate toward the opening of the scratch to close the gap. By taking images at the beginning and at different times during the experiments, the cell migration can be easily monitored, as cells move to the center of the wound to close the gap. The images can be quantified by ImageJ, or other image analysis software. Figure 1a illustrates migration of SKOV3 cells treated with IFNγ for up to 24 h; Fig. 1b shows the quantification of wound width of the obtained images. On average, this protocol can be accomplished within 3 days, depending on the cell type and condition; 1 or 2 days are required for cells to form monolayers, and 6–24 h are needed for cells to close the scratch.

3.1 Cell Culture and Wound Healing Assay

1. Plate 2 mL suspension of SKOV3 cells (5×10^5 cells/mL) in RPMI complete medium containing low serum in a 6-well plate. Incubate the plate in a humidified 5% CO_2 atmosphere at 37 °C for 24 h (*see* **Note 3**).
2. Use sterile 200 μL pipette tip to scratch the cell monolayer to generate the wound. Press the pipette tip firmly against the bottom of the well and make a vertical wound on the cell monolayer (*see* **Note 4**).
3. Carefully remove the medium and cell debris from the well (*see* **Note 5**).
4. Carefully add 2 mL of complete RPMI medium containing low serum and supplemented with control vehicle solution and 50 ng/mL IFNγ into the wells (*see* **Note 6**).
5. Take initial images of the wound under the microscope at 4× magnification.
6. Incubate the plate in a humidified 5% CO_2 atmosphere at 37 °C.
7. At 6, 12, and 24 h, take images of the wound under the microscope at 4× magnification (*see* **Note 7**).

3.2 Image Analysis

1. Open ImageJ software, click on the file, and open the image (*see* **Note 8**).
2. Rotate the image to make sure the scratch wound is vertical.
3. To measure the wound width, in the ImageJ main window, select *Straight* line and place it over the wound space horizontally.
4. Under "Analyze" tab, select "Measure" to measure the width of the wound and note the value.
5. Tabulate the quantified results of the wound closure over time in the form of a bar graph.

4 Notes

1. Serum induces cell proliferation; to reduce the serum-induced cell proliferation, we use RPMI complete medium containing only 1% serum. The serum concentration should be optimized for each particular cell type, to minimize cell proliferation.
2. Aliquot IFNγ in sterile microcentrifuge tubes and store at −80 °C to avoid repeated freeze-thaw cycles that might decrease IFNγ biological activity.
3. Depending on the cell type, different concentration of cells can be plated to get the cell monolayer.

4. Do not press the pipette tip too hard on the surface of the well. This might damage the coating on the well surface, thus affecting cell migration.
5. Slightly tilt the culture plate to remove the medium. Check under the microscope for any remaining cell debris. If needed, wash the well carefully with PBS to remove the cell debris.
6. Add medium to the side of the well to prevent the possibility of cell detachment.
7. Depending on the cell type and treatment(s) used, images can be taken at several time points.
8. ImageJ can be downloaded freely from (https://imagej.nih.gov/ij/download.html).

Acknowledgements

This work was supported by NIH grant CA202775 to I. Vancurova.

References

1. Ikeda H, Old LJ, Schreiber RD (2002) The roles of IFN gamma in protection against tumor development and cancer immunoediting. Cytokine Growth Factor Rev 13:95–109
2. Zaidi MR, Merlino G (2011) The two faces of interferon-γ in cancer. Clin Cancer Res 17:6118–6124
3. Mandai M, Hamanishi J, Abiko K et al (2016) Dual faces of IFNγ in cancer progression: a role of PD-L1 induction in the determination of pro- and antitumor immunity. Clin Cancer Res 22:2329–2334
4. Mojic M, Takeda K, Hayakawa Y (2017) The dark side of IFN-γ: its role in promoting cancer immunoevasion. Int J Mol Sci 19(1):E89. https://doi.org/10.3390/ijms19010089
5. Castro F, Cardoso AP, Gonçalves RM et al (2018) Interferon-gamma at the crossroads of tumor immune surveillance or evasion. Front Immunol 9:847
6. Zaidi MR (2019) The interferon-gamma paradox in cancer. J Interf Cytokine Res 9:30–38
7. Iwai Y, Ishida M, Tanaka Y et al (2002) Involvement of PD-L1 on tumor cells in the escape from host immune system and tumor immunotherapy by PD-L1 blockade. Proc Natl Acad Sci U S A 99:12293–12297
8. Loke P, Allison JP (2003) PD-L1 and PD-L2 are differentially regulated by Th1 and Th2 cells. Proc Natl Acad Sci U S A 100:5336–5341
9. Chinai JM, Janakiram M, Chen F et al (2015) New immunotherapies targeting the PD-1 pathway. Trends Pharmacol Sci 36:587–595
10. Boussiotis VA (2016) Molecular and biochemical aspects of the PD-1 checkpoint pathway. N Engl J Med 375:1767–1778
11. Azuma T, Yao S, Zhu G et al (2008) B7-H1 is a ubiquitous antiapoptotic receptor on cancer cells. Blood 111:3635–3643
12. Chang CH, Qiu J, O'Sullivan D et al (2015) Metabolic competition in the tumor microenvironment is a driver of cancer progression. Cell 162:1229–1241
13. Clark CA, Gupta HB, Sareddy G et al (2016) Tumor-intrinsic PD-L1 signals regulate cell growth, pathogenesis, and autophagy in ovarian cancer and melanoma. Cancer Res 76:6964–6974
14. Abiko K, Mandai M, Hamanishi J et al (2013) PD-L1 on tumor cells is induced in ascites and promotes peritoneal dissemination of ovarian cancer through CTL dysfunction. Clin Cancer Res 19:1363–1374

15. Abiko K, Matsumura N, Hamanishi J et al (2015) IFN-gamma from lymphocytes induces PD-L1 expression and promotes progression of ovarian cancer. Br J Cancer 112:1501–1509
16. Zou Y, Uddin MM, Padmanabhan S et al (2018) The proto-oncogene Bcl3 induces immune checkpoint PD-L1 expression, mediating proliferation of ovarian cancer cells. J Biol Chem 293:15483–15496
17. Liang CC, Park AY, Guan JL (2007) In vitro scratch assay: a convenient and inexpensive method for analysis of cell migration in vitro. Nat Protoc 2:329–333
18. Cory G (2011) Scratch-wound assay. Methods Mol Biol 769:25–30
19. Kramer N, Walzl A, Unger C et al (2013) In vitro cell migration and invasion assays. Mutat Res 752:10–24

Chapter 9

Interleukin-8-Induced Invasion Assay in Triple-Negative Breast Cancer Cells

Mohammad M. Uddin, Bijaya Gaire, Betsy Deza, and Ivana Vancurova

Abstract

The pro-inflammatory and pro-angiogenic chemokine interleukin-8 (IL-8, CXCL8) induces proliferation and invasion of solid tumor cells. In many types of solid cancer, including triple-negative breast cancer (TNBC), the IL-8 expression is induced by proteasome inhibition. In this chapter, we describe a protocol for the analysis of TNBC cell invasion induced by IL-8 in response to proteasome inhibition by bortezomib (BZ). Using this approach, we show that BZ increases the invasion ability of TNBC cells, and that the BZ-increased TNBC cell invasion is suppressed by IκB kinase (IKK) inhibition, which also decreases the IL-8 expression. The experimental protocol includes the cell invasion assay, microscopic evaluation of the invading cells, and quantitative analysis of the obtained images. This protocol should be applicable also for measurement of chemokine-induced tumor cell invasion in other types of cancer cells.

Key words Bortezomib, Cancer cell invasion, Chemokines, Interleukin-8, IκB kinase, Proteasome inhibition, Triple-negative breast cancer

1 Introduction

Interleukin-8 (IL-8, CXCL8) is a pro-angiogenic chemokine, which stimulates cancer progression by promoting tumor cell migration and invasion. The IL-8 expression is increased in many types of solid tumors, including triple-negative breast cancer (TNBC), and correlates with poor outcomes [1–6]. Although proteasome inhibition by bortezomib (BZ; Velcade; PS-341) and other proteasome inhibitors has been very effective in treating hematological malignancies, it has failed to show a significant clinical activity in solid tumors, including TNBC [7–14]. Interestingly, studies from our laboratory have shown that while BZ inhibits, or does not have any significant effect on the expression of most NFκB-regulated genes, it dramatically increases the IL-8 expression in prostate, ovarian, and TNBC cells [15–18]. These findings indicate that the BZ-induced IL-8 expression may represent one of the

Ivana Vancurova and Yan Zhu (eds.), *Immune Mediators in Cancer: Methods and Protocols*, Methods in Molecular Biology, vol. 2108, https://doi.org/10.1007/978-1-0716-0247-8_9, © Springer Science+Business Media, LLC, part of Springer Nature 2020

mechanisms responsible for the limited effectiveness of BZ, and other proteasome inhibitors, in the treatment of solid tumors.

We have recently demonstrated that proteasome inhibition by BZ induces the IL-8 expression in TNBC cells, resulting in their increased invasion ability [18]. Importantly, inhibition of IL-8 expression by IKK suppression decreases the BZ-induced invasion of TNBC cells [18]. In this chapter, we describe a protocol for quantitative analysis of the IL-8-mediated invasion of TNBC cells, MDA-MB-231. The main points of this protocol are: (1) invasion assay of MDA-MB-231 cells incubated in the presence of BZ, which induces the IL-8 expression; (2) microscopic evaluation of the invading cells; and (3) quantitative analysis of the obtained microscopic images using the image J software. The protocol should be easily modifiable to analyze cancer cell invasion in response to other chemokines as well.

2 Materials

2.1 Cell Culture

1. Triple-negative breast cancer MDA-MB-231 cells (American Type Culture Collection).
2. DMEM complete medium: DMEM supplemented with 10% fetal bovine serum (FBS) and 1% penicillin-streptomycin solution.
3. Serum-free DMEM medium: DMEM supplemented 1% penicillin-streptomycin solution.
4. 75 cm^2 Culture flasks.
5. Bortezomib stock solution: Dissolve bortezomib in dimethyl-sulfoxide (DMSO) to a final concentration of 10 μM. Store at −20 °C (*see* **Note 1**).
6. Bay 11-7082 stock solution: Dissolve Bay 11-7082 in DMSO to a final concentration of 10 mM. Store at −20 °C (*see* **Note 2**).
7. 0.25% Trypsin-EDTA.
8. Phosphate-buffered saline (PBS), pH 7.4.
9. 15 mL Centrifuge tubes.
10. 1.5 mL Micro-centrifuge tubes.
11. Trypan Blue solution.
12. Hemocytometer.
13. BioCoat™ Matrigel® Invasion Chambers.
14. 24-Well plate.

2.2 Cell Invasion Assay

1. Cotton swabs.
2. Forceps.

3. 100% Methanol (*see* **Note 3**).
4. 0.5% Crystal violet (*see* **Note 4**).
5. Scalpel (#11 blade).
6. Immersion oil.
7. Microscope slides.
8. Cover slips.
9. Microscope (with camera).

2.3 Image Analysis

1. ImageJ software.
2. Stage micrometer calibration slide.

3 Methods

In this section, we describe a protocol for quantitative analysis of the invasion ability of triple-negative breast cancer MDA-MB-231 cells. TNBC cells have increased invasion ability in the presence of the pro-angiogenic chemokine IL-8. The proteasome inhibitor BZ induces IKK-dependent IL-8 expression in TNBC cells, resulting in their increased invasion [18]. Inhibition of IKK activity by the IKK inhibitor Bay 11-7082 decreases IL-8 expression and TNBC cell invasion ability [18]. This protocol can be easily modified to measure invasion ability of other types of cancer cells as well. On average, this protocol can be accomplished within 2 days. Figure 1 illustrates the experimental setup. Figure 2 shows invasion of MDA-MB-231 cells in response to the BZ-induced IL-8.

3.1 Cell Culture

1. Grow TNBC MDA-MB-231 cells in a T75 flask in complete DMEM medium to a concentration of at least 0.1×10^6 cells/mL (*see* **Note 5**).
2. Remove media and wash attached cells with 5 mL of 1× PBS. After removing PBS, add 3 mL of 0.25% trypsin-EDTA to the flask and incubate at 37 °C until the cells detach. Neutralize trypsin by adding an equal volume of serum-free media (*see* **Note 6**).
3. Collect cells in a 15 mL tube and centrifuge at 130 × *g* for 5 min at 4 °C. Discard supernatant and resuspend cells in 4 mL of serum-free media.
4. To count the cells, transfer 50 μL of the above cell suspension into a 1.5 mL micro-centrifuge tube, and add 50 μL of 1× PBS and 100 μL of Trypan Blue solution. Mix well (*see* **Note 7**).
5. Add 10 μL of the Trypan Blue cell suspension obtained from **step 4** to each chamber of the hemocytometer.

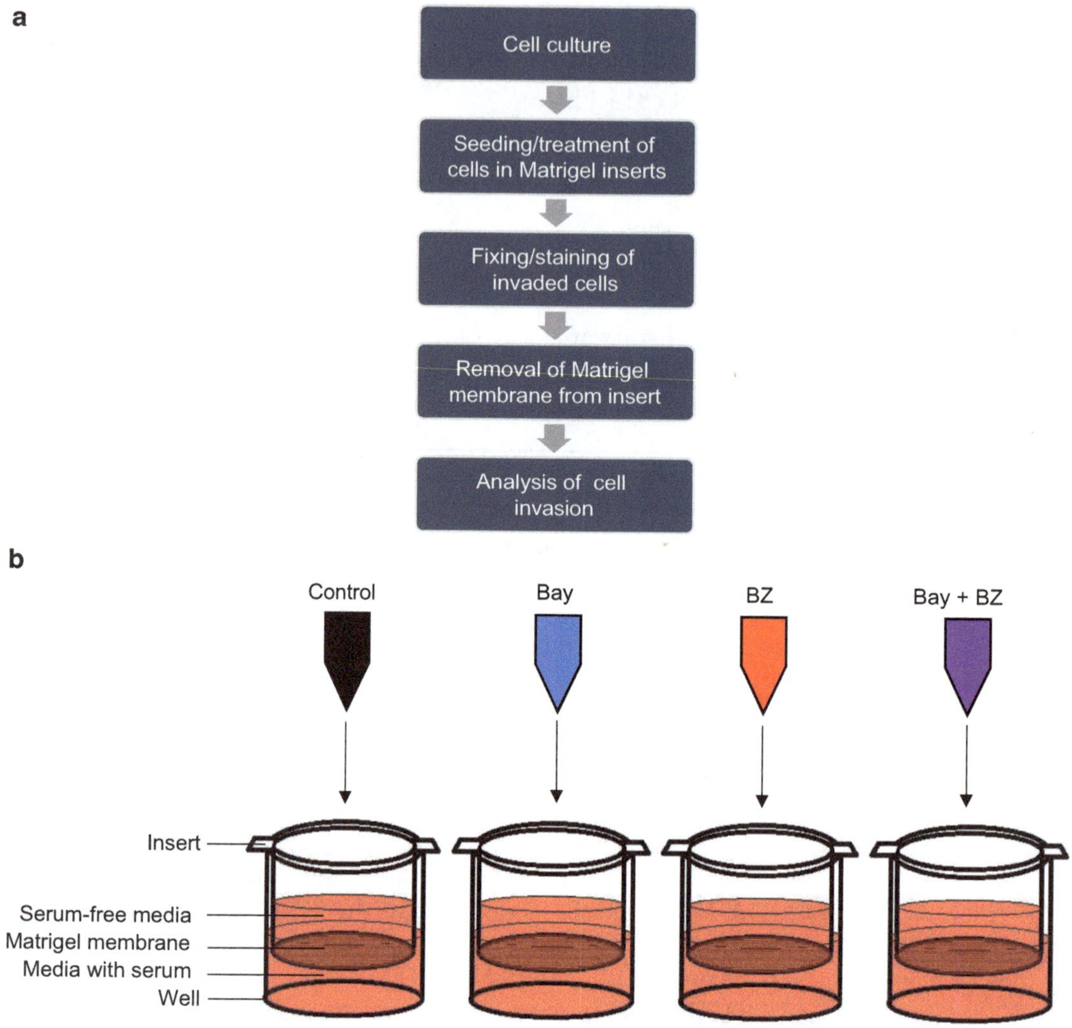

Fig. 1 Schematic illustration of the cell invasion protocol. (**a**) Illustrates the steps involved in the protocol. (**b**) Illustrates the experimental setup. In this experiment, cells were treated with control DMSO, 10 μM Bay 11-7082, and/or 10 nM BZ

6. Count the number of viable cells, and calculate the cell concentration using the following formula: Cell concentration = average cell count in four squares $\times 4 \times 10^4$ cells/mL.
7. Dilute the cell suspension obtained from **step 3** to a final concentration of 50,000 cells/mL using serum-free DMEM media.
8. Aliquot 1 mL of diluted cells into respective 1.5 mL microcentrifuge tubes (*see* **Note 8**).

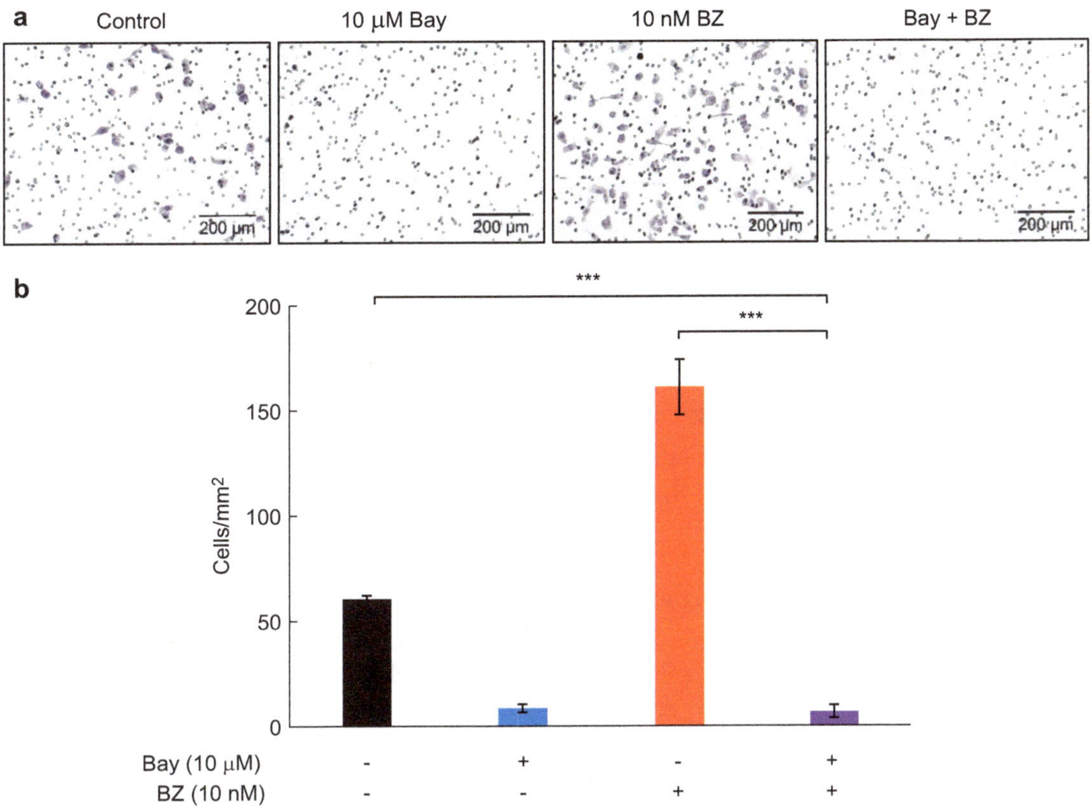

Fig. 2 IKK inhibition suppresses BZ-increased invasion of TNBC cells. (**a**) Shows the microscopic images of MDA-MB-231 cell invasion; cells that have invaded through the Matrigel are stained purple with crystal violet. (**b**) Represents a quantification of MDA-MB-231 cell invasion shown in (**a**). The data represent the mean $\pm$ SE ($n = 3$); asterisks denote a statistically significant change ($***$, $p < 0.001$) compared to control

3.2 Cell Invasion Assay

1. Rehydrate Matrigel inserts before starting the experiment (*see* **Note 9**).
2. To the micro-centrifuge tubes containing diluted cells from **step 8** (Subheading 3.1), add Bay 11-7082 to a final concentration of 10 μM (*see* **Note 10**).
3. Using sterile forceps, transfer inserts that will be used to empty wells.
4. To respective wells, add 0.75 mL of DMEM medium supplemented with 10% FBS (*see* **Note 11**).
5. Add 0.5 mL of diluted cells (with treatment) from micro-centrifuge tubes into respective inserts.
6. Using forceps, immediately transfer inserts into the wells containing media (*see* **Note 12**).
7. Incubate the plate in 37 °C humidified incubator for 12 h.
8. After 12 h, add BZ to a final concentration of 10 nM to the respective tubes and incubate for 12 h (*see* **Note 10**).

9. Prepare two beakers each containing 150 mL of deionized water.
10. Transfer inserts to empty wells, and remove media from existing wells.
11. To fix and stain the invasive cells, in a new 24-well plate, add 0.5 mL of 100% methanol to one set of wells, and 0.5 mL of 0.5% crystal violet to another set of wells.
12. Carefully remove media from inserts (*see* **Note 13**).
13. Gently but firmly scrub the inside membrane layer of the insert using a cotton swab soaked in PBS to remove the Matrigel and any non-invading cells. Repeat twice with fresh cotton swabs for each condition.
14. Immediately transfer the inserts using forceps into wells containing methanol for fixing. Incubate at room temperature for 2 min.
15. After incubation, transfer inserts into wells containing crystal violet for staining. Incubate at room temperature for 2 min.
16. Using forceps, wash inserts in a beaker containing deionized water. Repeat twice. Place wells inverted on a paper towel and allow to air-dry.
17. Once the inserts are dry, cut out the membrane using a blade (*see* **Note 14**).
18. Put a drop of immersion oil on a microscope slide, and then place the membrane, bottom side down, over it. Add another drop of immersion oil on top of the membrane, and cover with a cover slip.
19. Observe the slides under the microscope at 20× magnification. Save 5 field images per condition.

3.3 Image Analysis

1. Open images saved from microscope in ImageJ. Under "Plugins" tab, select "Cell Counter." Click "Initialize" and begin selecting invaded (stained) cells on the image.
2. Record the total number of invaded cells. Repeat for all saved fields and conditions.
3. To add a scale bar to images, open image saved from a stage micrometer calibration slide. Draw a straight line across a known length on the slide. Under "Analyze" tab, select "Set Scale" and fill out "Known distance" (with respect to the scale from the slide), "Unit of length," check "Global" box, and click "OK." Open image on which you want to add the scale bar. Under "Analyze" tab, select "Tools" and then "Scale Bar." Adjust parameters accordingly and select "OK."

4. Express the results as the number of invaded cells/mm^2 by calculating the total number of invaded cells per condition (from 5 selected areas), and dividing it by the total area of those 5 fields (*see* **Note 15**).

4 Notes

1. Bortezomib (MW 384.2) is a potent, specific, and reversible inhibitor of the 26S proteasome. Prepare a stock concentration of 10 μM BZ in DMSO, aliquot, and store at −80 °C. The final working concentration of BZ is 10 nM, depending on the cell type.
2. Bay 11-7082 (MW 207.25) is a broad-spectrum inhibitor of IKK. Prepare a stock concentration of 10 mM Bay in DMSO, aliquot, and store at −80 °C. The final working concentration of Bay is 10 μM, depending on the cell type.
3. Methanol is used as a fixation as well as a permeabilization reagent.
4. 0.5% Crystal violet is prepared in 25% methanol. It is used to stain invaded cells on the Matrigel.
5. 25,000 Cells are required per condition. For this experiment, a total of 100,000 cells are required.
6. Neutralize trypsin with serum-free media as soon as the cells start detaching. Incubation time for MDA-MB-231 cells is approximately 5 min; however, different cells may require different times. A prolonged incubation of cells with trypsin is toxic to the cells.
7. Make sure to mix cells evenly in the Trypan Blue solution by pipetting up and down. Uneven mixing results in incorrect cell counts.
8. In this experiment, we have four conditions (control, Bay, BZ, and Bay + BZ), so four 1.5 mL micro-centrifuge tubes are prepared.
9. Remove the transwell invasion plate (inserts and wells) from −20 °C freezer and allow it to equilibrate to room temperature. Add 0.5 mL of warmed-up (37 °C) serum-free DMEM media into respective inserts and wells, and rehydrate for 2 h in 37 °C humidified incubator. After 2 h, carefully remove the media from both the inserts and wells using a micro-pipetter.
10. In this experiment, cells are first treated with Bay 11-7082 for 12 h, followed by BZ for additional 12 h. Control untreated cells receive an equal volume of DMSO.

11. Chemoattractant (10% FBS) is added to the bottom well and is absent in the top insert. This will facilitate cell invasion from the insert toward the well through the Matrigel membrane.
12. Ensure that there are no air bubbles trapped between the insert and wells by tilting the inserts slightly while lowering them into the media.
13. The Matrigel membrane, while it is firmly attached to the bottom of the insert, is still susceptible to damage. Care must be taken when adding or removing media with a micropipettor.
14. Insert the blade at a corner of the inside radius of the upside-down insert, and carefully cut all the way around, leaving a small area uncut so that the membrane does not detach completely. Grabbing a corner of the membrane with forceps, the remaining point of attachment can then be cut.
15. The total area can be measured using the scale bar.

Acknowledgements

This work was supported by NIH grant CA202775 to I. Vancurova.

References

1. Waugh DJ, Wilson C (2008) The interleukin-8 pathway in cancer. Clin Cancer Res 14:6735–6741
2. Lazennec G, Richmond A (2010) Chemokines and chemokine receptors: new insights into cancer-related inflammation. Trends Mol Med 16:133–144
3. Freund A, Chauveau C, Brouillet JP, Lucas A, Lacroix M, Licznar A et al (2003) IL-8 expression and its possible relationship with estrogen-receptor-negative status of breast cancer cells. Oncogene 22:256–265
4. Freund A, Jolivel V, Durand S, Kersual N, Chalbos D, Chavey C et al (2004) Mechanisms underlying differential expression of interleukin-8 in breast cancer cells. Oncogene 23:6105–6114
5. Rody A, Karn T, Liedtke C, Pusztai L, Ruckhaeberle E, Hanker L et al (2011) A clinically relevant gene signature in triple negative and basal-like breast cancer. Breast Cancer Res 13:R97
6. Hartman ZC, Poage GM, den Hollander P, Tsimelzon A, Hill J, Panupinthu N et al (2013) Growth of triple-negative breast cancer cells relies upon coordinate autocrine expression of the proinflammatory cytokines IL-6 and IL-8. Cancer Res 73:3470–3480
7. Hideshima T, Richardson P, Chauhan D, Palombella VJ, Elliott PJ, Adams J et al (2001) The proteasome inhibitor PS-341 inhibits growth, induces apoptosis, and overcomes drug resistance in human multiple myeloma cells. Cancer Res 61:3071–3076
8. Richardson PG, Mitsiades C, Hideshima T, Anderson KC (2005) Proteasome inhibition in the treatment of cancer. Cell Cycle 4:290–296
9. Shah JJ, Orlowski RZ (2009) Proteasome inhibitors in the treatment of multiple myeloma. Leukemia 23:1964–1979
10. Kuhn DJ, Orlowski RZ (2012) The immunoproteasome as a target in hematologic malignancies. Semin Hematol 49:258–262
11. McConkey DJ, Zhu K (2008) Mechanisms of proteasome inhibitor action and resistance in cancer. Drug Resist Updat 11:164–179
12. Chen YJ, Yeh MH, Yu MC, Wei YL, Chen WS, Chen JY et al (2013) Lapatinib-induced NFκB activation sensitizes triple-negative breast cancer cells to proteasome inhibitors. Breast Cancer Res 15:R108

13. Petrocca F, Altschuler G, Tan SM, Mendillo ML, Yan H, Jerry DJ et al (2013) A genome-wide siRNA screen identifies proteasome addiction as a vulnerability of basal-like triple-negative breast cancer cells. Cancer Cell 24:182–196
14. Deshmukh RR, Kim S, Elghoul Y, Dou QP (2017) P-glycoprotein inhibition sensitizes human breast cancer cells to proteasome inhibitors. J Cell Biochem 118:1239–1248
15. Vu HY, Juvekar A, Ghosh C, Ramaswami S, Le DH, Vancurova I (2008) Proteasome inhibitors induce apoptosis of prostate cancer cells by inducing nuclear translocation of IκBα. Arch Biochem Biophys 475:156–163
16. Manna S, Singha B, Phyo SA, Gatla HR, Chang TP, Sanacora S et al (2013) Proteasome inhibition by bortezomib increases IL-8 expression in androgen-independent prostate cancer cells: the role of IKKα. J Immunol 191:2837–2846
17. Singha B, Gatla HR, Manna S, Chang TP, Sanacora S, Poltoratsky V et al (2014) Proteasome inhibition increases recruitment of IκB kinase β (IKKβ), S536P-p65, and transcription factor EGR1 to IL-8 promoter, resulting in increased IL-8 production in ovarian cancer cells. J Biol Chem 289:2687–2700
18. Uddin MM, Zou Y, Sharma T, Gatla HR, Vancurova I (2018) Proteasome inhibition induces IKK-dependent interleukin-8 expression in triple negative breast cancer cells: opportunity for combination therapy. PLoS One 13(8): e0201858. https://doi.org/10.1371/journal.pone.0201858

Chapter 10

Interleukin-8 Induces Proliferation of Ovarian Cancer Cells in 3D Spheroids

Mohammad M. Uddin, Bijaya Gaire, and Ivana Vancurova

Abstract

Ovarian cancer (OC) is the most common cause of cancer deaths among gynecological malignancies. OC ascites contain multicellular spheroid aggregates, which exhibit increased pro-survival signaling, invasive behavior, and chemotherapeutic resistance. OC cells are characterized by an increased expression of the pro-inflammatory and pro-angiogenic chemokine interleukin-8 (IL-8, CXCL8), which increases their survival and migration, thus contributing to OC metastasis and angiogenesis. While previous studies have shown that IL-8 increases proliferation of OC cells grown in monolayer cultures, the effect of IL-8 on proliferation of OC cells grown in 3D spheroids has not been investigated. The spheroid 3D culture assays have been particularly useful in translational research since they allow cell-to-cell interactions that resemble tumor growth in vivo, while allowing easy cell manipulations and visualization. Here, we used the 3D spheroid culture assay to investigate the effect of IL-8 on OC cell proliferation. Using this assay, our results show that IL-8 significantly increases proliferation of OC cells grown in 3D spheroids.

Key words Cancer cell proliferation, CXCL8, 3D culture, Interleukin-8, Ovarian cancer, Spheroid formation

1 Introduction

Ovarian cancer (OC) is the leading cause of death from all gynecologic malignancies. OC tumors and ascites contain both individual OC cells and multicellular spheroid 3D aggregates, which exhibit increased pro-survival signaling, invasive behavior, and chemotherapeutic resistance [1–4]. In addition, OC tumors and ascites are characterized by an increased expression of the pro-inflammatory and pro-angiogenic chemokine IL-8 (CXCL8), which confers a tremendous growth advantage to the malignant cells, and correlates with poor prognosis [5–8]. While previous studies have shown that IL-8 increases proliferation of OC cells grown in monolayer cultures [9–11], the effect of IL-8 on proliferation of OC cells grown in 3D spheroids has not been investigated. Unlike 2D monolayer culture assays, spheroids 3D culture assays allow

Ivana Vancurova and Yan Zhu (eds.), *Immune Mediators in Cancer: Methods and Protocols*, Methods in Molecular Biology, vol. 2108, https://doi.org/10.1007/978-1-0716-0247-8_10, © Springer Science+Business Media, LLC, part of Springer Nature 2020

cell-to-cell interactions that resemble tumor growth in vivo, while providing an environment that allows easy cell manipulations and visualization. Thus, experiments obtained using 3D culture assays provide results reflective of in vivo systems, being particularly useful in translational research.

In this chapter, we describe analysis of IL-8-induced proliferation of OC cells grown in 3D spheroids. Using the 3D spheroid assay, our results demonstrate that IL-8 significantly increases proliferation of OC cells. The protocol consists of IL-8-induced proliferation assay using 3D cell spheroids, microscopic evaluation of the spheroid growth, and quantitative analysis of the obtained images. Although in this chapter we used ovarian cancer SKOV3 cells, the assay can be modified for other types of cancer cells, and can be accomplished within 2 weeks, depending on the cell type.

2 Materials

2.1 Cell Culture

1. Ovarian cancer SKOV3 cells (American Type Culture Collection).
2. RPMI complete medium: RPMI medium supplemented with 10% fetal bovine serum (FBS), 2 mM glutamine, 1 mM sodium pyruvate, 10 mM HEPES, and 1% penicillin-streptomycin solution.
3. 75 cm^2 Culture flasks.
4. Phosphate-buffered saline (PBS), pH 7.4.
5. Recombinant human IL-8 protein. Dissolve IL-8 protein in PBS to a concentration of 1 and 5 mg/mL. Aliquot and store at −80 °C (*see* **Note 1**).
6. 0.25% Trypsin-EDTA.
7. 1.5 mL micro-centrifuge tubes.
8. Trypan Blue solution.
9. Hemocytometer.

2.2 3D Culture Spheroid Formation Assay

1. 3D culture 96-well spheroid formation plate (low adhesion surface 96-well plate).
2. 10× Spheroid formation extracellular matrix (ECM) (from 3D culture kit).
3. Invasion matrix (from 3D culture kit).
4. 1.5 mL Micro-centrifuge tubes.

2.3 3D Culture Proliferation Assay and Analysis

1. Prechilled P200 pipet tips.
2. RPMI medium containing 2× supplements: 20% FBS, 4 mM glutamine, 2 mM sodium pyruvate, 20 mM HEPES, and 2% penicillin-streptomycin solution.
3. Microscope with camera.
4. ImageJ software.

3 Methods

This chapter describes the protocol for quantitative analysis of the proliferative ability of ovarian cancer SKOV3 cells in a 3D spheroid culture. Chemokine IL-8 promotes proliferation in OC cells, which can be visualized by the change in size of spheroids treated with recombinant human IL-8 protein. This protocol can be easily modified to measure proliferative ability of other types of cancer cells as well. On average, this protocol can be accomplished within 11 days. Figure 1 illustrates the experimental setup. Figure 2 shows the obtained results; Fig. 2a shows that IL-8 promotes cell proliferation in 3D culture spheroids, and Fig. 2b represents the quantified images.

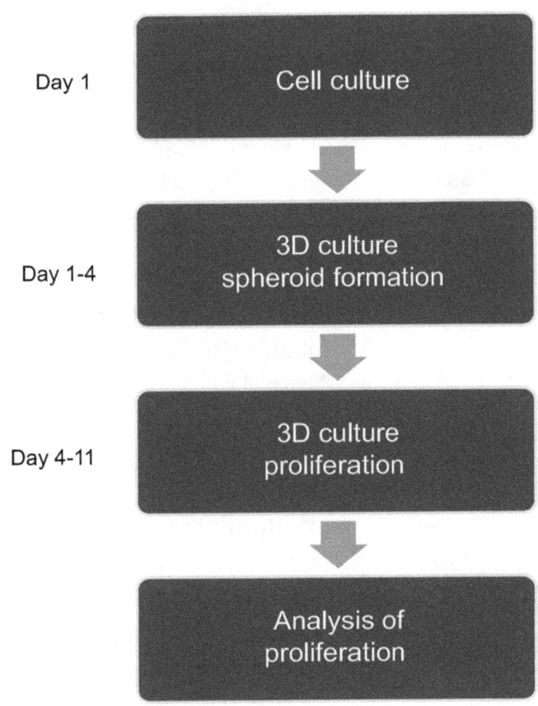

Fig. 1 Schematic illustration of the protocol

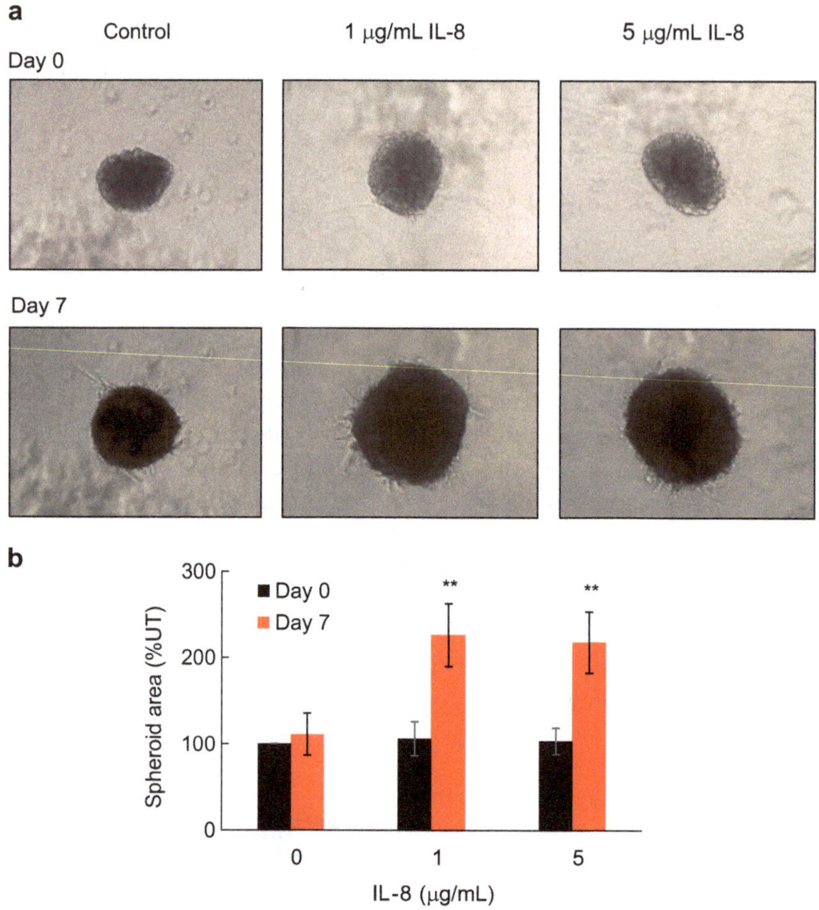

Fig. 2 IL-8 increases proliferation of ovarian cancer cells in 3D culture. (**a**) Images of 3D culture spheroids of SKOV3 cells incubated with recombinant IL-8 for 0 and 7 days. (**b**) Quantification of images shown in panel (**a**). The data represent the mean ± SE of three experiments; asterisks denote a statistically significant change compared to control

3.1 Cell Culture

1. Grow ovarian SKOV3 cells in a T75 flask in complete RPMI medium to a concentration of at least 1×10^6 cells/mL (*see* **Note 2**).
2. Remove media and wash attached cells with 5 mL of PBS. After removing PBS, add 3 mL of 0.25% trypsin-EDTA to the flask and incubate at 37 °C until the cells detach. Neutralize trypsin by adding equal volume of serum-free media (*see* **Note 3**).
3. Collect cells in a 15 mL tube and centrifuge at $120 \times g$ for 5 min at 4 °C. Discard supernatant and resuspend cells in 4 mL of media.
4. To count the cells, transfer 50 μL of the above cell suspension into a 1.5 mL micro-centrifuge tube, and add 50 μL of PBS and 100 μL of Trypan Blue solution. Mix well (*see* **Note 4**).

5. Add 10 μL of the Trypan Blue cell suspension obtained from **step 4** to each chamber of the hemocytometer.
6. Count the number of viable cells, and calculate the cell concentration using the following formula: Cell concentration = average cell count in four squares $\times$ 4 $\times$ 10^4 cells/mL.
7. Dilute the cell suspension obtained from **step 3** to a final concentration of 1 $\times$ 10^6 cells/mL using RPMI complete medium.

3.2 3D Culture Spheroid Formation Assay

1. Ensure that 10× spheroid formation ECM is thawed overnight before starting experiment (*see* **Note 5**).
2. Prepare cell suspension in 1× spheroid formation ECM using the following dilutions (*see* **Note 6**).

   For each condition, 3000 cells are required. The cell suspension dilution for one condition is as follows.

10× spheroid formation ECM	5 μL
Complete RPMI medium	42 μL
Cells (1 × 10^6 cells/mL)	3 μL
Total	50 μL

3. Add 50 μL of prepared cell suspension into respective wells of the 3D culture 96-well spheroid formation plate.
4. Centrifuge the plate at 200 × *g* for 3 min at room temperature. The purpose of this step is to pull the cells toward the center of the well to aid in spheroid formation (*see* **Note 7**).
5. Incubate the plate in 37 °C humidified incubator for 72 h.

3.3 3D Culture Proliferation Assay

1. Ensure that the invasion matrix is thawed before starting the experiment (*see* **Note 8**).
2. After incubation, remove the plate from incubator, and put on ice for 15 min to cool wells.
3. Keeping the plate on ice, add 50 μL of invasion matrix to the respective wells using prechilled P200 pipet tips (*see* **Note 9**).
4. Centrifuge the plate at 300 × *g* for 3 min at 4 °C. This is performed to remove any present bubbles, as well as to position the spheroids toward the center of the wells.
5. Following centrifugation, incubate the plates in 37 °C humidified incubator for 1 h. This is to allow the invasion matrix to properly form. During this period, the respective treatments can be prepared (*see* **Note 10**).

6. After incubation, add 100 μL of the RPMI medium containing 2× supplements, and any treatments to the respective wells (*see* **Note 11**).
7. Incubate the plates in 37 °C humidified incubator for the next 7 days, closely monitoring and saving images of the cell proliferation (*see* **Note 12**).

3.4 Image Analysis

1. Before quantifying images, the scale will need to be set. Open image saved from a stage micrometer calibration slide in ImageJ. Draw a straight line across a known length on the slide. Under "Analyze" tab, select "Set Scale" and fill out "Known distance" (with respect to the scale from the slide, in μm format), "Unit of length" (μm), check "Global" box, and click "OK."
2. Open images saved from microscope in ImageJ.
3. Convert image to an 8-bit image. Under "Image" tab, go to "Type" and select "8-bit."
4. To set image threshold, under "Image" tab, go to "Adjust" and select "Threshold." Adjust the slider so that the entire spheroid is selected. This is the area that will be measured. Click "Apply."
5. Using the "Oval" selection option, make a selection that covers just the spheroid, while excluding any other pixels from the measurement.
6. To measure the area, under "Analyze" tab, select "Analyze Particles." Check the box "Summarize" and click "OK." Record down the "Total Area" (in μm^2). Repeat for all images.
4. Express the spheroid area results as a percentage of control in the form of a bar graph.

4 Notes

1. Human IL-8 protein (MW 8 kDa) is a cytokine that promotes chemotaxis. Prepare stock concentrations of 1 mg/mL and 5 mg/mL in PBS, aliquot, and store at −80 °C. The final working concentration of recombinant IL-8 protein is 1 μg/mL and 5 μg/mL, depending on the cell type.
2. 3000 Cells are required per condition. This particular experiment includes three conditions run in triplicates; that means the total of 27,000 cells.
3. Neutralize trypsin with serum-free media as soon as the cells start detaching. Incubation time for SKOV3 cells is approximately 5 min, but can vary across different cell lines. Longer incubation of cells with trypsin is toxic to the cells.

4. Make sure to mix cells evenly in the Trypan Blue solution by pipetting up and down. Uneven mixing results in incorrect cell counts.
5. 10× Spheroid formation ECM medium should be thawed on ice overnight in a 4 °C refrigerator prior to the start of the experiment.
6. For three conditions in triplicates, 1 mL of diluted cell suspension is to be prepared in 1.5 mL micro-centrifuge tubes.
7. Use plate carrier adapter for centrifuging the 96-well plate. Set breaking speed for centrifuge to a minimal, so as to minimize agitation of cells at the end of the centrifugation.
8. Invasion matrix should be thawed on ice in a 4 °C refrigerator prior to the start of the experiment. Invert the invasion matrix to homogenize the solution, being careful not to produce any bubbles in the process.
9. Samples and solutions should be at 4 °C working conditions. Plates can be placed on ice or an ice-pack, and P200 pipet tips should be prechilled in −20 °C freezer prior to use.
10. Up to this point, the total volume in the well is 100 μL. To compensate, 100 μL of RPMI medium containing 2× supplements and 2× working concentrations of recombinant human IL-8 protein is added.
11. In this experiment, we used treatment with recombinant human IL-8.
12. In this experiment, we used 20× magnification.

Acknowledgements

This work was supported by NIH grant CA202775 to I. Vancurova.

References

1. Shield K, Ackland ML, Ahmed N, Rice GE (2009) Multicellular spheroids in ovarian cancer metastases: biology and pathology. Gynecol Oncol 113:143–148
2. Zietarska M, Maugard CM, Filali-Mouhim A, Alam-Fahmy M, Tonin PN, Provencher DM et al (2007) Molecular description of a 3D in vitro model for the study of epithelial ovarian cancer (EOC). Mol Carcinog 46:872–885
3. Watters KM, Bajwa P, Kenny HA (2018) Organotypic 3D models of the ovarian cancer tumor microenvironment. Cancers (Basel) 10(8): E265. https://doi.org/10.3390/cancers10080265
4. Moffitt L, Karimnia N, Stephens A, Bilandzic M (2019) Therapeutic targeting of collective invasion in ovarian cancer. Int J Mol Sci 20: E1466
5. Xu L, Fidler IJ (2000) Interleukin 8: an autocrine growth factor for human ovarian cancer. Oncol Res 12:97–106
6. Huang S, Robinson JB, Deguzman A, Bucana CD, Fidler IJ (2000) Blockade of NFκB signaling inhibits angiogenesis and tumorigenicity of human ovarian cancer cells by suppressing expression of VEGF and IL-8. Cancer Res 60:5334–5339

7. Merritt WM, Lin YG, Spannuth WA, Fletcher MS, Kamat AA, Han LY et al (2008) Effect of interleukin-8 gene silencing with liposome-encapsulated small interfering RNA on ovarian cancer cell growth. J Natl Cancer Inst 100:359–372
8. Pecot CV, Rupaimoole R, Yang D, Akbani R, Ivan C, Lu C et al (2013) Tumour angiogenesis regulation by the miR-200 family. Nat Commun 4:2427. https://doi.org/10.1038/ncomms3427.
9. Wang Y, Xu RC, Zhang XL, Niu XL, Qu Y, Li LZ et al (2012) Interleukin-8 secretion by ovarian cancer cells increases anchorage-independent growth, proliferation, angiogenic potential, adhesion and invasion. Cytokine 59:145–155
10. Singha B, Gatla HR, Manna S, Chang TP, Sanacora S, Poltoratsky V et al (2014) Proteasome inhibition increases recruitment of IκB kinase β (IKKβ), S536P-p65, and transcription factor EGR1 to interleukin-8 (IL-8) promoter, resulting in increased IL-8 production in ovarian cancer cells. J Biol Chem 289:2687–2700
11. Gatla HR, Zou Y, Uddin MM, Vancurova I (2017) Epigenetic regulation of interleukin-8-expression by class I HDAC and CBP in ovarian cancer cells. Oncotarget 8:70798–70810

Chapter 11

Detection of Ferroptosis by BODIPY™ 581/591 C11

Alejandra M. Martinez, Ahryun Kim, and Wan Seok Yang

Abstract

Ferroptosis is a distinctive form of regulated cell death that is driven by lethal accumulation of lipid peroxides in plasma membranes. Failure to control ferroptosis has been implicated in multiple pathological conditions including cancer development, neurodegeneration, renal injury, ischemia/reperfusion injury, and T-cell immunity. Here we describe a method to detect ferroptosis by determining the amount of lipid peroxides in cellular membranes using BODIPY-C11 probe and flow cytometry. Putative role of ferroptosis in immune modulatory cells can be determined using the same method.

Key words Ferroptosis, Lipid peroxides, BODIPY-C11, Erastin, Flow cytometry

1 Introduction

Ferroptosis is a regulated form of cell death that is driven by lethal accumulation of lipid peroxides within cells [1]. It is a nonapoptotic form of cell death that requires accessible cellular iron to drive the uncontrolled generation of lipid peroxidation. Ferroptosis was originally identified from an effort to develop an anticancer drug targeting RAS-mutated cancer cells using a chemical genetics approach [2, 3]. Since then, evidence has been increased about the role of ferroptosis in various pathophysiological conditions such as heart, kidney, or brain injuries [1, 3].

The role of ferroptosis in the immune system has not been tested formally. However, the lipid peroxide damages on the plasma membrane will impair its barrier function, and many cellular components will be released outside of cells. These molecules are recognized by neighboring immune cells as damage-associated molecular patterns (DAMPs), which triggers inflammation and immune responses [4, 5]. Indeed, inhibition of ferroptosis using ferrostatin-1 (Fer-1), a specific inhibitor of ferroptosis, prevented upregulation of chemokines and cytokines upon folic acid-induced kidney injury in mice [6]. Moreover, specific deletion of Gpx4 gene

Ivana Vancurova and Yan Zhu (eds.), *Immune Mediators in Cancer: Methods and Protocols*, Methods in Molecular Biology, vol. 2108, https://doi.org/10.1007/978-1-0716-0247-8_11, © Springer Science+Business Media, LLC, part of Springer Nature 2020

in mouse T-cells failed to protect the animals from parasite infections revealing an essential role of Gpx4 in T-cell immunity [7].

Specific inducers of ferroptosis such as erastin and RSL3 increase cellular levels of lipid peroxides while specific inhibitors of ferroptosis such as Fer-1 and liproxstatin-1 act as lipophilic antioxidants and thus lower cellular levels of lipid peroxides [2, 8, 9]. Therefore, determination of lipid peroxide level is an essential method in analyzing ferroptosis in biological samples.

Cellular lipid peroxide levels can be assayed by immunostaining [10], colorimetric assay [11], or flow cytometry assay [12]. Among these, flow cytometry-based assay is highly sensitive, measures lipid peroxide levels in live cells, and is easy to carry out. This chapter describes the use of BODIPY™ 581/591 C11 dye and flow cytometry to determine the level of lipid peroxides in live cells. Although this protocol uses erastin and HT-1080 cells, the gold-standard reagents in analyzing ferroptosis, the same protocol can be readily applied to other pairs of immune modulators and immune cells where the involvement of ferroptosis is speculated.

2 Materials

1. HT-1080 cells (ATCC® CCL-121): A human fibrosarcoma cell line.
2. Growth medium: DMEM, 1× MEM nonessential amino acids, 1× Penicillin-Streptomycin, 10% fetal bovine serum (*see* **Note 1**).
3. Trypsin-EDTA.
4. HBSS.
5. 10 mM Erastin (MilliporeSigma, E7781) stock in DMSO (*see* **Notes 2** and **3**).
6. 1.5 mM BODIPY™ 581/591 C11 (Invitrogen™ D3861) stock in 100% ethanol (*see* **Note 4**).
7. Flow cytometer (Millipore Guava® easyCyte™ or equivalent instrument).
8. Cell strainer: nylon mesh with 40 μm size.

3 Methods

3.1 Erastin Treatment

1. The day before erastin treatment, seed 1.7×10^5 HT1080 cells per well in a 6-well plate (*see* **Note 5**). Label three wells as "no staining," "no erastin," and "5 μM erastin," respectively (*see* **Note 6**).

2. Next day, prepare three 15 mL falcon tubes and label them as "no staining," "no erastin," and "5 μM erastin."
3. Add 2 mL of growth media to each 15 mL tube.
4. Add 1 μL of 10 mM erastin to 2 mL of media in "5 μM erastin" tube and 1 μL of DMSO to "no erastin" tube.
5. Take out the 6-well plate with HT1080 cells from the tissue culture incubator and replace media with 2 mL of media in the 15 mL tube prepared above.
6. Return the 6-well plate with HT1080 cells to the tissue culture incubator and wait until cells undergo ferroptosis by erastin (*see* **Note 7**).

3.2 BODIPY-C11 Staining

1. Power on and warm up the FACS machine. Also, warm up the growth media and HBSS.
2. Six hours after treatment, take out the 6-well plate with HT1080 cells from tissue culture incubator.
3. Add 2 μL of 1.5 mM BODIPY-C11 stock solution to "no erastin" and "5 μM erastin" wells. DO NOT add BODIPY-C11 to the "no staining" well (*see* **Notes 8** and **9**).
4. Mix well by shaking and rocking the 6-well plate.
5. Return the 6-well plate to the tissue culture incubator and stain HT-1080 cells with BODIPY-C11 for 20 min.

3.3 Detection of Lipid-ROS by Flow Cytometry

1. Prepare three empty 15 mL tubes and label them as "no stain," "no erastin," and "5 μM erastin."
2. Take out the 6-well plate with stained HT-1080 cells from tissue culture incubator.
3. Transfer media from each well to the corresponding 15 mL tubes in **step 1** (*see* **Note 10**).
4. Wash cell monolayer with 1 mL HBSS; do not discard HBSS wash.
5. Transfer the HBSS wash to the same 15 mL tubes in **step 3** (*see* **Note 11**).
6. Add 0.5 mL trypsin to each well and return the 6-well plate to the tissue culture incubator.
7. After 1 min, take out the plate and harvest all cells using 1 mL of HBSS/media solution in the 15 mL tube in **step 5**.
8. Centrifuge all 15 mL tubes at 216 × *g* for 4 min.
9. Remove supernatant and wash cell pellet using 2 mL HBSS (*see* **Note 12**).
10. Centrifuge 15 mL tubes at 216 × *g* for 4 min.
11. Remove supernatant and resuspend cell pellet with 500 μL HBSS (*see* **Note 13**).

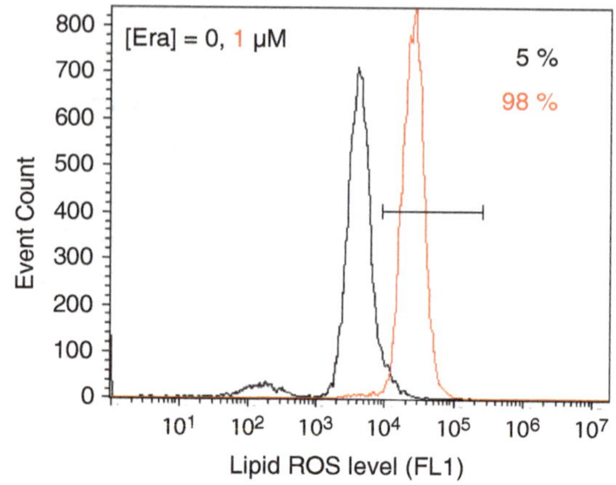

Fig. 1 Ferroptosis induction by erastin treatment in HT-1080 cells accompanied massive generation of lipid peroxides as assessed by BODIPY-C11 staining and flow cytometry analysis. HT-1080 cells were treated with 1 μM of erastin or DMSO for 6 h and harvested to determine lipid peroxide level as described in the text

12. Bring samples in 15 mL tube to the flow cytometry machine.
13. Pass the cell suspension through nylon mesh (40 μm, cell strainer) to remove cell aggregates (*see* **Note 14**).
14. Run flow cytometry machine and analyze data. A typical result is shown in Fig. 1 (*see* **Note 15**).

4 Notes

1. Serum contains many metabolites and antioxidants whose concentration varies a lot among different batches. Therefore, we recommend checking the lot number of the serum and using the same lot throughout the experiments in order to obtain consistent results in ferroptosis sensitivity.
2. For long-term storage, store the erastin powder in a jar with Drierite® granules at −80°.
3. Use of anhydrous DMSO reduces oxidative damage to the erastin and increases stability of erastin DMSO stock solution. Store the 10 mM stock solution at −20°.
4. Store the dissolved BODIPY-C11 stock solution at −20°.
5. As each cell line has different cell size, one should test different cell seeding numbers to find the optimal cell seeding condition.
6. Do not forget to prepare the unstained sample. This sample is required for adjusting flow cytometer settings and producing a control data for assessing cell intrinsic autofluorescence.

7. HT-1080 cells start to die by ferroptosis after 6 h of erastin treatment. As each cell line responds differently to erastin, one needs to determine optimal time point and concentration before carrying out BODIPY-C11 staining experiment.
8. Rock and shake the 6-well plate gently to ensure even distribution of BODIPY-C11 solution in the culture. Alternatively, you can prepare 2 mL of culture media with 1.5 μM BODIPY-C11 dye in a 15 mL falcon tube and replace the culture media with the BODIPY-C11 containing media.
9. It is recommended to test different concentrations of BODIPY-C11 to find the best signal-to-noise ratio in flow cytometry when using a different cell line. HT-1080 cells showed best signal-to-noise ratio when 1.5 μM of BODIPY-C11 was used.
10. Some cells are detached and floating as ferroptosis goes. We want to collect all cells including floating cells in the well.
11. Again, we want to collect all cells including floating cells in the well.
12. This washing is required for removing excessive BODIPY-C11 from cells.
13. The volume of HBSS in this step needs to be determined empirically for different cell lines.
14. This filtration step is necessary to prevent clogging of flow cytometer.
15. Run the "no stain" sample first and adjust FL1 gaining value such that you see the median peak around 10^1 values on the *x*-axis. Then, run "DMSO" sample and confirm that you see increase in FL1 signal. After that, run "erastin" sample to see a shift of histogram to the right side of *x*-axis (*see* Fig. 1), which indicates an increase in BODIPY-C11 signal and represents an increase in lipid peroxide level.

Acknowledgements

This work was supported by National Institute of Health Grants 1SC2NS104275 to W.S.Y.

References

1. Stockwell BR, Friedmann Angeli JP, Bayir H, Bush AI, Conrad M, Dixon SJ, Fulda S, Gascon S, Hatzios SK, Kagan VE, Noel K, Jiang X, Linkermann A, Murphy ME, Overholtzer M, Oyagi A, Pagnussat GC, Park J, Ran Q, Rosenfeld CS, Salnikow K, Tang D, Torti FM, Torti SV, Toyokuni S, Woerpel KA, Zhang DD (2017) Ferroptosis: a regulated cell death nexus linking metabolism, redox biology, and disease. Cell 171 (2):273–285. https://doi.org/10.1016/j.cell.2017.09.021
2. Dixon SJ, Lemberg KM, Lamprecht MR, Skouta R, Zaitsev EM, Gleason CE, Patel DN, Bauer AJ, Cantley AM, Yang WS, Morrison B 3rd, Stockwell BR (2012) Ferroptosis: an

iron-dependent form of nonapoptotic cell death. Cell 149(5):1060–1072. https://doi.org/10.1016/j.cell.2012.03.042

3. Yang WS, Stockwell BR (2016) Ferroptosis: death by lipid peroxidation. Trends Cell Biol 26(3):165–176. https://doi.org/10.1016/j.tcb.2015.10.014
4. Seong SY, Matzinger P (2004) Hydrophobicity: an ancient damage-associated molecular pattern that initiates innate immune responses. Nat Rev Immunol 4(6):469–478. https://doi.org/10.1038/nri1372
5. Krysko DV, Agostinis P, Krysko O, Garg AD, Bachert C, Lambrecht BN, Vandenabeele P (2011) Emerging role of damage-associated molecular patterns derived from mitochondria in inflammation. Trends Immunol 32 (4):157–164. https://doi.org/10.1016/j.it.2011.01.005
6. Martin-Sanchez D, Ruiz-Andres O, Poveda J, Carrasco S, Cannata-Ortiz P, Sanchez-Nino MD, Ruiz Ortega M, Egido J, Linkermann A, Ortiz A, Sanz AB (2017) Ferroptosis, but not necroptosis, is important in nephrotoxic folic acid-induced AKI. J Am Soc Nephrol 28 (1):218–229. https://doi.org/10.1681/ASN.2015121376
7. Matsushita M, Freigang S, Schneider C, Conrad M, Bornkamm GW, Kopf M (2015) T cell lipid peroxidation induces ferroptosis and prevents immunity to infection. J Exp Med 212 (4):555–568. https://doi.org/10.1084/jem.20140857
8. Yang WS, Sriramaratnam R, Welsch ME, Shimada K, Skouta R, Viswanathan VS, Cheah JH, Clemons PA, Shamji AF, Clish CB, Brown LM, Girotti AW, Cornish VW, Schreiber SL, Stockwell BR (2014) Regulation of ferroptotic cancer cell death by GPX4. Cell 156(1-2):317–331. https://doi.org/10.1016/j.cell.2013.12.010
9. Friedmann Angeli JP, Schneider M, Proneth B, Tyurina YY, Tyurin VA, Hammond VJ, Herbach N, Aichler M, Walch A, Eggenhofer E, Basavarajappa D, Radmark O, Kobayashi S, Seibt T, Beck H, Neff F, Esposito I, Wanke R, Forster H, Yefremova O, Heinrichmeyer M, Bornkamm GW, Geissler EK, Thomas SB, Stockwell BR, O'Donnell VB, Kagan VE, Schick JA, Conrad M (2014) Inactivation of the ferroptosis regulator Gpx4 triggers acute renal failure in mice. Nat Cell Biol 16(12):1180–1191. https://doi.org/10.1038/ncb3064
10. Uchida K, Szweda LI, Chae HZ, Stadtman ER (1993) Immunochemical detection of 4-hydroxynonenal protein adducts in oxidized hepatocytes. Proc Natl Acad Sci U S A 90 (18):8742–8746
11. Yagi K (1998) Simple assay for the level of total lipid peroxides in serum or plasma. Methods Mol Biol 108:101–106. https://doi.org/10.1385/0-89603-472-0:101
12. Drummen GP, van Liebergen LC, Op den Kamp JA, Post JA (2002) C11-BODIPY (581/591), an oxidation-sensitive fluorescent lipid peroxidation probe: (micro)spectroscopic characterization and validation of methodology. Free Radic Biol Med 33(4):473–490

Chapter 12

Methods for Studying TNFα-Induced Autophagy

Sheyda Najafi, Ehab M. Abo-Ali, and Vikas V. Dukhande

Abstract

Autophagy is an evolutionarily conserved cellular mechanism in eukaryotes that plays an important role in the maintenance of cellular homeostasis. The autophagy process maintains protein homeostasis by recycling damaged organelles and degrading many long-lived proteins in conjunction with the ubiquitin-proteasome system. Cytokines are low-molecular-weight secreted proteins that regulate a broad range of biological activities. For instance, pro-inflammatory cytokines such as tumor necrosis factor-α (TNFα) induce inflammation, autophagy, and apoptotic cell death. In this chapter, we discuss experimental techniques such as immunoblotting and fluorescence microscopy that can be utilized to measure autophagy in response to TNFα treatment.

Key words Apoptosis, Autophagy, Bafilomycin A1, Chloroquine, Fluorescence microscopy, Immunoblotting, LC3, p62, TNFα

1 Introduction

Tumor necrosis factor-α (TNFα) is a pro-inflammatory cytokine that is known to induce inflammation, autophagy, and apoptosis [1]. TNFα was discovered as a factor released by host cells in response to endotoxin treatment in *Mycobacterium bovis* [BCG]-infected mice; subsequently, its antitumor properties were observed [2]. TNFα is a protein produced mainly by activated macrophages and monocytes, T lymphocytes, natural killer cells, endothelial cells, and fibroblasts [3]. Membrane-bound TNFα is cleaved by a metalloprotease enzyme called TNFα-converting enzyme to form soluble TNFα, which is a trimeric protein that activates TNFα receptors (TNFR1 and TNFR2).

Protein degradation pathways such as autophagy and the ubiquitin-proteasome system help maintain cellular homeostasis. Three major subtypes of autophagy have been recognized that includes macroautophagy (referred to as autophagy hereafter), microautophagy, and chaperone-mediated autophagy [4]. Autophagy is an adaptive process in which cytosolic contents such as

Ivana Vancurova and Yan Zhu (eds.), *Immune Mediators in Cancer: Methods and Protocols*, Methods in Molecular Biology, vol. 2108, https://doi.org/10.1007/978-1-0716-0247-8_12,

proteins, damaged organelles, and even pathogens are engulfed by a selection membrane to form autophagosomes, which subsequently fuse with lysosomes for degradation by lysosomal enzymes [5]. Autophagy, a well-known physiological response to starvation, helps maintain cell survival through recycling of the cellular cargo and is implicated in a wide range of physiological functions [6, 7]. Autophagy proceeds through multiple consecutive steps including: (1) the formation of a primary isolation membrane to encompass a portion of the cytoplasm; (2) expansion of the primary membrane; (3) the maturation of the double-membranous autophagosome; and (4) fusion of an autophagosome with lysosome [8, 9].

The process of autophagy relies on a set of conserved gene products known as the autophagy-related (Atg) proteins that are needed for the formation of isolation membrane and autophagosomes. The majority of the Atg proteins such as Atg13, Atg14, Atg101, Atg12, Atg16L1, ULK1/2, and Beclin 1 are observed in the isolation membrane but not in the final autophagosome [10]. Microtubule-associated protein light chain 3 (LC3) is shown to localize on the inner surface of the mature autophagosomal membranes and is a widely used marker for monitoring autophagosome formation. After its synthesis, LC3 is modified at its carboxy-terminus by the cysteine protease Atg4 to form LC3-I, which is then conjugated with phosphatidylethanolamine to form the lipidated LC3-II. Following the fusion of an autophagosome with a lysosome, Atg4 cleaves LC3-II in the outer leaflet of the membrane while the remainder of the polypeptide in the inner membrane is degraded by lysosomal enzymes. The protein expression of LC3-I and LC3-II can be assessed using antibodies against LC3 and the amount of LC3-II correlates with the number of cellular autophagosomes. In addition, the maturation of autophagosomes can be detected by fluorescence microscopy using cellular transfection with a plasmid containing GFP-tagged LC3. Cytoplasmic punctate structures (fluorescent dots) that are observed under the microscope indicate the presence of mature autophagosomes. The number of LC3 puncta per transfected cell can be used as an accurate measure of autophagosome number. However, an increase in the number of autophagosomes is not necessarily indicative of the normal autophagic process and could reflect a defect or block in autophagosomal formation or maturation [11, 12].

In contrast to the static analysis of autophagy, which can result in errors in data interpretation, autophagic flux is a preferred way to investigate the dynamic process of autophagosome formation, the transport of autophagic cargo to the lysosome, and the final degradation of this cargo in the lysosome. One of the major techniques used to measure autophagic flux is the monitoring of LC3 turnover. In vitro studies have shown that reagents such as chloroquine and bafilomycin A1, which inhibit acidification inside the lysosome and autophagosome-lysosome fusion, respectively, prevent LC3-II degradation and lead to LC3-II accumulation in autophagosomes [13]. Therefore, the difference in the amount of LC3-II in the presence and absence of lysosomal inhibitors reflects the amount of LC3 that is delivered to the lysosome [14]. Another substrate for autophagy that can be used to assess autophagic flux is p62 (also known as sequestosome 1, SQSTM1). p62 is a multifunctional protein that is essential to the formation of ubiquitinated aggregates that are cleared by autophagy [15]. p62 is incorporated selectively into autophagosomes via direct interaction with LC3 and is ultimately degraded by autophagy [16]. p62 has also been shown to interact with ubiquitin chains on proteins and to deliver ubiquitinated substrates to the proteasome [17]. Oxidative stress, chemical inducers of autophagy, and pathways such as Ras/MAPK and JNK/c-Jun can affect intracellular p62 levels by regulating its transcription [18]. In addition, starvation-induced autophagy and inhibition of proteasomal activity play a role in modulating p62 levels [19]. Moreover, the transcription of both p62 and LC3 can be regulated during autophagy [20], which may compromise the interpretation of p62 and LC3 levels as markers of autophagic flux. Considering these limitations, the combination of autophagic flux assessment along with other experimental methods is recommended [11, 21, 22].

It is also important to delineate the autophagic effects of TNFα from its effects on inflammation and apoptosis. There are two major modes of apoptotic cell death: the extrinsic and intrinsic pathways [23]. The extrinsic pathway is stimulated by binding of the Fas ligand to the Fas death receptor (CD95), leading to the activation of pro-caspase-3, an effector protein that executes a cell death program. It has been well established that TNFα induces the extrinsic pathway of apoptosis by binding to TNFR1 (CD120a), which belongs to the same superfamily as the Fas death receptor. In contrast, the intrinsic pathway is activated via cellular triggers (such as hypoxia and DNA damage) that generate mitochondrial stress and also lead to activation of pro-caspase-3 [24].

In the following sections, we discuss the protocols used in our laboratory to measure autophagy using immunoblotting and fluorescence microscopy techniques. Specifically, we demonstrate TNF-α-induced autophagy in HeLa cells using steady-state and flux measurements of the autophagic markers LC3 and p62.

2 Materials

All reagents and solutions are stored according to the manufacturer's instructions.

2.1 Cell Culture

1. HeLa: human cervical cancer cells (ATCC Number: CCL-2).
2. DMEM high glucose: Dulbecco's Modified Eagle Medium, 4.5 g/L glucose, 4 mM L-glutamine, 5% fetal bovine serum, 100 μg/mL penicillin/streptomycin/amphotericin B. Store at 4 °C.
3. Phosphate-buffered saline (PBS, pH 7.3): 140 mM NaCl, 2.6 mM KCl, 2 mM Na_2HPO_4, 1.45 mM KH_2PO_4. Store at 4 °C.
4. Opti-MEM (1×) medium (Thermo Fisher Scientific, 31985070). Store at 4 °C.
5. 3 mM Bafilomycin A1 (ApexBio, A8627) in DMSO. Store at −20 °C.
6. 50 mM Etoposide (ApexBio, A1971) in DMSO. Stored at −20 °C.
7. 100 μg/mL recombinant Human TNFα (PeproTech, 300-01A): 50 μg lyophilized form in 3 mM sodium phosphate, pH 8.0 and 20 mM NaCl. Reconstitute in water and store aliquots at −20 °C.
8. 125 mM Chloroquine (Alfa Aesar, J6445914) in sterile water. Stored at −20 °C.
9. Poly-D-Lysine (Millipore Sigma P6407): 0.1 mg/mL solution in sterile water (*see* **Note 1**). Store at 4 °C.
10. Transfection reagent: Transit-LT1 (Mirus Bio, MIR2300). Store at 4 °C.
11. Plasmid DNA for transfection: pEGFP-LC3 (human) was a gift from Dr. Toren Finkel (Addgene plasmid #24920). Plasmid DNA in sufficient quantity was prepared in TE buffer using PureLink HiPure Plasmid Maxiprep Kit (K210007).
12. Trypan blue stain (Invitrogen, T10282): 0.4% w/v, stored at room temperature.
13. Cell culture dishes: diameter 100 mm.
14. Cell counting chamber slides for Countess (Invitrogen, C10228).
15. Cell-counter instrument (Countess II, Life Technologies).
16. CO_2 incubator: set to 5% CO_2 and 37 °C.

2.2 Cell Lysis

1. Protease inhibitor cocktail (PIC) (Sigma-Aldrich, P8340).
2. Modified RIPA buffer: 50 mM Tris pH 8, 150 mM NaCl, 1% v/v NP40, 10% w/v glycerol, 10 mM NaF, 0.4 mM EDTA.
3. *N*-Ethylmaleimide (NEM) (Sigma-Aldrich, E3876).
4. 4× SDS-PAGE dye: 1 M Tris–HCl pH 6.8, 10% w/v SDS, 40% w/v glycerol, 10% v/v β-mercaptoethanol, 0.5 M EDTA, 0.05% w/v bromophenol blue.

2.3 Gel Electrophoresis and Immunoblotting

1. BIO-RAD Mini PROTEAN® Tetra Cell blotting apparatus.
2. BIO-RAD Mini-PROTEAN® TGX™ Precast gels (4561085): 4–15%, 12-well comb.
3. SDS-PAGE running Buffer (10×): diluted tenfold in water, the solution yields 0.025 M Tris, 0.192 M glycine, 0.1% SDS, pH 8.5.
4. Transfer buffer: 25 mM Tris base and 192 mM glycine, 20% (v/v) methanol, SDS 10%, pH 8.3.
5. Protein standards (BIO-RAD, Precision Plus Protein Standards Dual Color, 161-0374).
6. Tris-buffered saline (TBS): 50 mM Tris–HCl, pH 7.5, 150 mM NaCl.
7. TBS-T: TBS with 0.1% (v/v) Tween-20.
8. Blocking solution: TBS-T, 5% (w/v) milk powder.
9. Antibody diluent solution: TBS-T.
10. PVDF blotting membrane (GE Healthcare, 10600023): 0.45 μm pore size.
11. Whatman filter paper.
12. ImageJ software (https://imagej.nih.gov/ij/); National Institute of Health.

2.4 Antibodies

1. Anti-LC3 antibody (Sigma-Aldrich, L8918): 1:1000 dilution in TBS-T.
2. Anti-SQSTM1/p62 antibody (Cell Signaling, 80255): 1:1000 dilution in TBS-T.
3. Goat anti-mouse HRP-conjugated secondary antibody (BIO-RAD, 1705047): 1:7000 dilution in TBS-T.
4. Goat anti-rabbit IgG HRP-conjugated secondary antibody (Invitrogen, 65-6120): 1:7000 dilution in TBS-T.
5. β-Actin mouse antibody (Proteintech, 60008-1): 1:4000 dilution in TBS-T.

2.5 Immunoblot Detection

1. Supersignal West Pico Luminescent Enhancer Solution (Thermo Scientific, 1856136).
2. Supersignal West Pico Stable Peroxide Solution (Thermo Scientific, 1856135).
3. Supersignal West Femto Luminescent Enhancer Solution (Thermo Scientific, 1859022).
4. Supersignal West Femto Stable Peroxide Solution (Thermo Scientific, 1859023).
5. Chemiluminescence detection instrument (Azure Biosystems, C500).
6. CSeries capture software (Azure Biosystems, C500).

2.6 Fluorescence Microscopy

1. Tissue culture 24-well plates.
2. Glass coverslips: diameter 18 mm.
3. Fixation solution: 3.7% v/v formaldehyde in PBS; prepare fresh solution before use.
4. DNA staining solution (Dapi Fluoromount-G, SouthernBiotech, 0100-20): Store at 4 °C protected from light.
5. Microscope slides 76 × 26 mm with frosted ends.
6. Fluorescence microscope and instrument software (Evos FL Auto, Life Technologies).
7. ImageJ software (https://imagej.nih.gov/ij/); National Institute of Health.

3 Methods

All procedures are carried out according to the manufacturer's instructions unless otherwise stated.

3.1 Cultivation of Cells

1. Grow HeLa cells in 20 mL DMEM high glucose medium at 37 °C in an incubator providing humidity and 5% CO_2 in T-75 flasks.
2. Subculture cells when they become confluent (every 3–5 days, *see* **Notes 2** and **3**).

3.2 Seeding Cells for Protein Expression Experiments

1. Perform cell seeding in biosafety cabinets using sterile equipment and reagents, which should be pre-warmed to 37 °C prior to use.
2. Aspirate the culture medium from cells and gently wash the cells with 5 mL sterile PBS (1×) solution.
3. Detach the adherent cells using incubation with 700 μL trypsin for 3–5 min at 37 °C in a cell culture incubator.
4. Add 5–10 mL of culture medium to inhibit trypsin activity.
5. Centrifuge the cells at 450 × *g* for 5 min at room temperature.
6. Remove the supernatant and resuspend the cell pellet in 2 mL culture medium.
7. Determine HeLa cell viability by adding 20 μL of trypan blue dye to 20 μL of cell suspension in a separate microcentrifuge tube and transfer (10 μL of this mixture) to a Countess cell counter slide.
8. Follow the Countess II instrument prompts to obtain the count of live and dead cells (*see* **Note 4**).

9. Seed 1.4×10^6 HeLa cells into a 100 mm cell culture dish containing 10 mL media and allow the cells to attach under normal growth conditions at 37 °C with 5% CO_2 overnight.

3.3 Cell Treatment

1. Perform the cell treatments in biosafety cabinets.
2. Change the media 24 h after plating.
3. Treat HeLa cells with TNFα at concentrations of 2, 10, 50, and 100 ng/mL for 12–16 h in the presence or absence of 300 nM bafilomycin A1 (*see* **Note 5**). Bafilomycin A1 is added to HeLa cells 4 h prior to lysis step as per the experimental setup (*see* **Note 6**).
4. As a positive control for the autophagosome accumulation, one group was treated with chloroquine (50 and 125 μM) for 12 h. The concentration and timing for TNFα treatment in our experiments were carefully designed to favor induction of autophagy rather than apoptosis.

3.4 Harvesting of the Cells

1. Cell harvesting can be done on a regular laboratory bench.
2. Perform all the cell lysis steps on ice to prevent protein degradation.
3. Protein lysates from HeLa cells are prepared in modified RIPA lysis buffer containing 1× protease inhibitor cocktail and 5 mM *N*-ethylmaleimide (*see* **Note 7**).
4. Aspirate the medium and wash the cells with 5 mL TBS.
5. Add 200 μL of lysis buffer to the dish. The cells are then scraped from the dishes using a cell scraper and the cell lysate transferred into a 1.5 mL microcentrifuge tube.
6. Centrifuge the lysate at 10,000 × *g* for 10 min at 4 °C.
7. Collect the supernatant and place in a tube on ice and discard the pellet. The amount of total protein in your samples can be measured by protein assay methods such as the Bradford method or the bicinchoninic acid (BCA) assay.
8. Add 100 μL of 4× SDS-PAGE dye to the supernatant and heat the samples at 95 °C for 10 min.
9. Analyze the samples (after being cooled to room temperature) immediately with immunoblotting or store the samples at −20 °C for later use.

3.5 Gel Electrophoresis

1. Load equal amounts (in μg) of protein lysate on an SDS-polyacrylamide (SDS-PAGE) 4–15% gradient gel.
2. Separate the proteins electrophoretically at 120 V for 1 h or until the bromophenol blue dye reaches the bottom of the gel. In the case of low-molecular-weight proteins, make sure to end the electrophoresis before the expected size proteins run off the gels (*see* **Note 8**).

3. To prepare for the electrophoretic transfer of the proteins to a PVDF blotting membrane, equilibrate two sponges, two Whatman filter papers, and a PVDF membrane for a few min with transfer buffer and subsequently transfer to holder cassettes. Soak the PVDF membrane in methanol for a few seconds before equilibration in transfer buffer (*see* **Note 9**). The order of the materials in the holder cassette (starting from the negative electrode) is as follows: a thick sponge, Whatman filter paper, gel, PVDF membrane, Whatman filter paper, and a thick sponge. While assembling the stack, make sure to remove any air bubbles with a roller.
4. Close the holder cassette and pack it inside the blotting apparatus in the correct orientation to ensure the proper transfer of proteins to the membrane.
5. Place the blotting apparatus inside an ice-filled tray and place an ice pack inside the transfer apparatus.
6. Perform the transfer at 100 V for 1 h.
7. After transfer, the membrane is removed from the cassette and blocked with blocking solution (20 mL of 5% w/v non-fat dry milk in TBS-T) for at least 1 h at room temperature on a horizontal shaker in a clear plastic box.
8. Remove the blocking solution from the cassette and incubate the blot with the corresponding primary antibody solution (10 μL of antibody in 10 mL TBS-T) at 4 °C overnight on a horizontal shaker at low speed (*see* **Note 10**).
9. On the next day, wash the blots with 20 mL TBS-T three times for 10 min each on a horizontal shaker at high speed (80 rpm, VWR rocking platform, *see* **Note 11**).
10. Incubate the blots with the secondary antibody diluted in TBS-T with milk (3 μL of antibody in 20 mL of TBS-T with 1% w/v milk) for 1 h at room temperature on the shaker with low speed.
11. Wash the blots with 20 mL TBS-T three times for 15 min each time at high speed (80 rpm, VWR rocking platform) to prevent nonspecific antibody binding (*see* **Note 12**).
12. For chemiluminescent detection of proteins, add 300 μL of a chemiluminescent substrate on the blot (volume of the substrate depends on the size of your blot).
13. Perform detection with a lower sensitivity substrate (SuperSignal West Pico) first and enhance the sensitivity to a higher sensitivity substrate (SuperSignal West Femto), if necessary. Place the blots in a detection instrument (Azure Biosystems) and detect the chemiluminescence from the bands of interest using the CSeries capture software.

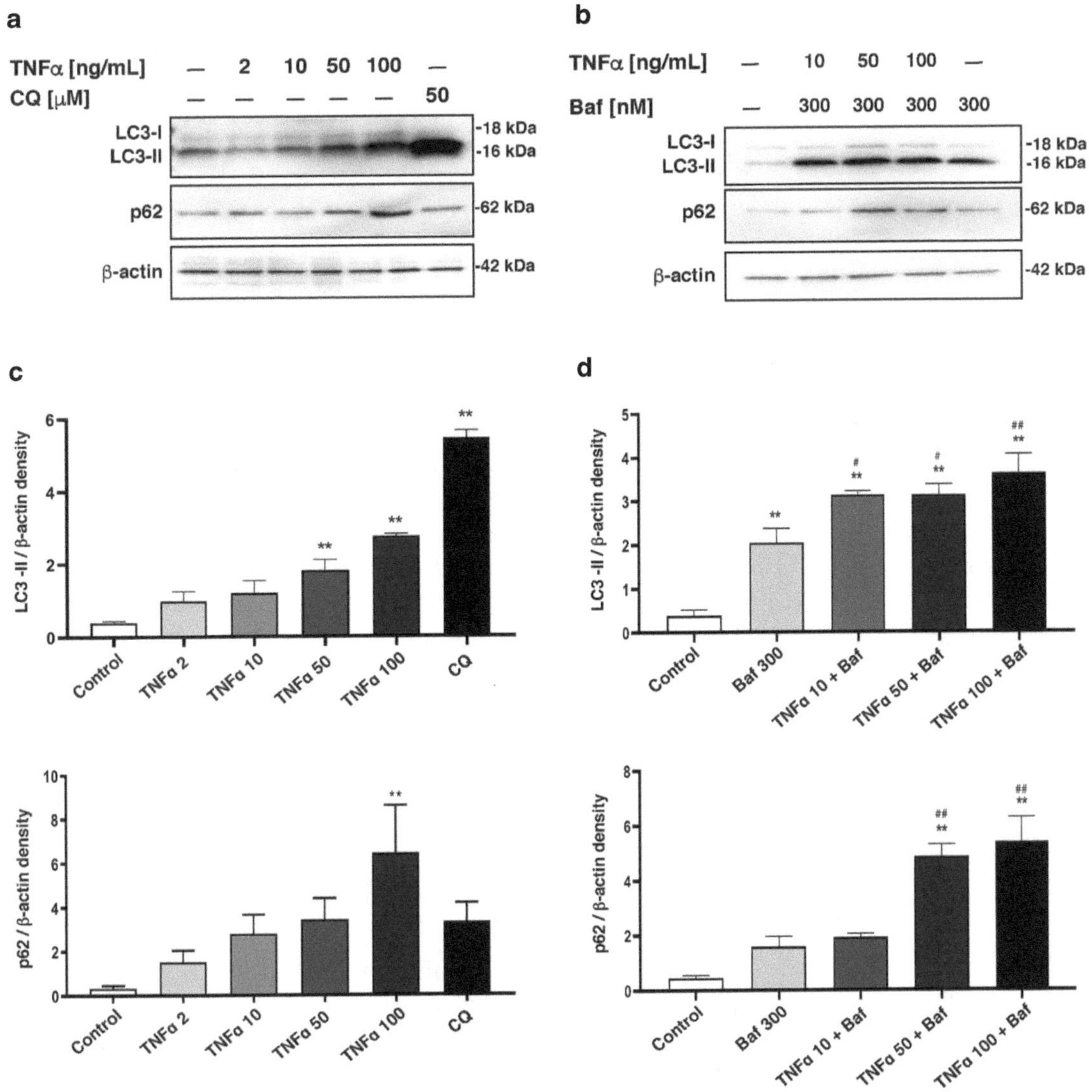

Fig. 1 Western blot analysis of autophagic markers in HeLa cells. Protein expression of LC3 and p62 was analyzed by Western blotting in HeLa cells (**a**) treated with indicated concentrations of TNFα or chloroquine and (**b**) treated with combinations of indicated concentrations of TNFα and bafilomycin A1. β-Actin was used as a loading control. (**c**, **d**) Quantification of image densities of LC3II/β-actin and p62/β-actin in treatment groups is shown in (**a**, **b**), respectively. Data are presented as mean ± SEM. The statistical analysis was performed using one-way ANOVA and (**c**) Dunnett's post hoc test or (**d**) post hoc Tukey ($n = 4$; comparison with control group $*p \leq 0.05$, $**p \leq 0.01$; comparison with bafilomycin A1-treated group $^{\#}p \leq 0.05$, $^{\#\#}p \leq 0.01$)

14. Use ImageJ software to quantify the densities of detected protein bands on the blot and normalize against β-actin bands (*see* **Notes 13** and **14**) (Fig. 1).

3.6 Seeding Cells for Fluorescence Microscopy

1. Perform the following steps in a biosafety cabinet.
2. Place sterile glass coverslips in each well of a 24-well plate using sterile forceps.
3. Coat each glass coverslip with 200 μL of 0.1 mg/mL sterile solution of poly-D-lysine; incubate for 2–4 h. Make sure to cover the glass coverslips in their entirety with this solution.
4. Aspirate the poly-D-lysine solution from the wells and wash the coverslips with 500 μL of autoclaved deionized water. Gently shake the plate to distribute water evenly.
5. Aspirate the water from the wells and seed 5×10^4 cells in a 24-well plate containing the coverslips and 500 μL media to perform immunofluorescence analysis.
6. Incubate the cells in an incubator with normal growth conditions at 37 °C with 5% CO_2 overnight.

3.7 Transient Transfection

1. On the second day, the cells grown on the coverslips are transfected with plasmid DNA (pEGFP-LC3) using the transfection reagent TransIT LT1 and Opti-MEM reduced-serum medium according to the manufacturer's protocol (Mirus Bio) (*see* **Notes 15** and **16**).
2. The following are recommended starting conditions for DNA transfection with TransIT-LT1 in the 24-well plates that were used in our experiments (*see* **Notes 17** and **18**):
   TransIT-LT1: 1.5 μL per well.

   DNA (pEGFP-LC3, 1 μg/μL stock): 0.5 μL/well.

   Serum-free medium (Opti-MEM): 50 μL/well.
3. Prepare the transfection solution in a sterile 1.5 mL microcentrifuge tube at room temperature.
4. Add the transfection reagent to Opti-MEM medium and incubate the solution for 5 min.
5. After addition of the DNA, the final solution should be mixed thoroughly by flicking the bottom of the tube five times to form transfection complexes containing DNA (pEGFP-LC3).
6. Incubate the mixture at room temperature for 30 min.
7. Pipette the mixture and add dropwise in the wells of the 24-well plate containing HeLa cells grown on the surface of the glass coverslips.
8. Shake the plate gently and incubate at 37 °C with 5% CO_2 for 12 h to allow transfection to occur (*see* **Note 19**).

3.8 Cell Treatment

1. Twelve hours after transfection, treat HeLa cells with TNFα at the concentrations of 2, 10, 50, and 100 ng/mL for 16 h in the presence or absence of 300 nM bafilomycin A1 (bafilomycin A1 is added 4 h prior to fixation).

2. As a positive control for LC3 puncta formation, treat one group with chloroquine (50–125 μM) for 12 h.

3.9 Fluorescence Microscopy

1. 12–16 h after treatment of HeLa cells in a 24-well plate, aspirate the medium from wells and wash the wells with 500 μL of ice-cold sterile 1× PBS twice.
2. Add 300 μL of fixative solution (3.7% v/v formaldehyde in ice-cold 1× PBS) and incubate for 10 min at 4 °C (*see* **Note 20**).
3. Aspirate the fixative solution and wash the wells containing coverslips with 200 μL of 1× PBS three times.
4. In the final step, wash the coverslips with autoclaved water two to three times to prevent PBS crystallization in the mounting medium.
5. Add 5 μL of DAPI Fluoromount on a frosted microscope slide to stain the nuclei and to use as a mounting medium.
6. Lift up the coverslips from the wells using a sharp, bent needle and pick up the coverslip gently using thin-tipped forceps.
7. Transfer the coverslip to the microscope slide using the forceps with the coverslip side containing cells facing down onto the DAPI Fluoromount reagent. Up to three coverslips can be placed on one microscope slide.
8. Seal the coverslips on the slide with black nail enamel.
9. Incubate for 15 min at room temperature in the dark to allow the enamel to dry.
10. Place the microscope slides containing coverslips (with the coverslips facing down) on the EVOS Vessel Holder adapter plate, which holds two 25 mm × 75 mm slides, in the EVOS FL Auto microscope.
11. Obtain all images with a 40× (AMEP 4699) and a 100× (AMEP 4696) plan fluorite objective using GFP and DAPI channels.
12. Adjust the exposure time and light intensity to acquire a strong signal without saturating the intensity to obtain an optimum contrast between the signal and the background fluorescence.
13. Quantify LC3 fluorescent puncta using ImageJ software. After selecting the cells to be analyzed and thresholding the region of interest for minimum and maximum pixel values using the Threshold function, use the ImageJ software to employ the Measure Particles algorithm to record EGFP-LC3 puncta number, area, and size (Fig. 2).
14. Displayed results can be transferred to a Microsoft Excel sheet for further statistical analysis (*see* **Notes 21** and **22**).

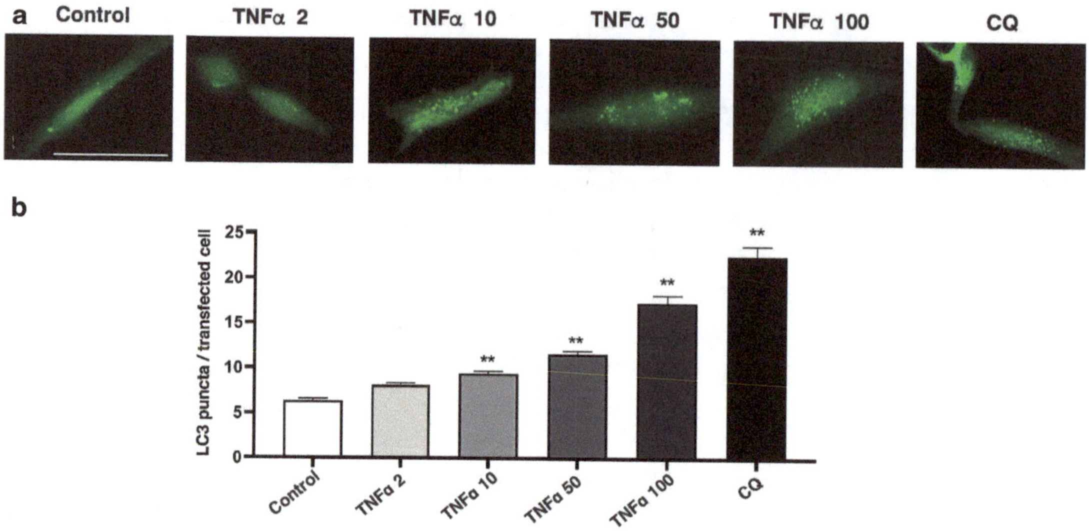

Fig. 2 Detection of autophagy in HeLa cells using fluorescence microscopy. (**a**) Representative images of HeLa cells expressing EGFP-LC3 treated with indicated concentrations of TNFα or 125 μM chloroquine taken using a 100× oil immersion objective. Scale bar 100 μm. (**b**) Quantification of the LC3 puncta per transfected cell following 12 h treatment with the indicated concentrations of TNFα or 125 μM chloroquine. Data are presented as mean ± SEM. The statistical analysis was performed using one-way ANOVA and Dunnett's post hoc test ($n > 100$, $*p \leq 0.05$, $**p \leq 0.01$)

3.10 Analysis of Autophagic Flux

1. Autophagic flux can be assessed by analyzing the protein expression of LC3-II and p62/SQSTM1, and by examining the amount of EGFP-LC3 using fluorescence microscopy following treatment with TNFα, and co-treatment with bafilomycin A1.
2. Bafilomycin A1 was added at a final concentration of 300 nM to HeLa cells 4 h prior to lysis (immunoblotting experiments) or fixation (fluorescence microscopy experiment) in both the experimental groups (Fig. 3).

4 Notes

1. Poly-D-Lysine is used to promote the adhesion of cells to the glass coverslips. The polycationic structure of the molecules interacts with the anionic sites on the cells allowing efficient attachment of cells to the cover slips.
2. Passage the cells at least twice after thawing them from liquid nitrogen to give the cells time to recover and return to the normal growth state before their use in any experiments.
3. The cells should not have a high passage number. The growth rate and morphology of cells can change at high passage numbers.

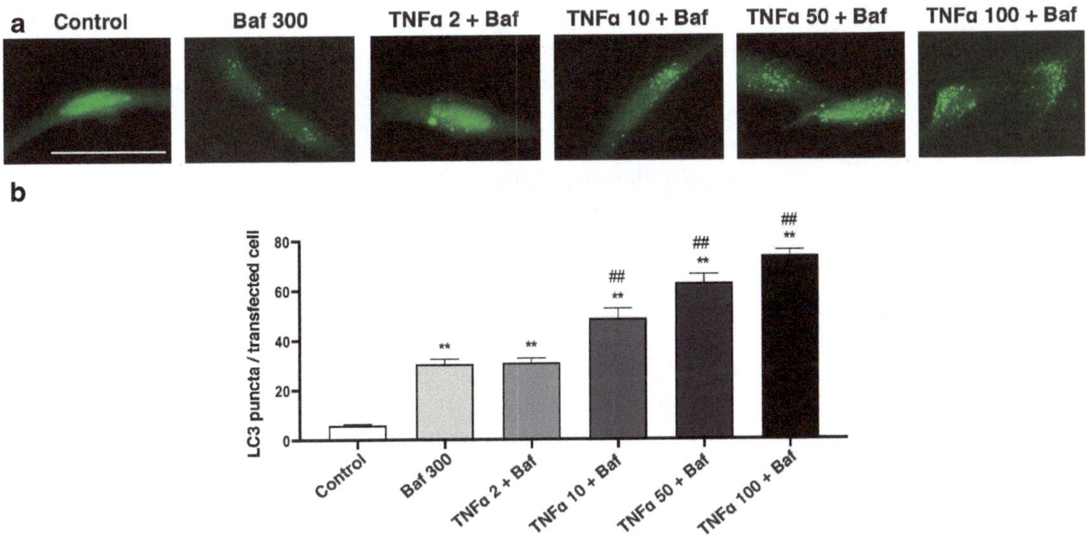

Fig. 3 Assessment of autophagy flux in HeLa cells using bafilomycin A1 treatment and fluorescence microscopy. (**a**) Representative images of HeLa cells treated with indicated concentrations of TNFα (16 h) and 300 nM bafilomycin A1 (Baf, 4 h prior to fixation) taken using a 100× oil immersion objective. Scale bar 100 μm. (**b**) Quantification of LC3 puncta per transfected cell after treatment of HeLa cells with the indicated concentrations of TNFα and 300 nM bafilomycin-A1. Data are presented as mean ± SEM. The statistical analysis was performed using one-way ANOVA and post hoc Tukey ($n > 100$; comparison with control group $*p \leq 0.05$, $**p \leq 0.01$; comparison with bafilomycin A1-treated group $^{\#}p \leq 0.05$, $^{\#\#}p \leq 0.01$)

4. Healthy cells are at least 90% live when counted on the Countess slide using trypan blue dye, and healthy cells should be used for experiments.
5. TNFα in high concentrations and for longer treatment periods can induce apoptosis, so the concentration and timing of TNFα treatment employed will dictate the occurrence of autophagy and apoptosis.
6. Several methods are available to assess autophagic flux such as bafilomycin A1 treatment or use of plasmids that fluoresce differently when associated with autophagosomes and lysosomes. The application and limitations of each of these methods may be different in various cell types and in different experimental setups; thus, a combination of assays is recommended to monitor autophagic flux.
7. During the cell lysis process, proteolysis and denaturation can begin, which can be slowed down if the cell culture dishes are kept on ice and protease inhibitors are used in the lysis mixture. We also used *N*-ethylmaleimide in the lysis mixture as an alkylating compound that reacts with protein sulfhydryl groups to prevent disulfide bond formation and thereby inhibiting cysteine enzymes.

8. In our experiment, gradient gels were preferred for detection of the desired proteins because proteins with close low molecular weights (LC3-I and LC3-II) separate more appropriately on a gradient gel. In addition, the gradient in pore size facilitates separation of a broad range of molecular weights [25]. Alternatively, gels with higher polyacrylamide concentration than normal such as 13% SDS-PAGE gels can also be used.
9. Due to the hydrophobic nature of the PVDF blotting membrane, it should be soaked in methanol before equilibration in transfer buffer.
10. During incubation of the PVDF membrane with the antibody, the side of the membrane facing gel should be facing up in the Western blot boxes.
11. During immunoblotting, several steps need incubation of the blot on a shaker. When incubating with primary and secondary antibody, the appropriate speed (not too fast or too slow) will allow the antibody to bind uniformly and will help reduce nonspecific binding.
12. Do not use saturated images to compare band densities in Western blot analysis as that will result in inaccurate interpretation of data.
13. Commercial LC3 antibodies generally show greater affinity for LC3-II, so the ratio of LC3-I and LC3-II does not represent the actual ratio of cytosolic and membrane-bound LC3 [26]. In addition, LC3-I can show a very faint signal depending on the antibody used and cell type. Therefore, LC3-I levels or the ratio of LC3-II to LC3-I is not a reliable way to quantify LC3-II. Instead, it is suggested to compare the amount of LC3-II with the expression of abundant proteins such as tubulin or β-actin [27].
14. The actual molecular weight of LC3-II is greater than LC3-I because of conjugation with phosphatidylethanolamine. However, LC3-II travels faster than LC3-I on a gel due to hydrophobicity. Thus, the apparent molecular weight of LC3-II and LC3-I are 14 kDa and 16 kDa, respectively [12].
15. For transfection, follow the transfection reagent protocol and optimize the transfection conditions in your experiment considering the cell type, concentration of DNA, and transfection reagent.
16. During transfections, use high-quality plasmid DNA with an appropriate concentration. High DNA and transfection reagent amounts can influence the viability of cells.
17. TransIT-LT1 is a broad-spectrum transfection reagent that can be used in various cell types. However, it is critical to optimize the ratio of TransIT-LT1 to DNA for each cell type.

18. Determination of optimal cell density is carried out to achieve high transfection efficacy. Highly confluent cells do not take up plasmid DNA efficiently. In our experiments, transfections were performed when HeLa cells were ~70% confluent.
19. Some cells that are difficult to transfect such as primary fibroblasts require the use of alternate plasmid delivery methods like electroporation.
20. Fixation of cells with formaldehyde can lead to disruption of nucleic acids. Fixation at low temperature (4 °C) helps to maintain subcellular structures.
21. For statistical analysis of puncta per cell, it is appropriate to quantify the average number of EGFP-LC3 puncta per cell in all cells. In this experiment, at least 100 cells were considered for each group for the quantification of puncta taken with a 40× objective. Images taken with a 100× plan fluorite oil immersion objective show better visualization of punctate structures and were therefore used as representative images.
22. Although the number of puncta are considerably enhanced after autophagy induction, few puncta are observed even under normal conditions. Thus, the percentage of cells with EGFP-LC3 puncta is not an appropriate autophagic marker because transfection efficiency could be very high in many cell types.

Acknowledgments

Research reported in this chapter was supported by an award from the National Institute of General Medical Sciences of the National Institutes of Health under Award Number SC2GM125550 to VVD and by the College of Pharmacy and Health Sciences, St. John's University startup fund to VVD.

References

1. Chu L-Y, Hsueh Y-C, Cheng H-L, Wu KK (2017) Cytokine-induced autophagy promotes long-term VCAM-1 but not ICAM-1 expression by degrading late-phase IκBα. Sci Rep 7:12472. https://doi.org/10.1038/s41598-017-12641-8
2. Carswell EA, Old LJ, Kassel RL et al (1975) An endotoxin-induced serum factor that causes necrosis of tumors. Proc Natl Acad Sci U S A 72:3666–3670. https://doi.org/10.1073/pnas.72.9.3666
3. Sedger LM, McDermott MF (2014) TNF and TNF-receptors: from mediators of cell death and inflammation to therapeutic giants - past, present and future. Cytokine Growth Factor Rev 25:453–472. https://doi.org/10.1016/j.cytogfr.2014.07.016
4. Ravikumar B, Sarkar S, Davies JE et al (2010) Regulation of mammalian autophagy in physiology and pathophysiology. Physiol Rev 90:1383–1435. https://doi.org/10.1152/physrev.00030.2009
5. Ryter SW, Cloonan SM, Choi AMK (2013) Autophagy: a critical regulator of cellular metabolism and homeostasis. Mol Cells 36:7–16. https://doi.org/10.1007/s10059-013-0140-8

6. Eskelinen E-L, Saftig P (2009) Autophagy: a lysosomal degradation pathway with a central role in health and disease. Biochim Biophys Acta 1793:664–673. https://doi.org/10.1016/j.bbamcr.2008.07.014
7. Mizushima N, Komatsu M (2011) Autophagy: renovation of cells and tissues. Cell 147:728–741. https://doi.org/10.1016/j.cell.2011.10.026
8. Yoshii SR, Mizushima N (2017) Monitoring and measuring autophagy. Int J Mol Sci 18:1865. https://doi.org/10.3390/ijms18091865
9. Mizushima N, Levine B, Cuervo AM, Klionsky DJ (2008) Autophagy fights disease through cellular self-digestion. Nature 451:1069
10. Longatti A, Tooze SA (2009) Vesicular trafficking and autophagosome formation. Cell Death Differ 16:956–965. https://doi.org/10.1038/cdd.2009.39
11. Mizushima N, Yoshimori T, Levine B (2010) Methods in mammalian autophagy research. Cell 140:313–326. https://doi.org/10.1016/j.cell.2010.01.028
12. Kabeya Y, Mizushima N, Ueno T et al (2000) LC3, a mammalian homologue of yeast Apg8p, is localized in autophagosome membranes after processing. EMBO J 19:5720–5728. https://doi.org/10.1093/emboj/19.21.5720
13. Tanida I, Minematsu-Ikeguchi N, Ueno T, Kominami E (2005) Lysosomal turnover, but not a cellular level, of endogenous LC3 is a marker for autophagy. Autophagy 1:84–91
14. Rubinsztein DC, Cuervo AM, Ravikumar B et al (2009) In search of an autophagomometer. Autophagy 5:585–589. https://doi.org/10.4161/auto.5.5.8823
15. Lamark T, Kirkin V, Dikic I, Johansen T (2009) NBR1 and p62 as cargo receptors for selective autophagy of ubiquitinated targets. Cell Cycle 8:1986–1990. https://doi.org/10.4161/cc.8.13.8892
16. Bjorkoy G, Lamark T, Brech A et al (2005) p62/SQSTM1 forms protein aggregates degraded by autophagy and has a protective effect on huntingtin-induced cell death. J Cell Biol 171:603–614. https://doi.org/10.1083/jcb.200507002
17. Myeku N, Figueiredo-Pereira ME (2011) Dynamics of the degradation of ubiquitinated proteins by proteasomes and autophagy: association with sequestosome 1/p62. J Biol Chem 286:22426–22440. https://doi.org/10.1074/jbc.M110.149252
18. Puissant A, Fenouille N, Auberger P (2012) When autophagy meets cancer through p62/SQSTM1. Am J Cancer Res 2:397–413
19. Liu WJ, Ye L, Huang WF et al (2016) p62 links the autophagy pathway and the ubiquitin-proteasome system upon ubiquitinated protein degradation. Cell Mol Biol Lett 21:29. https://doi.org/10.1186/s11658-016-0031-z
20. He C, Klionsky DJ (2009) Regulation mechanisms and signaling pathways of autophagy. Annu Rev Genet 43:67–93. https://doi.org/10.1146/annurev-genet-102808-114910
21. Klionsky DJ, Abeliovich H, Agostinis P et al (2008) Guidelines for the use and interpretation of assays for monitoring autophagy in higher eukaryotes. Autophagy 4:151–175
22. Krieg S, Lüscher B, Vervoorts J, Dohmen M (2018) Studying the role of AMPK in autophagy. In: Neumann D, Viollet B (eds) AMPK: methods and protocols. Springer New York, New York, NY, pp 373–391
23. Fulda S, Debatin KM (2006) Extrinsic versus intrinsic apoptosis pathways in anticancer chemotherapy. Oncogene 25:4798–4811. https://doi.org/10.1038/sj.onc.1209608
24. Ouyang L, Shi Z, Zhao S et al (2012) Programmed cell death pathways in cancer: a review of apoptosis, autophagy and programmed necrosis. Cell Prolif 45:487–498. https://doi.org/10.1111/j.1365-2184.2012.00845.x
25. Walker JM (1984) Gradient SDS polyacrylamide gel electrophoresis. Methods Mol Biol 1:57–61. https://doi.org/10.1385/0-89603-062-8:57
26. Mizushima N, Yoshimori T (2007) How to interpret LC3 immunoblotting. Autophagy 3:542–545
27. Jiang P, Mizushima N (2015) LC3- and p62-based biochemical methods for the analysis of autophagy progression in mammalian cells. Methods 75:13–18. https://doi.org/10.1016/j.ymeth.2014.11.021

Chapter 13

Isolation of Antibody Binders to MISIIR from a Phage Display Library by Sorting

Andy Qingan Yuan

Abstract

Cell surface antigens represent the most common targets for antibody-based cancer therapy. Isolation of lead antibodies to these membrane targets from antibody repertoires, such as immunized or naïve phage display libraries, has been a challenging task, which is an outstanding issue when soluble portion of the target(s) is not available, and/or a naïve phage display library is used. Common cell-based panning methods often encounter numerous difficulties, including high background and loss of cells during repeated washes. Here we described a novel FACS sorter-based protocol to isolate single-chain Fv molecules specific for defined antigen MSIIR expressed on stably transformed mammalian cells, and screening of unique binders to the tumor target.

Key words Phage display, Biopanning, Antibody, Sorting, Single-chain Fv (scFv)

1 Introduction

Antibodies targeting relevant cancer cell surface antigens are playing an increasingly important role in cancer diagnosis and therapy [1–3]. More recent generations of MAbs entering clinical trials are derived from naïve phage display of human immunoglobulin variable domains in single-chain Fv (scFv) or Fab formats [4]. When using human naïve phage display scFv library, straightforward biopannings (solid phase, solution phase) are used to isolate specific clones when purified soluble target is available and there is good consistence between the soluble portion and the membrane counterpart [5]. While solid phase panning is generally effective, it often yields clones to epitopes that are either not exposed due to protein conformation or not accessible due to steric hindrance by other components in the cell membrane [6].

When cells expressing the chosen target must be used as "bait" to isolate binders from phage display library, undesired binders to the common and uncommon cell surface proteins often obscure the panning process [7]. Solutions have been tested to tackle this

Ivana Vancurova and Yan Zhu (eds.), *Immune Mediators in Cancer: Methods and Protocols*, Methods in Molecular Biology, vol. 2108, https://doi.org/10.1007/978-1-0716-0247-8_13, © Springer Science+Business Media, LLC, part of Springer Nature 2020

issue, including an initial blocking step against a normal cell population to deplete undesired clones prior to panning against the tumor cell line of interest [8] and stripping unwanted phage from the cell surface prior to recovering the selected phage to isolate those that target internalized antigens [9, 10]. Cell-based panning strategies could potentially yield antibody clones with a higher specificity and accessibility for the desired target if the background could be curtailed [11]. However, the current methodologies involve tedious and complicated optimization of choosing appropriate cell lines, the number of cell number used, incubation duration, washing stringency, etc. to achieve acceptable signal/noise ratio and decent positive yield [12].

We described here a novel method to overcome the obstacles to cell-based panning that are mentioned above. A human Müllerian inhibiting substance (MIS) type II receptor (MISIIR), which is also known as the anti-Müllerian hormone (AMH) receptor type II (AMHRII), was used as a target antigen to demonstrate the method. MISIIR is involved in the regression of the female Müllerian duct during the normal development of the male reproductive system (reviewed in ref. [13]) and is reported to be expressed in more than 50% of human ovarian carcinomas ascites cells [14] with a very limited distribution pattern in normal female tissues [15–17]. This makes MISIIR an attractive target for antibody-based intervention of ovarian cancer. Even with purified target (MISIIR-Fc) available, our initial attempts yielded several clones failed to bind to native MISIIR on the surface of tumors cells in flow cytometry assays. To overcome this obstacle, we developed the cell sorter-based methodology described here.

2 Materials

Prepare all solutions using ultrapure water (prepared by purifying deionized water, to attain a sensitivity of 18 MΩ-cm at 25 °C) and analytical grade reagents. Prepare and store all reagents at room temperature (unless indicated otherwise). Diligently follow all waste disposal regulations when disposing waste materials. We do not add sodium azide to reagents.

2.1 Phage Display Antibody Library

YUAN-FCCC phage display library (*see* **Note 1**).

2.2 Soluble Protein Target

MISIIR-Fc (*see* **Note 2**).

2.3 Target-Expressing Cell Line

1. PDisplay (Invitrogen, Cat# V660-20).
2. HEK-293 (ATCC, Cat# CRL-1573).

3. cDNA encoding the chosen target: MISIIR ECD.
4. Construct that express the target on the cell membrane: pDisplay-MISIIR ECD.
5. Fugene 6 (Roche Diagnostics).
6. G418 antibiotic (Cellgro, Cat# MT-30-234-CR).
7. Penicillin-streptomycin and L-glutamine.
8. Anti-HA, fluorescein-conjugated, clone 3F10 (Roche Diagnostics GmBH).
9. FBS, 10% female (Biotechnics Research Inc.).
10. Hanks's Balanced Salt Solution (HBSS, Thermo Fisher Scientific).

2.4 Phage Library/ Cell Incubation and Sorting

1. Target-expressing cell line, or HEK-MISIIR(+) cells in the protocol, prepared as following methods.
2. HEK-293, which is target (MISIIR) negative, or HEK-MISIIR (−) cells in the protocol, prepared as following methods.
3. Cell Tracker Green (Invitrogen, Cat# C2102).
4. Log-phase TG1: fresh colony of TG1 is prepared by stripping TG1 glycerol stock to a M9 minimal media (MM) plate (Cat# M1289-04, Teknova).
5. Phosphate-buffered saline (PBS).
6. Hanks's Balanced Salt Solution (HBSS, Invitrogen).
7. 50 mM EDTA.
8. Cell strainer (Cat# 352340, BD Falcon™, BD Bioscience).
9. OPTI-MEM®I (Cat# 22600-050, Invitrogen).
10. 4% MPBS (4% w/v fat-skimmed milk powder in PBS).
11. FACSVantage SE cell sorter (Becton-Dickson).
12. TEA (triethylamine, Cat# 90337, Sigma).

2.5 Monophage ELISA

1. Target protein of your choice, or MISIIR-Fc protein in this protocol.
2. 0.1 M Sodium bicarbonate (pH 9.6).
3. M13KO7 helper phage (Invitrogen, Cat#18311-019).
4. ELISA microplate, high binding (Nunc Maxisorp).
5. Anti-M13 mouse antibody, HRP conjugated.
6. PBS containing 0.05% Tween 20 (PBST).
7. 1-Step Turbo HRP substrate (Invitrogen).
8. 2YT-AG: 2YT contains 100 μg/mL ampicillin and 2% glucose.
9. 2YT-AK: 2YT contains 100 μg/mL ampicillin and 30 μg/mL kanamycin.

10. Stop Solution: 2 M H_2SO_4.
11. Photometer Absorbance Reader (A_{600nm}).
12. ELISA Absorbance Reader (A_{450nm}).

2.6 scFv and/or scFv-Fc Expression, Purification, and Binding Analysis

1. phagemid that contains scFv genes from the phage display library (pAK100-lnk in this protocol).
2. Restriction enzymes and modification enzymes (SfiI, EcoRI, HindIII, T4 DNA ligase, NEB).
3. TG1 chemical-competent cells (made in-house, or commercially available).
4. pCYN2 [18] (scFv expression vector that contains pLac promoter).
5. HEK293 cells.
6. pHingstuffer [19] (scFv-Fc mammalian expression vector).
7. Ni-NTA agarose (Qiagen) for scFv affinity purification.
8. Protein A beads (GE healthcare, Lifesciences) for scFv-Fc purification.
9. BIAcore 1000 (GE Healthcare, Lifesciences).
10. LB broth.
11. IPTG(Sigma), 1 M stock solution.
12. 293 Freestyle media (Invitrogen).
13. 1 M Imidazole (Sigma).
14. Lysis Buffer: 50 mM NaH_2PO_4, 300 mM NaCl, 10 mM imidazole, pH 8.0.
15. Wash Buffer: 50 mM NaH_2PO_4, 300 mM NaCl, 20 mM imidazole, pH 8.0.
16. Elution buffer for scFvNi-NTA purification: 50 mM NaH_2PO_4, 300 mM NaCl, 250 mM imidazole, pH 8.0.

2.7 SDS-PAGE

1. NuPAGE 4–12% Bis-Tris Protein Gel (Thermo Fisher Scientific).
2. NuPAGE LDS Sample Buffer, NuPAGE Sample Reducing Agent (Thermo Fisher Scientific).
3. NuPAGE MES SDS Running Buffer (Thermo Fisher Scientific).
4. Novex Sharp Prestained Protein standard (Thermo Fisher Scientific).
5. Xcell SureLock mini-cell (Invitrogen).
6. SimplyBlue safe stain (Thermo Fisher Scientific).

2.8 Flow Cytometry Analysis of Antibody Binding to Cells

1. Target-expressing cell line (engineered MISIIR-expressing cell line and natural MISIIR-expressing cell line AN3Ca in this protocol; ATCC, Manassas, VA).
2. Negative cell line (HEK293 cells in this protocol).
3. FACS buffer (1% BSA in PBS, 0.02% NaN_3).
4. Alexa-488 anti-His antibody (Thermo Fisher Scientific).
5. FITC-labeled anti-human IgG MAb (Biosource, Camarillo, CA).
6. Cell strainer.
7. FACscan flow cytometer (Becton & Dickson).
8. CellQuest Pro software program (Becton & Dickson).

3 Methods

Carry out all procedures at room temperature unless otherwise specified.

3.1 Prepare Engineering Cell Line to Express the Target

1. Subclone the cDNA encoding the chosen target, MISIIR ECD, into pDisplay by site-directed restriction cloning to obtain pDisplay-MISIIR. Confirm the correct clone by DNA sequencing of the insert fragment.
2. Transfect linearized pDisplay-MISIIR and empty pDisplay into HEK-293 cells, respectively.
3. Select stable transfectants with 1000 μg/mL G418 antibiotic.
4. Enrich the subpopulation that expresses high levels of MISIIR ECD, about 5% of the total population, by cell sorting on a FACS-VantageSE/DiVa instrument, using fluorescein-conjugated anti-HA antibody 3F10.
5. Grow the enriched HA-positive subpopulation and name as HEK-MISIIR(+).
6. For the empty vector, survival cells under G418 were collected, which is named as HEK-MISIIR(−).
7. Grow and maintain both HEK-MISIIR(+) and HEK-MISIIR (−) cell lines in DMEM supplemented with 10% female FBS, G418 (1000 μg/mL), penicillin-streptomycin, and L-glutamine in 5% CO_2 incubator at 37 °C.

3.2 Cell Labeling

1. The day before sorting, inoculate one TG1 colony from freshly prepared plate to 2 mL 2YT media. Grow at 37 °C, 180 rpm, overnight.
2. Grow negative cells HEK-MISIIR(−) in DMEM supplemented with 10% female FBS, G418 (1000 μg/mL), penicillin-streptomycin, and L-glutamine in 5% CO_2 incubator at 37 °C to 70% confluence. Prepare at least 20 million cells for one sorting.

3. Grow HEK-MISIIR(+) in DMEM supplemented with 10% female FBS, G418 (1000 μg/mL), penicillin-streptomycin, and L-glutamine in 5% CO_2 incubator at 37 °C to 70% confluence. About five million target-expressing cells are needed.
4. Wash the cell layer once with PBS to remove nonadherent cells and harvest by incubation in Hanks's Balanced Salt Solution containing EDTA (1 mM).
5. Pass the cells through a cell strainer to obtain single cell suspension and count the cells.
6. Dilute the cell into 1.2×10^6 cells/mL with prewarmed staining solution (serum-free DMEM containing 10 nM Cell Tracker green BODIFY) for 20 min at 37 °C (*see* **Note 3**).
7. Replace staining solution by 1 mL prewarmed (37 °C) serum-free OPTI-MEM medium and incubate cells for an additional 30 min at 37 °C.
8. Wash cells once in 1 mL PBS and block cells in 1 mL of 4% MPBS (4% w/v fat-skimmed milk powder in PBS) at room temperature for 30–60 min.

3.3 Phage/Cell Incubation and Sorting

1. Collect and count HEK-MISIIR(−) cells (the negative cells) as in Subheading 3.2, **steps 4** and **5**. Prepare at least 20 million single cell suspension for one sorting. Resuspend the cells in 4–5 mL 4% MPBS at room temperature by gentle rotating for 1 h. Take out one million cells as negative sample to serve following sorting setting.
2. Thaw one aliquot of an antibody phage display library of your choice (YUAN-FCCC library in this protocol) on ice. 100 μL, starting titer of 1×10^{12} cfu of antibody phage library solution is recommended (*see* **Note 4**).
3. Add the thawed phage library solution to blocked 20 million negative cells, continue to incubate at room temperature by gentle rotating for 1 h.
4. Grow 30 mL of TG1 (1:100) from the overnight culture to log-phase (OD_{600} is 0.5–0.7).
5. Add 20,000 stained HEK-MISIIR(+) cells to the above step cell/phage mixture, incubated on a rotator at room temperature for another 2 h. Save the rest labeled cells as positive sample in sorting gate setting (*see* **Note 5**).
6. Spin down the incubation mixture to collect pellet ($500 \times g$, 5 min), which is resuspended at 2×10^7 cells/mL in PBS.
7. On a FACS machine, use negative and 488 nm positive samples to set the gate (Fig. 1). Collect labeled HEK-MISIIR(+) cells on fluorescence at 488 nm in an Eppendorf tube containing 100 μL PBS to prevent desiccation. It takes about 4–5 h to finish the sorting. Expect to recover 50–70% of the labeled cells.

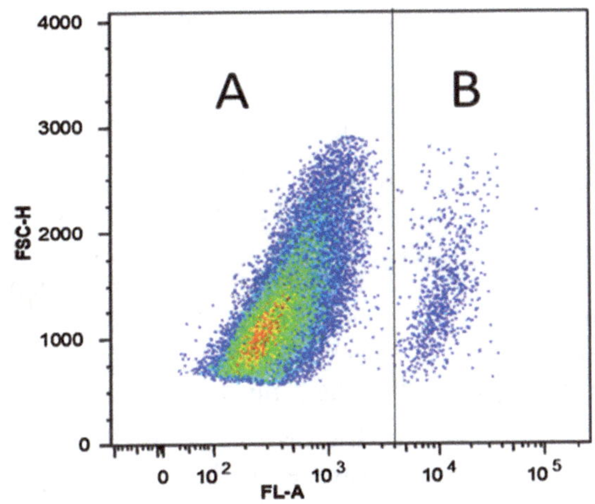

Fig. 1 Flow cytometry-based separation of stained and unstained cells. HEK-MISIIR(+) cells stained with the vital dye CellTracker Green were well separated (**b**, right) from unstained negative HEK-MISIIR(−) cells (**a**, left) by flow cytometry, even if it only accounts for around 0.02% of the total population

8. Elute bound phage by adding 800 μL fresh-made 100 mM TEA to the collected cell solution, mix, and incubate at RT for 10 min.
9. Neutralize the solution with 500 μL Tris·HCl (1 M, pH 7.4). Take half of the neutralized phage solution to infect 10 mL log-phase TG1. Place the culture at 37 °C for 30 min without shaking.
10. Spin down the infected TG1 at 6000 × *g*, 10 min. Resuspend the pellet in 500 μL media and spread to a 2YT-AG plate (if the phagemid contains β-lactase gene) and incubate at 30 °C, overnight (*see* **Note 6**).
11. Scrape bacterial lawn from the plates, then freeze it with 10% glycerol as seed and/or use it as inoculum for further rounds of phage preparation (*see* **Note 7**).

3.4 Monophage ELISA, PCR Fingerprint, and scFv Expression

1. Coat soluble target, MISIIR ECD-Fc, to the ELISA plate to primarily confirm the identity of any potential hits (*see* **Notes 8** and **9**).
2. Amplify the scFv genes of ELISA-positive clones by PCR using corresponding primers. Categorize the PCR product by PCR fingerprinting (RFLP) to reveal the gel electrophoresis pattern (*see* **Note 10**).
3. Identify unique antibody clones by DNA sequencing analysis.
4. Subclone the genes for the scFv from the pAK100-lnk phagemid to any *E. coli* expression vector under the promoter of Lac, such as pCYN2.

5. Express soluble scFv in *E. coli* TG1. Isolate soluble scFv from the periplasmic space and purify by Ni-NTA agarose affinity chromatography and high-performance liquid chromatography (HPLC) (*see* **Note 11**).
6. Carry out the binding of scFv and scFv-Fc to purified MISIIR ECD-Fc by surface plasmon resonance on a BIAcore1000.

3.5 FACS Confirmation of Hit Clones to Native Membrane MISIIR (See Note 12)

1. Harvest AN3Ca, a human endometrial adenocarcinoma cell line, expressing MISIIR (2×10^5) and HEK293 cells (negative cells) from logarithmically growing cultures and wash cells with FACS buffer.
2. Incubate cells with 1 μg/mL of scFv or scFv-Fc and for 30 min on ice, wash twice with FACS buffer and then incubate with either Alexa-488 anti-His antibody (for scFv samples) or FITC-labeled anti-human IgG MAb (for scFv-Fc samples).
3. Analyze binding to cells by flow cytometry on FACscan flow cytometer and use CellQuest Pro software program to analyze the data.

4 Notes

1. In the protocol a large naïve human single chain variable fragment (scFv) phage display library, the YUAN-FCCC phage display library [20] is used. Alternatively, any customer-built [25] or commercially available phage display libraries, as well as immunized library, can be used as the antibody repertoire. The bigger the library size, the higher the chance of success in panning. It is better to check the phage antibody titer and store the library aliquots at −80 °C in a solution of 15% glycerol.
2. In the protocol MISIIR-Fc is used [20]. Purified soluble target protein provides "cross-examine" of the specificity of binder isolated through cell-based panning, and robust monophage ELISA method can be used to screen hits. Most target can be purchased commercially. If not, one can express it in-house by a variety of approaches, such as Fc-fusion, if the extracellular domain (ECD) is from a single-pass type I receptor. Fc fusion is the preferred choice since it offers native folding and easy purification.
3. Labeling target-expressing cells with fluorescence dye rather than target itself offers unmodified "bait" for potential binders. Even though there is a tag (HA-tag in pDisplay vector), anti-tag antibody may still hinder the binding of phage antibodies to the target. Because the chosen dye (BODIPY Green) demonstrate very strong fluorescence intensities, it makes easy to separate labeled cells from the vast negative cells.

4. The size matters when a naïve antibody phage display library is chosen as the antibody source. Typically, the colony-forming unit should be over 1×10^{10}. For an immunized antibody library, the size can be significantly small (over 1×10^7 cfu should be fine).
5. It is very important to use high ratio of negative cell/positive cells in the method to improve positive screen rate. However, the high density of cell slurry tends to settle down easily. To avoid tubing stuck by the cell pellet, it is highly recommended to gently flick the sample tube every 3 min. One can divide the total cell samples into a few vials and take turn to use the vials during sorting. The resting samples are kept on ice.
6. Spreading a series of dilutions to plate is recommended to get total count of output and well-isolated colonies.
7. We observed neither clone enrichment nor positive rate of additional sorting. One reason could be the use of very few labeled cells, which was outnumbered by binders in the latter rounds of sorting.
8. It is great and very convenient to have purified target protein prepared (or purchased) before using the cell-based panning method. Purified protein offers very low background signal in monophage ELISA, which helps to determine positive hits. On the other hand, it demonstrates the specificity of the binders. For multi-span membrane receptor such as GPCRs, it is very challenging to obtain purified protein. Detailed standard procedure can be found in previous publications [20, 21].
9. We prefer to generate an engineered cell line, under the promoter of pCMV, to highly express the extracellular domain (ECD) of a membrane receptor. The empty-vector transfected same cell line offers great negative control and complete depletion of unwanted binders. One must prove that the engineered cell line expresses functional ECD before using it in the sorting panning. Alternative way of generating a pair of cell line is, one can use gene-editing approach (such as CRISPR) to knockout the wild-type-expressing cell line, which express the chosen target, to obtain negative cell line. The unmodified cell line serves as positive cells.
10. Detailed standard procedure for RFLP can be found in previous publication [22].
11. Detailed procedure for hit clone expression and purification can be found in previous publication [23]. Alternatively, a procedure with minor modifications as shown for scFv-Fc [20] can be used. The size and integrity of the resulting scFv and scFv-Fc need to be assayed by SDS-PAGE [24].

12. Even monophage ELISA on purified target yield positive binding, and the hits were derived from cell-based panning, one still needs to verify the binding of hits on target-expressing cell line, particularly on native target-expressing cell line.

References

1. Carter P, Smith L, Ryan M (2004) Identification and validation of cell surface antigens for antibody targeting in oncology. Endocr Relat Cancer 11:659–687
2. Ross JS, Schenkein DP, Pietrusko R, Rolfe M, Linette GP, Stec J, Stagliano NE, Ginsburg GS, Symmans WF, Pusztai L et al (2004) Targeted therapies for cancer 2004. Am J Clin Pathol 122:598–609
3. Adams GP, Weiner LM (2005) Monoclonal antibody therapy of cancer. Nat Biotechnol 23:1147–1157
4. Winter G, Griffiths AD, Hawkins RE, Hoogenboom HR (1994) Making antibodies by phage display technology. Annu Rev Immunol 12:433–455
5. Coomber DW (2002) Panning of antibody phage-display libraries. Standard protocols. Methods Mol Biol 178:133–145
6. Nagy P, Friedlander E, Tanner M, Kapanen AI, Carraway KL, Isola J, Jovin TM (2005) Decreased accessibility and lack of activation of ErbB2 in JIMT-1, a herceptin-resistant, MUC4-expressing breast cancer cell line. Cancer Res 65:473–482
7. Krag DN, Shukla GS, Shen GP, Pero S, Ashikaga T, Fuller S, Weaver DL, BurdetteRadoux S, Thomas C (2006) Selection of tumor-binding ligands in cancer patients with phage display libraries. Cancer Res 66:7724–7733
8. Rajotte D, Arap W, Hagedorn M, Koivunen E, Pasqualini R, Ruoslahti E (1998) Molecular heterogeneity of the vascular endothelium revealed by in vivo phage display. J Clin Invest 102:430–437
9. Poul MA, Becerril B, Nielsen UB, Morisson P, Marks JD (2000) Selection of tumor specific internalizing human antibodies from phage libraries. J Mol Biol 301:1149–1161
10. Heitner T, Moor A, Garrison JL, Marks C, Hasan T, Marks JD (2001) Selection of cell binding and internalizing epidermal growth factor receptor antibodies from a phage display library. J Immunol Methods 248:17–30
11. Hoogenboom HR, Lutgerink JT, Pelsers MM, Rousch MJ, Coote J, Van Neer N, De Bruine A, Van Nieuwenhoven FA, Glatz JF, Arends JW (1999) Selection dominant and nonaccessible epitopes on cell-surface receptors revealed by cell-panning with a large phage antibody library. Eur J Biochem 260:774784
12. Watters JM, Telleman P, Junghans RP (1997) An optimized method for cell-based phage display panning. Immunotechnology 3:21–29
13. Nef S, Parada LF (2000) Hormones in male sexual development. Genes Dev 14:3075–3086
14. Masiakos PT, MacLaughlin DT, Maheswaran S, Teixeira J, Fuller AF Jr, Shah PC, Kehas DJ, Kenneally MK, Dombkowski DM, Ha TU et al (1999) Human ovarian cancer, cell lines, and primary ascites cells express the human Mullerian inhibiting substance (MIS) type II receptor, bind, and are responsive to MIS. Clin Cancer Res 5:3488–3499
15. He WW, Gustafson ML, Hirobe S, Donahoe PK (1993) Developmental expression of four novel serine/threonine kinase receptors homologous to the activin/transforming growth factor-beta type II receptor family. Dev Dyn 196:133–142
16. Baarends WM, van Helmond MJ, Post M, van der Schoot PJ, Hoogerbrugge JW, de Winter JP, Uilenbroek JT, Karels B, Wilming LG, Meijers JH et al (1994) A novel member of the transmembrane serine/threonine kinase receptor family is specifically expressed in the gonads and in mesenchymal cells adjacent to the mullerian duct. Development 120:189–197
17. Teixeira J, He WW, Shah PC, Morikawa N, Lee MM, Catlin EA, Hudson PL, Wing J, Maclaughlin DT, Donahoe PK (1996) Developmental expression of a candidate mullerian inhibiting substance type II receptor. Endocrinology 137:160–165
18. Schier R, Marks JD, Wolf EJ, Apell G, Wong C, McCartney JE, Bookman MA, Huston JS, Houston LL, Weiner LM et al (1995) In vitro and in vivo characterization of a human anti-c-erbB-2 single-chain Fv isolated from a filamentous phage antibody library. Immunotechnology 1:73–81
19. Gould LH, Sui J, Foellmer H, Oliphant T, Wang T, Ledizet M, Murakami A, Noonan K, Lambeth C, Kar K et al (2005) Protective and therapeutic capacity of human single-chain

Fv-Fc fusion proteins against West Nile virus. J Virol 79:14606–14613

20. Yuan QA, Simmons HH, Robinson MK, Russeva M, Marasco WA, Adams GP (2006) Development of engineered antibodies specific for the Mullerian inhibiting substance type II receptor: a promising candidate for targeted therapy of ovarian cancer. Mol Cancer Ther 5:2096–2105
21. Kingsbury GA, Junghans RP (1995) Screening of phage display immunoglobulin libraries by anti-M13 ELISA and whole phage PCR. Nucleic Acids Res 23:2563–2564
22. Marks JD, Hoogenboom HR, Bonnert TP, McCafferty J, Griffiths AD, Winter G (1991) By-passing immunization. Human antibodies from V-gene libraries displayed on phage. J Mol Biol 222:581–597
23. Adams GP, Schier R, Marshall K, Wolf EJ, McCall AM, Marks JD, Weiner LM (1998) Increased affinity leads to improved selective tumor delivery of single-chain Fv antibodies. Cancer Res 58:485–490
24. Matson CF (1965) Polyacrylamide gel electrophoresis. A simple system using gel columns. Anal Biochem 13:294–304
25. Rothe C, Urlinger S, Löhning C, Prassler J, Stark Y, Jäger U, Hubner B, Bardroff M, Pradel I, Boss M, Bittlingmaier R, Bataa T, Frisch C, Brocks B, Honegger A, Urban M (2008) The human combinatorial antibody library HuCAL GOLD combines diversification of all six CDRs according to the natural immune system with a novel display method for efficient selection of high-affinity antibodies. J Mol Biol 376(4):1182–1200

Chapter 14

Measuring Chimeric Antigen Receptor T Cells (CAR T Cells) Activation by Coupling Intracellular Cytokine Staining with Flow Cytometry

Chong Xu and Yibo Yin

Abstract

*C*himeric *a*ntigen *r*eceptor *T* cells (CAR T cells) therapy is one kind of immunotherapy that has revolutionally changed the landscape of immunotherapy and been approved by the FDA from 2017 for several blood malignancies. To bring new CAR T cells to clinic, every new CAR need to test in vitro for antigen recognition, tumor cell killing capacity, and off-target cytotoxicity effect. Detecting the secretion of cytokines upon engagement of CAR T cells with tumor antigens is routinely applied to assess these CAR functions. Here we describe coupling of intracellular cytokine staining and multicolor flow cytometry to measure CAR T cells activation upon antigen stimulation.

Key words Chimeric antigen receptor T cells, CAR T cells, Intracellular cytokine staining, Flow cytometry, T cell activation, Immunotherapy

1 Introduction

Immunotherapy is a group of therapies involving any aspects of human innate and adaptive immunity to fight against viruses, bacteria, foreign immunogens, and tumors [1, 2]. While B cell-mediated humoral adaptive immunity has been widely applied in clinic, the other branch of T cell-mediated adaptive immunity has attracted intensive attention in recent years and achieved tremendous success in treating several blood malignancies and gained FDA approval from 2017 [3–5]. Chimeric antigen receptor T cells (CAR T cells) as the major players impose several advantages compared to other traditional immunotherapies: (a) personalized because they were the product of individual patient's own T cells; (b) target specific because its single-chain variable fragment (scFv) moiety was selected against tumor-specific or tumor-enriched antigens; (c) can be manipulated in vitro and proliferated to tens of billions cells; and (d) can be once-for-life time treatment because some

Ivana Vancurova and Yan Zhu (eds.), *Immune Mediators in Cancer: Methods and Protocols*, Methods in Molecular Biology, vol. 2108, https://doi.org/10.1007/978-1-0716-0247-8_14, © Springer Science+Business Media, LLC, part of Springer Nature 2020

CAR T cells can maintain memory characteristics and live as long as the recipient [6–8].

To conduct CAR T therapy, patient's T cells were collected and genetically engineered in the laboratory to express CAR, which can recognize specific antigen(s) on tumor cells and kill them. Currently the mainstream design on a functional CAR composes an scFv as the extracellular domain fused with CD8 or CD28 transmembrane domain followed by 4-1BB (CD137) or CD28 costimulatory domain and CD3ζ ITAM domain [6–9]. Upon activation after antigen encounter, phosphorylation of the CD3ζ ITAM domain initiates a series of downstream signaling pathways and mediates CAR T cell's anti-tumoral effects by sensitizing tumor cells through the release of cytokines, secreting perforin and granzymes to destroy the integrity of target cell's membrane, and forming the Fas and Fas ligand complex to activate caspases, which induce apoptosis in the target cell [10, 11].

During CAR T development, researchers need to determine one or a few suitable scFvs to incorporate to the CAR for future clinical development if a pool of scFvs were available [7, 9, 12]. Mainly, antigen on-target recognition and killing capacity of a particular scFv are scored by measuring how much cytokines the CAR T cells can release upon activation by their targets. There are several methods commonly used to detect secreted cytokines by activated T cells, such as ELISA and ELISpot assay [13]. We couple intracellular cytokines staining with Flow Cytometry because not only we can measure several cytokines simultaneously and quantitatively, but also measure them on single-cell level [7–9].

2 Materials

2.1 Special Consumables and Hardware

1. 96-Well round-bottom cell culture microplate.
2. Bio-Rad™ Titertube® Micro Test tubes.
3. Multichannel pipettes.
4. Reservoir.

2.2 Medium, Reagents, Buffer, and Antibodies

1. Intracellular cytokine staining (ICCS) medium: RPMI-1640 medium supplemented with 10% FBS, 1 μL/mL GolgiPlug™ (BD, Cat. No. 555029), and 0.7 μL/mL GolgiStop™ (BD, Cat. No. 554724) (*see* **Note 1**).
2. PMA: 1 mg/mL stock solution, used at a final concentration of 0.1 μg/mL.
3. Ionomycin: 1 mg/mL stock solution, used at a final concentration of 1 μg/mL.
4. Phosphate-buffered saline (PBS).

5. Flow cytometry staining (FACS) buffer: PBS supplemented with 2% fetal bovine serum (FBS).
6. Dead cell staining buffer: LIVE/DEAD™ Fixable Violet Dead Cell Stain Kit (Invitrogen, Cat. No. L34064).
7. Cell surface staining antibodies: anti-CD3-BV605 (BioLegend, Cat. No. 317322) and anti-CD8-FITC (BioLegend, Cat. No. 344704).
8. Intracellular cytokine staining antibodies: anti-Interferon gamma-PE (anti-IFNγ, BioLegend, Cat. No. 506507), anti-Tumor necrosis factor alpha-BV650 (anti-TNFα, BioLegend, Cat. No. 502938), anti-Interleukin 2-PerCP-eF710 (anti-IL-2, ThermoFisher, Cat. No. 46-7029-42).
9. FIX & PERM™ Cell Permeabilization Kit (Invitrogen, Cat. No. GAS003) (*see* **Note 1**).
10. BD™ Vortex CompBeads Negative Control, Anti-Mouse and Anti-Rat/Hamster Ig, κ beads.

3 Methods

3.1 Coculture

1. Planning the coculture of CAR T cells with target cells in 96-well round-bottom microplate (Fig. 1).
2. Newly rested CAR T cells, or overnight recovery frozen CAR T cells are diluted to 2×10^6 cells/mL in ICCS assay medium (*see* **Notes 2** and **3**).

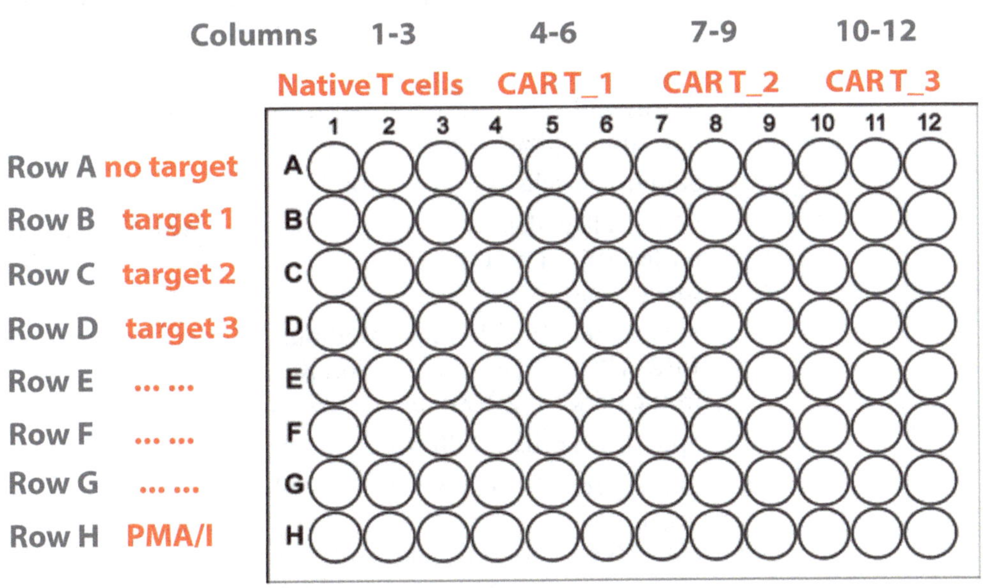

Fig. 1 Setting up coculture in 96-well plates. Each type of target cells was seeded in different rows with no target negative control and PMA/Ionomycin positive control. Each type of CAR T cells or their corresponding non-transduced T cells were seeded in three columns as triplicates

3. Target cells are also resuspended in ICCS assay medium to 2×10^6 cells/mL (*see* **Note 4**).
4. Seed 100 μL effector cell suspension (non-transduced T cells or CAR T cells) and 100 μL target cell suspension in each test well as outlined in Fig. 1; pipette gently up and down four or five times to mix them thoroughly. In no target wells add 100 μL ICCS assay medium instead of target cells, and in PMA/Ionomycin wells add 100 μL PMA/Ionomycin containing ICCS assay medium instead of target cells to reach 200 μL total volume per well.
5. Keep the plate in incubator for 4–16 h at 37 °C with 5% CO_2.

3.2 Cell Surface and Intracellular Staining

1. After desired incubation time, remove the plate from incubator and spin down the cells at 500 × *g* for 5 min and discard supernatants (*see* **Note 5**).
2. Resuspend cell pellets with 200 μL PBS per well. Spin down the cells at 500 × *g* for 5 min and discard supernatants.
3. During centrifuge, prepare Dead cell staining buffer by adding 1 μL of LIVE/DEAD™ Fixable Violet Dead Cell Stain to 10 mL PBS.
4. After centrifuge, resuspend cell pellets with 100 μL Dead cell staining buffer. Keep at room temperature for 20–30 min and avoid light (*see* **Notes 6** and 7).
5. Spin down cells at 500 × *g* for 5 min and discard supernatants.
6. During centrifuge, prepare surface staining master mix as the following formula: 0.6 μL of anti-CD3 antibody and 0.5 μL anti-CD8 antibody in 50 μL FACS buffer per well (*see* **Notes 6** and 7).
7. Resuspend cell pellets with 50 μL cell surface staining master mix and incubate at 4 °C for 30 min in the dark.
8. Spin down cells at 500 × *g* for 5 min and discard supernatants.
9. Wash cell pellets once by resuspending with 200 μL FACS buffer, spin down the cells at 500 × *g* for 5 min, and discard supernatants.
10. Fix cell pellets with 50 μL Medium A of the Invitrogen FIX & PERM™ Cell Permeabilization Kit, keep at room temperature in the dark for 20–30 min (*see* **Notes 6** and 7).
11. Spin down cells at 500 × *g* for 5 min and discard supernatants.
12. During centrifuge, prepare intracellular cytokine master staining mix as the following formula: 1 μL anti-IL-2 antibody, 2 μL anti-TNFα antibody, and 1 μL anti-IFNγ antibody in 96 μL Medium B of the Invitrogen FIX & PERM™ Cell Permeabilization Kit for each well (*see* **Notes 6** and 7).

13. Resuspend cell pellets with 100 μL intracellular staining master mix, and keep at room temperature for 30 min in the dark.
14. Spin down cells at 500 × *g* for 5 min and discard supernatants.
15. Wash cell pellets by resuspending with 200 μL FACS buffer, spin down cells at 500 × *g* for 5 min, and discard supernatants.
16. Resuspend cells with 200 μL FACS wash buffer, transfer to Titertube® Micro Test tubes, and keep at 4 °C in the dark until performing Flow cytometry analysis (*see* **Note 8**).

3.3 Flow Cytometry Analysis

1. Prepare compensation beads for all fluorophores used in staining with unstained control following manufacturer's recommendations (*see* **Notes 9** and **10**).
2. Process compensation with beads on flow cytometer according to manufacturer's instructions.
3. Run samples on flow cytometer after compensation panel defined, gate on live, single-cell lymphocytes and CD3-positive lymphocytes (Fig. 2a–c).
4. Analyze the percentage of cytokine-positive cells in total T cells (Fig. 2d–f) (*see* **Note 11**).

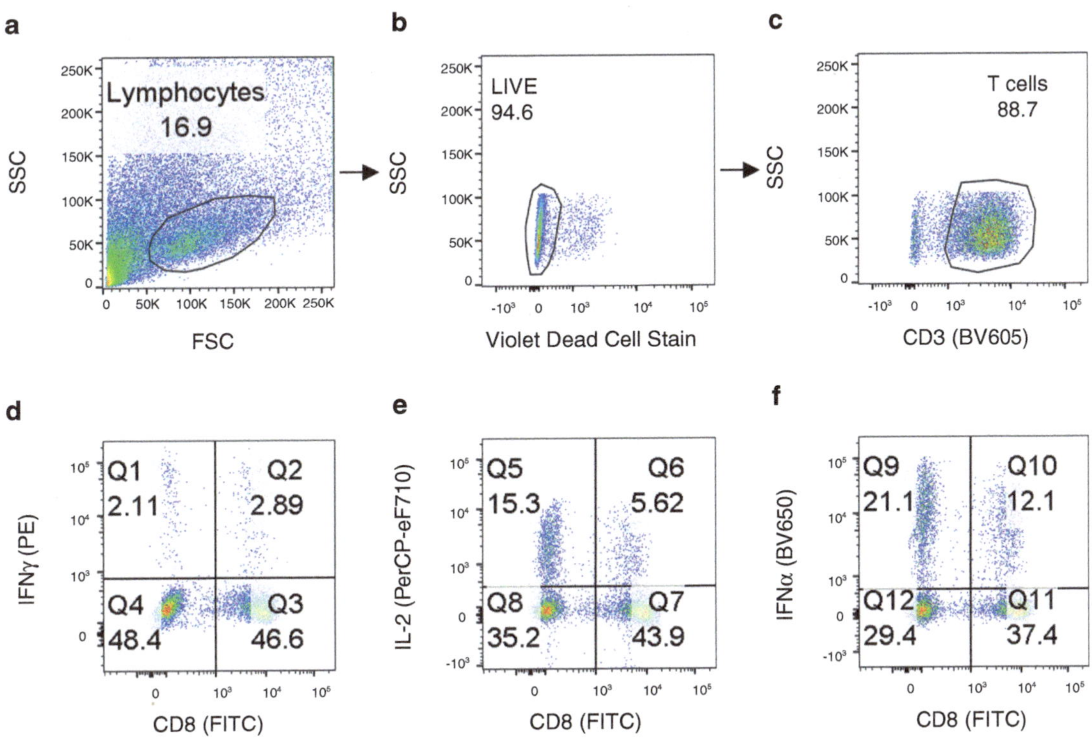

Fig. 2 Gating strategy of intracellular cytokine staining. Gating on lymphocytes (**a**) based on FSC and SSC, then →live cells (**b**) →CD3-positive cells (**c**). Cytokine staining results shown as the percentage of IFNγ-positive T cells (**d**), IL-2-positive T cells (**e**) and TNFα-positive T cells (**f**) in total T cells

4 Notes

1. GolgiPlug™ and GolgiStop™ can be substituted with other protein transport inhibitors containing Brefeldin A and Monensin from other manufacturers. The FIX & PERM™ Cell Permeabilization Kit can also be replaced by other cell fixation and permeabilization reagents.
2. CAR T cells should be resting from active proliferation first before conducting this kind of coculture killing assay to avoid residual cytokine production during CAR T cell production from nontarget-specific anti-CD3/anti-CD28 activation.
3. If frozen CAR T cells were cultured for this assay, they need to be cultured for at least overnight to regain active metabolic state and allow CAR expressing on T cell surface again.
4. Target cells should also be actively culturing before mixing with CAR T cells. If target cells are adherent cells, nonenzymatic dissociation methods should be used to detach them from the surface of the culture vessel to avoid target antigen loss due to cleavage. We routinely use Gibco® Versene Solution to detach lightly adherent cells. However, if strongly adherent cells have to be used and enzymatic dissociation method is the only option, these cells should incubate with their appropriate culture medium in conical tube in incubator at 37 °C with 5% CO_2 for a few hours to allow target antigen re-expression on cell surface before carrying out the coculture assay.
5. Standard sterile techniques are applied during culture cells handling in tissue culture hood. However, the rest of the assay can be performed on regular bench after culture medium was removed.
6. Master mix should be made for Dead cell staining, cell surface staining, cell fixation, and intracellular staining, and aliquot to test wells using multichannel pipette. Usually we prepare the master mix at least enough for 110% of test wells.
7. Incubation with fluorophore-conjugated dyes and antibodies must be carried out in the dark and avoid prolonged exposure to light to prevent photobleach effect on cells; wrapping the plate with foil sheet is sufficient to achieve protection from light exposure.
8. If samples were not assayed right after staining, they must be stored at 4 °C in the dark until use. The samples could be still acceptable up to a week before analyzing on flow cytometer; however, ideally the samples should be analyzed within 48 h after staining is done.

9. The Violet Live-Dead dye is not an antibody and cannot be used for making compensation control. Any antibody conjugated with Pacific Blue fluorophore that has the same excitation and emission spectrum must be used for making compensation control.
10. Compensation beads should be fixed with Buffer A of the Invitrogen FIX & PERM™ Cell Permeabilization Kit after incubation with antibodies.
11. Per flow cytometer limitation and assay design, we detect three most important cytokines only. Furthermore, we had also included CD107a and Granzyme B staining in our assay panel which are excellent indicators of activated cytotoxic CD8+ lymphocyte degranulation and perforin-granzyme-mediated killing [14]. In this case, anti-CD107a antibody and anti-Granzyme B antibody must be added to ICCS medium and intracellular cytokine staining buffer, respectively [9]. Researchers should consider their available resources to optimize their staining strategy.

References

1. Khalil DN, Smith EL, Brentjens RJ et al (2016) The future of cancer treatment: immunomodulation, CARs and combination immunotherapy. Nat Rev Clin Oncol 13:273–290
2. Rosenberg SA, Restifo NP (2015) Adoptive cell transfer as personalized immunotherapy for human cancer. Science 348:62–68
3. Yang XH (2017) A new model T on the horizon? Cell 171:1–3
4. Porter DL, Levine BL, Kalos M et al (2011) Chimeric antigen receptor-modified T cells in chronic lymphoid leukemia. N Engl J Med 365:725–733
5. Maude SL, Frey N, Shaw PA et al (2014) Chimeric antigen receptor T cells for sustained remissions in leukemia. N Engl J Med 371:1507–1517
6. Maus MV, June CH (2016) Making better chimeric antigen receptors for adoptive T-cell therapy. Clin Cancer Res 22:1875–1884
7. Maude SL, Barrett DM, Rheingold SR et al (2016) Efficacy of humanized CD19-targeted chimeric antigen receptor (CAR)-modified T cells in children and young adults with relapsed/refractory acute lymphoblastic leukemia. Blood 128:217
8. Johnson LA, Scholler J, Ohkuri T et al (2015) Rational development and characterization of humanized anti-EGFR variant III chimeric antigen receptor T cells for glioblastoma. Sci Transl Med 7:275ra22
9. Yin Y, Boesteanu AC, Binder ZA et al (2018) Checkpoint blockade reverses Anergy in IL-13Rα2 humanized scFv-based CAR T cells to treat murine and canine gliomas. Mol Ther Oncolytics 11:20–38
10. Benmebarek MR, Karches CH, Cadilha BL et al (2019) Killing mechanisms of chimeric antigen receptor (CAR) T cells. Int J Mol Sci 20:E1283
11. Janeway CA Jr, Travers P, Walport M et al (eds) (2001) Immunobiology: the immune system in health and disease, 5th edn. Garland Publishing, New York, NY
12. Begent RH, Verhaar MJ, Chester KA et al (1996) Clinical evidence of efficient tumor targeting based on single-chain Fv antibody selected from a combinatorial library. Nat Med 2:979–984
13. Leehan KM, Koelsch KA (2015) T cell ELISPOT: for the identification of specific cytokine-secreting T cells. Methods Mol Biol 1312:427–434
14. Betts MR, Koup RA (2004) Detection of T-cell degranulation: CD107a and b. Methods Cell Biol 75:497–512

Chapter 15

Analysis of Interleukin-4-Induced Class Switch Recombination in Mouse Myeloma CH12F3-2 Cells

Wenjun Wu, Zhihui Xiao, Deon Buritis, and Vladimir Poltoratsky

Abstract

Affinity maturation of B lymphocytes is a process that includes somatic hypermutation and class switch recombination. Class switch recombination is a fundamental factor of the human adaptive immunity. The perturbation of this process has an adverse effect on human health, and results in global chromosome rearrangements and cell transformation. Evaluation of the class switch recombination efficiency is an important component of laboratory diagnosis of immunotoxic components. Here we describe a method for testing the efficiency of the class switch recombination. Cultivation of mouse myeloma CH12F3-2 cell line with anti-CD40 antibodies, transforming growth factor beta, and recombinant interleukin-4 (IL-4) triggers a cascade of signal transduction network events that lead to switching the immunoglobulin isotypes from IgM to IgA. This chapter describes the methodology of class switch recombination assay for assessment of the effect of environmental pollutants in toxicological laboratory diagnostics.

Key words Interleukin-4, Class switch recombination, Cadmium toxicity, Flow cytometry, Real-time PCR, NF-κB signaling, STAT6 signaling, SMAD signaling

1 Introduction

Adaptive immune response is the third line of defense of the immune system. After being activated by antigen and T helper cells, B cells modify the DNA segments encoding the variable and constant parts of immunoglobulins to improve recognition and effective functions of antibodies. In humoral immune response, the isotype switching modulates ability of antibody to interact with complement complex and isotype-specific surface receptors. Switching of the IgM class to IgG is required for neonatal immunity, complement activation, and Fc receptor phagocyte response; switching to IgA for mucosal immunity; and switching to IgE for immunity against helminthes and type I hypersensitivity [1–6].

In vivo T cell-dependent class switch recombination (CSR) in B cells is induced by activation of the CD40 B cell receptor with T cell CD195 (CD40L) and activation of the B cell surface receptors by

Ivana Vancurova and Yan Zhu (eds.), *Immune Mediators in Cancer: Methods and Protocols*, Methods in Molecular Biology, vol. 2108, https://doi.org/10.1007/978-1-0716-0247-8_15, © Springer Science+Business Media, LLC, part of Springer Nature 2020

cytokines secreted by CD4 T cells. In vitro switching of IgM to IgA CSR in B cells can be triggered by activation of CD40 with anti-CD40 antibodies, transforming growth factor beta (TGFβ) and interleukin-4 receptor (IL-4R) with recombinant IL-4 and TGFβ, respectively [7–11].

Activation of IL-4R triggers signal transduction pathway that leads to phosphorylation, dimerization, and translocation of the transcriptional factor STAT6 to the nucleus. In the nucleus, STAT6 is activated by proteolysis, and, in consort with other activation nuclear factors, participates in the expression of IgA silent transcript promoter and activation-induced cytosine deaminase (AID) [12–14]. It is believed that initiation of the silent transcription remodels the chromatin and exposes the ssDNA sites for AID-mediated deamination of the deoxycytosines [15, 16] (Fig. 1).

Interaction of CD40 with CD195 triggers the signal transduction pathway that leads, through TNF-Receptor Associated Factors (TRAFs), TRAF2 to TRAF6-mediated signaling, to activation and translocation of NFκB to the nucleus [17, 18]. Activation NFκB is required for AID expression [11–13] (Fig. 1). In transforming growth factor-β (TGFβ) pathway, serine-threonine receptor kinases oligomerize and phosphorylate cytoplasmic signaling molecules Smad 3. Phosphorylated subunits form a complex with Smad 4 and translocate in the nucleus. Phosphorylated Smad 3/4 complex recognize binding sites located in AID enhancer and in ICα germinal silent transcript upstream elements and initiate DNA transcription [11, 19, 20] (Fig. 1).

Initiation of the sterile RNA transcript of GC-rich switched regions upstream of IgH chain C regions Cμ, Cγ, Cε, and Cα is believed to provide ssDNA regions acceptable to AID. AID deaminates deoxycytidine (dC) to form DNA lesion, deoxyuracil (dU) [15, 16, 21, 22]. Proteins of the base excision repair cascade excise dU from DNA and produce single-strand DNA breaks. Mismatch repair (MMR) proteins produce double-strand DNA breaks that initiate recombination between switched regions upstream of Cμ and other activated C regions (Fig. 2).

Aligning of the recombinant target sequences during CSR could lead to the gross chromosomal rearrangements, activation of oncogenes, and cancer transformation [23]. In Burkitt's cell lymphoma (BL) c-myc gene is targeted to the constantly activated promoter located in IgH locus [24]. Continuous expression of the myc oncogene results in uncontrolled division of transformed B cells, leading to impaired immunity and often fatal consequences, if left untreated. While in the endemic, African, type of BL, translocation of c-myc gene into Ig locus is driven by improper V(D)J recombination, in the sporadic, American, type of BL translocation is driven by improper CSR [25, 26]. Translocations of another BCL6 oncogene into IgH locus is one of the most common genetic abnormalities in non-Hodgkin's lymphoma of B cell type [27, 28].

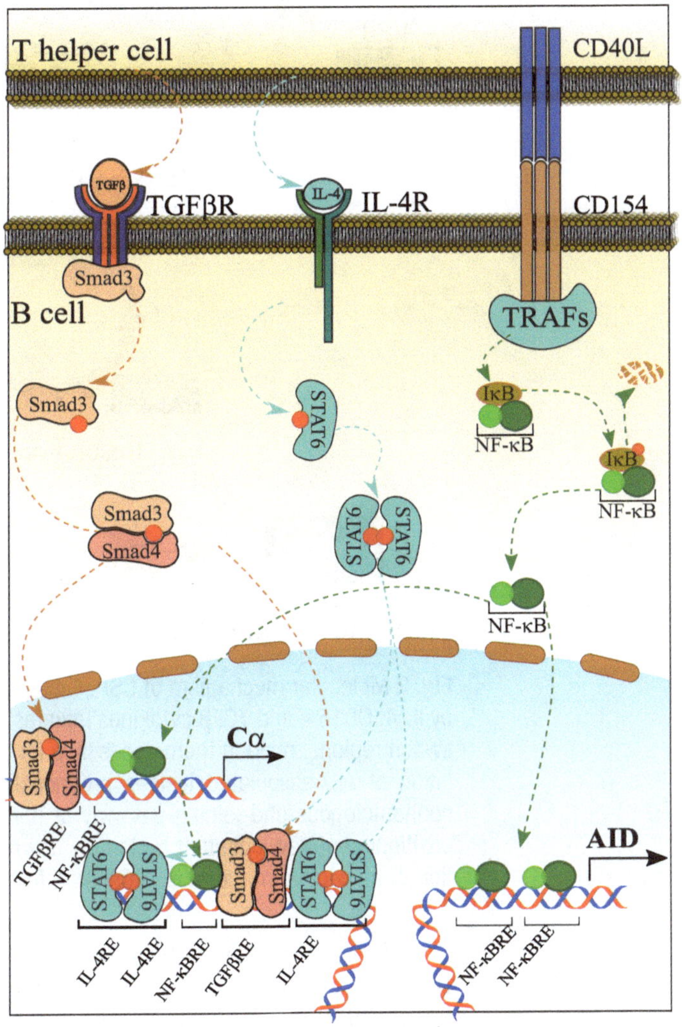

Fig. 1 CSR signal transduction pathways. T helper cells activate CSR in B cells by crosslinking of NF-κB, Smad3/4, and Stat6 pathways. TGFβ forms a complex with type I and type II serine-threonine kinase receptors. Receptors phosphorylate Smad 3. Phosphorylated Smad3 forms a dimer with coSmad subunit (Smad 4) and migrates to the nucleus where it interacts with TGFβ responsive element (TGFβRE) located within cytokine/ activation-inducible promoter upstream of intronic switch region (Sα) and enhancer of AID. Interaction of IL-4 receptor with IL-4 ligand initiates a phosphorylation cascade that phosphorylates STAT6 protein. Phosphorylated STAT6 forms a dimer that migrates to nucleus and interacts with IL-4 responsive element (IL-4RE) located within the AID enhancer. Crosslinking of CD40 by CD154 on TH cells initiates the formation of TNF-Receptor Associated Factor (TRAF) adaptor proteins complex that initiates a phosphorylation cascade that inactivates IκB inhibitor and leads to nuclear translocation of NF-κB transcriptional factors. In nucleus, they interact with NF-κB responsive elements (NF-κBRE) located within enhancer and promoter of AID. The NF-κBRE were identified within the cytokine/activation-inducible promoter upstream of intronic switch region (Sα) but their role in enhancing transcriptional activity in this locus are not clear

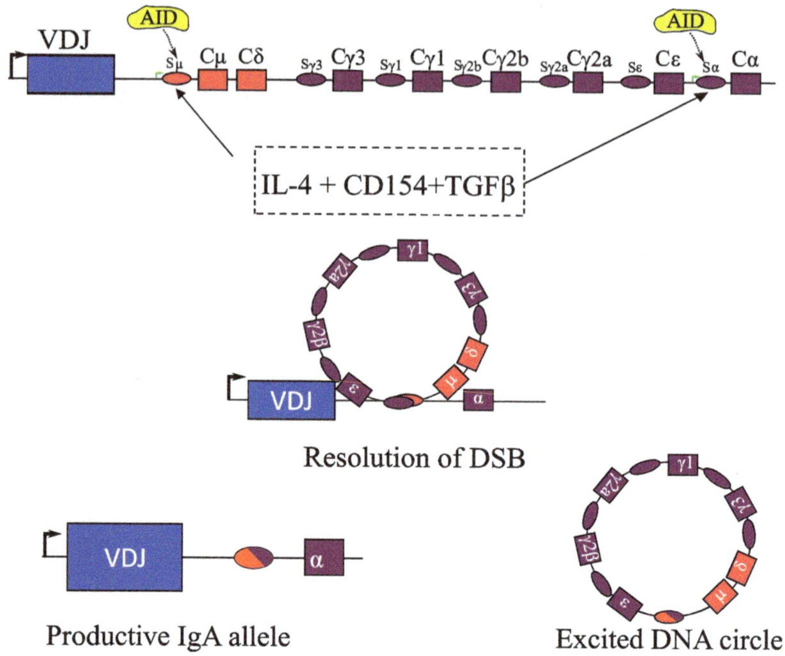

Fig. 2 Molecular mechanism of CSR. Crosslinking of the B cell surface receptors by IL-4, CD154, and TGFβ cytokines initiates chromatin remodeling of Sμ and Sα switch regions, making them accessible for AID-induced deamination. Accumulation of AID-associated lesions produce DSB. Error-prone repair of DSB by nonhomologous end-joining pathway or homologous recombination resulted in positioning of new constant region Cα downstream the V(D)J exons and formation of a switch circle that is eliminated further

Here, we provide the protocol for testing the efficiency of the IgM to IgA class switched recombination utilizing a mouse myeloma cell line CH12F3-2 as a model system.

2 Materials

2.1 Cell Culture

1. Mouse myeloma CH13F3-2 cells (*see* **Note 1**).
2. Complete RPMI medium: RPMI supplemented with 10 mM Hepes, pH 7.5, 10% fetal bovine serum (FBS, heat inactivated), 2 mM L-glutamine, 5% NCTC 109, 50 μM β-mercaptoethanol, 50 μg/mL penicillin, and 50 μg/mL streptomycin (*see* **Note 2**).
3. Hausser™ Bright-Line™ Phase hemocytometer.
4. Trypan Blue dye.
5. Functional grade purified anti-mouse CD40 antibodies.
6. Recombinant mouse IL-4 protein (mIL-4).

7. Recombinant human TGFβ1 protein.
8. 75 cm^2 culture flasks and 6-well plates.

2.2 Flow Cytometry

1. Goat anti-mouse IgM-Texas Red conjugate.
2. Phycoerythrin (PE)-conjugated anti-mouse IgA clone 11-44-2.
3. BD Cytofix/Cytoperm Solution.
4. 10× BD Perm/Wash™ buffer (BD Biosciences).
5. Paraformaldehyde 10% aqueous solution.
6. 10× Phosphate-buffered saline (PBS), pH 7.4: Dissolve 8.0 g NaCl, 1.44 g Na_2HPO_4, 0.24 g KH_2PO_4, and 0.2 g KCl in 100 mL of deionized water, adjust pH to 7.4, and sterilize buffer through 0.2 μm filter.
7. BD Accuri™ C6 Plus Flow Cytometer.

2.3 Real-Time PCR

1. TRIzol reagent.
2. Chloroform.
3. Ethanol.
4. Nuclease-free water.
5. Sterile, nuclease-free 1.7 mL polypropylene microcentrifuge tubes.
6. M-MLV reverse transcriptase.
7. Oligo dT primer.
8. dNTP mix (10 mM dATP, 10 mM dTTP, 10 mM dGTP, and 10 mM dCTP).
9. DNase I, RNase free.
10. RNaseOUT ribonuclease inhibitor.
11. SYBR Select Master Mix.
12. IhMf, IhAr, AIDf, AIDr, GAPDHf, GAPDHr primers (Table 1).
13. NanoDrop Spectrophotometer.
14. Agilent AriaMx Real-time PCR system.

2.4 Sequence Analysis of Switch Region

1. QuickExtract DNA Extraction solution.
2. Phusion High-Fidelity PCR Master Mix with HF Buffer.
3. Bio-Rad T100 Thermal Cycler.
4. Smf and Saf primers (Table 1).

Table 1
Oligonucleotide sequences used as primers in this study

	Oligonucleotide name	Sequence (5′ → 3′)
1	IhMf	AACTGCAGCAGCCTGGGACTGAACTG
2	IhAr	GAGCTGGTGGGAGTGTCAGTG
3	AIDrtf	CACCATGGACAGCCTTCTGATGAAGCAA
4	AIDrtr	TCAAAATCCCAACATACGAAATGC
5	GAPDHf	ACTGTGCCGTTGAATTTGCC
6	GAPDHr	TGTGAACGGATTTGGCCGTA
7	Smf	AACTCTCCAGCCACAGTAATGACC
8	Saf	GAGCTCGTGGGAGTGTCAGTG

3 Methods

In this section, we describe the method for quantification of the CSR in mouse myeloma B cells. The method is based on activation of the CD40, TGFβ, and IL4R surface receptors on B cells. Activation of CD40, the member of the tumor necrosis factor superfamily, is caused by crosslinking with antibodies against this receptor.

3.1 Cell Culture

1. Grow mouse myeloma CH12F3-2 cells in complete RPMI medium to a concentration 2×10^5 cells/mL in a 5% CO_2 humidified tissue culture incubator at 37 °C (*see* **Note 3**).
2. Count cells stained with Trypan Blue with hemocytometer and split them (1×10^4 cells/well) into 5 wells of a 6 well-plate (*see* **Note 4**).
3. Add recombinant human TGFβ to a final concentration of 1 ng/mL to wells number 2 and 5.
4. Add anti-mouse CD40 antibody to a final concentrations of 2 μg/mL to wells number 3 and 5.
5. Add recombinant mouse IL-4 to a final concentration of 10 ng/mL to wells number 4 and 5 (*see* **Note 5**).
6. Incubate the plate for 4 days in a 5% CO_2 humidified tissue culture incubator at 37 °C.
7. After 72 h, wash cells with fresh media and analyze the efficiency of the CSR by flow cytometry or real-time PCR.

3.2 Flow Cytometry

1. Collect cells from **step** 7, Subheading 3.1, by centrifugation at $600 \times g$ for 5 min. Pour off supernatant and resuspend the cell pellet in 250 μL of Cytofix/Cytoperm solution. Incubate cells for 20 min at room temperature. Put aside 50 μL of the cell suspension to use as an unstained cell control.

2. Wash cells twice with 1 mL of Perm/Wash buffer diluted 1/10 in distilled water.
3. Stain ~10^6 cells with 2 μL of anti-mouse IgA-PE conjugate in 50 μL of diluted Perm/Wash buffer.
4. Tap tubes to mix and incubate the cells for 30 min at 4 °C in the dark (*see* **Note 6**).
5. Wash cells twice with 1 mL of diluted Perm/Wash buffer.
6. Pour off supernatant and resuspend pellets in 100 μL of 4% paraformaldehyde in PBS.
7. Incubate for 10–20 min at 4 °C in the dark.
8. Wash cells twice with 1 mL of diluted Perm/Wash buffer.
9. Analyze using flow cytometry analyzer and appropriate controls to set gates.
10. The efficiency of CSR is calculated by dividing the number of IgA-positive cells in well number 5 to the number of IgA-positive cells in well number 1 and multiplying the obtained number by 100 (Fig. 3a).

3.3 Real-Time PCR

3.3.1 RNA Isolation

1. For RNA isolation, collect cells from **step** 7, Subheading 3.1, by centrifugation at 600 × *g* for 5 min at room temperature in 1.7 mL polypropylene microcentrifuge tubes. Discard supernatant.
2. Add 0.5 mL of TRIZOL Reagent and thoroughly mix with cells. Incubate homogeneous sample for 5 min (*see* **Note** 7).
3. Add 100 μL of chloroform, cap sample tube securely, and vortex for 15 s. Incubate sample for 5 min and centrifuge at 12,000 × *g* for 15 min at room temperature.
4. Collect aqueous upper phase without disturbing the white interphase and place in fresh polypropylene microtube.
5. Add 250 μL of isopropanol and mix. Incubate mix at room temperature for 10 min and precipitate RNA by centrifuging the sample at 12,000 × *g* for 10 min at 4 °C.
6. Discard supernatant, and wash pellets with 1 mL of 75% ethanol. Spin at 5500 × *g* for 5 min at 4 °C.
7. Discard supernatants, remove all leftover ethanol, air-dry the pellets for 2 min, and dissolve RNA in 50 μL of nuclease-free water.
8. Measure RNA concentration with NanoDrop Spectrophotometer (*see* **Note 8**).
9. Use samples immediately for cDNA synthesis or store at −70 °C.

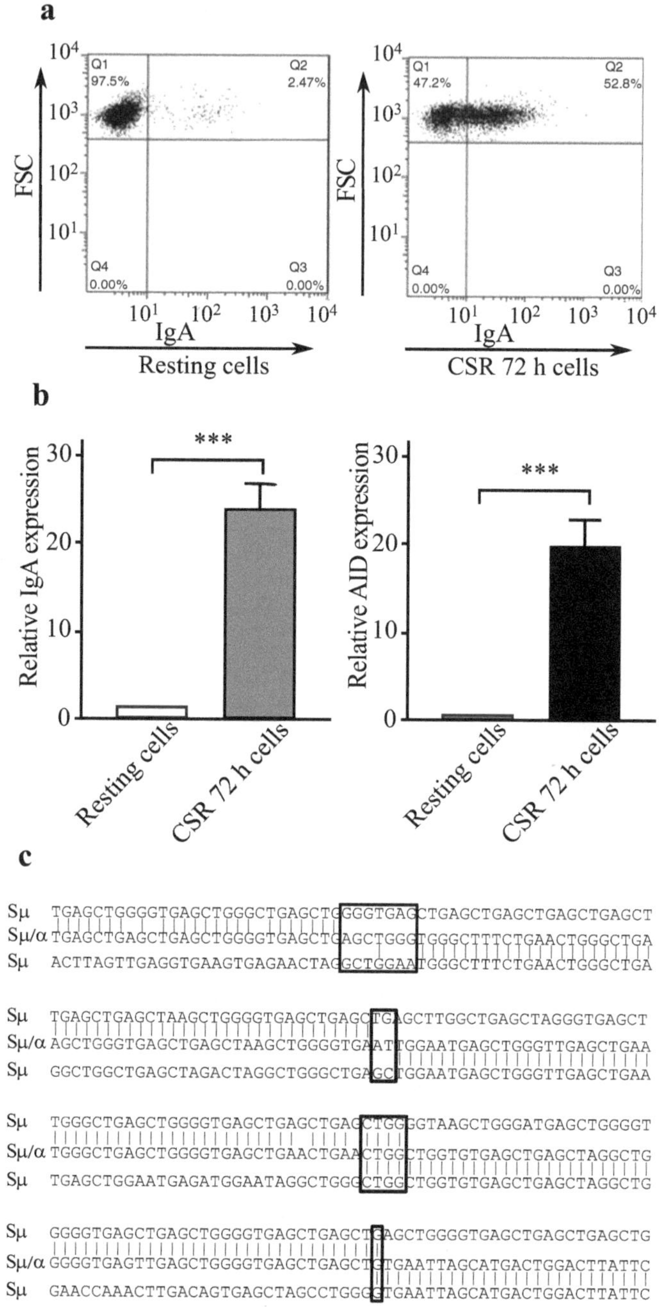

Fig. 3 Flow cytometry and real-time PCR evaluations of class switch recombination. (**a**) Flow cytometry analysis. Representative flow cytometry scatter plot showing the IgA-positive CH12F3 cells after treatment for 72 h with anti-mouse CD40 antibody, IL-4 and TGFβ recombinant proteins (CSR 72 h cells) compared to the untreated CH12F3 control cells (Resting cells). Cells were stained using anti- IgA antibody. (**b**) Relative IgA and AID expression. Real-time PCR analysis of IgA and AID genes relative expression in CH12F3 cells treated

3.3.2 cDNA Synthesis

1. To remove traces of contaminated DNA, mix 10 μL of RNA sample isolated at stage in Subheading 3.3, **step 8**, 2.5 μL of 10× reaction buffer for DNAse I with $MgCl_2$, 1 μL of DNase I/RNase free, and 10.5 μL of nuclease-free water.
2. Incubate for 30 min at 37 °C, add 10 μL of 12.5 mM EDTA, and inactivate DNase by incubating samples at 75 °C for 15 min.
3. Mix 2 μg of sample RNA with 1 μL 10 mM dNTP Mix and 1 μL of Oligo$(dT)_{12-18}$ (0.5 μg/μL) and add nuclease-free water to 12 μL. Incubate the mixture at 70 °C for 3 min, quick chill on ice, and incubate on ice for 10 min.
4. Collect the content of the tube by brief centrifugation and add 4 μL of 5× First-Strand Buffer, 2 μL of 0.1 mM DTT, and 1 μL of RNaseOUT ribonuclease inhibitor.
5. Gently mix the content of the tube, briefly spin it, and place in PCR heating block preheated to 37 °C; incubate for 2 min. Add 1 μL of M-MLV and incubate at 37 °C for 50 min.
6. Inactivate reaction by heating at 70 °C for 15 min.
7. Use samples immediately for RT-PCR analysis or store at −70 °C.

3.3.3 Real-Time PCR

1. Set up the experiment and the following PCR program on Agilent AriaMx Real-Time PCR system. Using different PCR instrument might require modification of the PCR protocol.
2. Mix 10 μL of SYBR Select Master Mix with 1 μL of 5 mM forward primer, 1 μL of 5 mM reverse primer, 1 μL of cDNA sample, and 7 μL of nuclease-free water. Use IgMf and IhAr primers for amplification of IgA mRNA, AIDrtf and AIDrtr for amplification of AID, and GAPDHf and GAPDHr for amplification of GAPDH (Table 1).
3. Set up PCR protocol starting with one cycle of DNA denaturation and enzyme activation for 10 min at 95° C, followed by 40 cycles of denaturation at 95 °C for 10 s, and annealing and extension together at 60 °C for 1 min. One melting cycle is

Fig. 3 (continued) with anti-mouse CD40 antibody, IL-4 and TGFβ recombinant proteins (CSR 72 h cells) versus untreated CH12F3 control cells (Resting cells). (**c**) Alignment of the germline Sμ and Sα DNA sequences with the recombined Sμ/α switch region. Upper sequence is represented by CH12F3 germline Sμ switch region; lower sequence is represented by CH12F3 germline Sα region. The middle sequences are represented by amplified Sμ/α switch region of four individual clones isolated from the IgA-positive population of CH12F3 cells treated with anti-mouse CD40 antibody, IL-4 and TGFβ recombinant proteins for 72 h. Identical nucleotides and overlapped regions are marked with vertical lines and boxes, respectively

added to the end of amplification with incubation at 95 °C for 30 s, followed with 65 °C for 30 s, then back to 95 °C for 30 s. Gene-specific primers for real-time PCR are listed in Table 1. GAPDH primer is set as the internal control. Relative mRNA levels are calculated based on the mRNA level of the internal control, GAPDH.

4. Analyze results using Aria Mx software package (Fig. 3b).

3.4 Sequence Analysis of CSR Region

3.4.1 Isolation of Individual Clones

1. Wash cells obtained at stage in Subheading 3.1, **step 7**, with 1 mL of PBS and spin at 600 × *g* for 5 min at room temperature. Pour off supernatant and resuspend the cell pellets in 1 mL of complete RPMI solution.
2. Count cells stained with Trypan Blue using hemocytometer.
3. Prepare cells suspensions in complete RPMI media at concentrations 500, 50, and 5 cells/mL, respectively.
4. Fill the sterile dispensing trays with 20 mL of appropriate cell suspension and disperse 200 μL cell suspension aliquots into three 96-well plates.
5. Incubate for 5–10 days. Observe each well under inverted microscope after 5–7 days of incubation. Mark all wells that contain just a single colony.

3.4.2 Isolation of DNA from Individual Clones

1. Transfer single colonies isolated in **step 5**, Subheading 3.4.1, into 200 μL PCR tubes. In addition, collect ~10^4 untreated cells for isolation of nonrecombinant control DNA.
2. Collect cells by spinning tubes for 5 min at 600 × *g* at room temperature and discard the supernatant.
3. Add 50 μL of QuickExtract DNA Extraction solution per tube. Mix for 15 s.
4. Place tubes in PCR heating block and incubate them at 65 °C for 6 min, followed by 2 min incubation at 98 °C. Cool the DNA samples to room temperature.
5. DNA samples can be utilized immediately in PCR reaction, or stored at −20 °C for 2 weeks. For longer periods, store DNA samples at −70 °C.

3.4.3 Amplification of CSR Region

1. Prepare reactions in PCR tubes by combining 2 μL of sample DNA, 1 μL of 10 μM forward (IhMf), 1 μL of 10 μM reverse (IhAr) primers mix (Table 1), 10 μL of 2× Phusion Master Mix, and 4 μL of nuclease-free water (*see* **Note 9**).
2. Gently mix, briefly centrifuge, and place PCR tubes in PCR heating block preheated to 98 °C (*see* **Note 10**).
3. Amplify PCR reaction samples using the following Thermocycling conditions: initial denaturation at 98 °C for 1 min,

followed by 35 cycles of denaturing at 98 °C for 10 s, annealing at 63 °C for 30 s, and extension at 72 °C for 1 min. After final cycle, incubate samples for final extension at 72 °C for additional 5 min.

4. Purify the products using the QIAquick PCR purification protocol according to the manufactures recommendations, and sequence using a local provider. Prepare samples using the local provider's recommendations. Use IhMf and IhAr primers as sequencing primers to sequence PCR product from 5′ and 3′ termini, respectively (Table 1.)
5. Analyze obtained sequences with the BLAST Sequence Analysis Tool using the nucleotides application (Fig. 3c).

4 Notes

1. Mouse myeloma CH12F3 is a fast-growing suspension cell line that must be passaged at a 1:10 ratio twice a week. Cells start losing viability at high density (>1 × 10^6 cells/mL). Cells were kindly provided by Dr. Matthew D. Scharff from Albert Einstein College of Medicine, Bronx, NY.
2. Cells must be grown in a 5% CO_2 humidified atmosphere at 37 °C. Medium must be supplemented with Hepes to increase the maximum buffering range of the medium, and β-mercaptoethanol to minimize B lymphocytes clamping. The complement system in FBS must be inactivated by incubating serum at 56 °C for 30 min. You can also use commercial heat-inactivated serum.
3. Cells undergo spontaneous CSR and therefore after long cultivation require isolation of the fresh individual clones. It is a good practice to grow individual clones and freeze them in sufficient amount and to work with freshly thawed clones.
4. Mix cell suspension with Trypan Blue. Count the unstained cells in the chamber; dead cells will be stained blue. The ratio of the uncolored to blue cells should be more than 95%. Cultures that contain significant number of dead cells will not perform well in this assay.
5. It is a good practice to add additional control treatments, such as treating the cells with only anti-CD40 or mIL-4. These cells should demonstrate minimal CSR.
6. To prevent photobleaching minimize exposure of the fluorophore to direct light and incubate samples in dark box.
7. RNA isolation contains hazardous material, like phenol and chloroform. It is recommended to do all steps in the chemical hood and use safe-loc or screw cap centrifuge tubes. Use only

polypropylene tubes, because polyethylene tubes will be melted by chloroform. You can also use commercial Qiagen RNeasy Mini Kit for RNA purification.

8. For pure RNA 260/280 ratio of absorbance should be ~2.0 and 260/230 ratio should be in the range 2.0–2.2.

9. The best results were achieved when we were using the Phusion High Fidelity DNA polymerase. To minimize optimizations steps, use The Phusion High-Fidelity PCR master mix with HF buffer.

10. Overlay PCR reaction samples with the mineral oil if PCR machine is not equipped with the heating lead.

References

1. Carroll MC, Isenman DE (2012) Regulation of humoral immunity by complement. Immunity 37(2):199–207. https://doi.org/10.1016/j.immuni.2012.08.002
2. Kawakami T, Galli SJ (2002) Regulation of mast-cell and basophil function and survival by IgE. Nat Rev Immunol 2(10):773–786. https://doi.org/10.1038/nri914
3. Macpherson AJ, Geuking MB, McCoy KD (2012) Homeland security: IgA immunity at the frontiers of the body. Trends Immunol 33 (4):160–167. https://doi.org/10.1016/j.it.2012.02.002
4. Nimmerjahn F, Ravetch JV (2011) Fcgammars in health and disease. Curr Top Microbiol Immunol 350:105–125. https://doi.org/10.1007/82_2010_86
5. Pabst O (2012) New concepts in the generation and functions of IgA. Nat Rev Immunol 12(12):821–832. https://doi.org/10.1038/nri3322
6. Roopenian DC, Akilesh S (2007) FcRn: the neonatal Fc receptor comes of age. Nat Rev Immunol 7(9):715–725. https://doi.org/10.1038/nri2155
7. Nakamura M, Kondo S, Sugai M, Nazarea M, Imamura S, Honjo T (1996) High frequency class switching of an IgM+ B lymphoma clone CH12F3 to IgA+ cells. Int Immunol 8 (2):193–201
8. Pene J, Rousset F, Briere F, Chretien I, Paliard X, Banchereau J, Spits H, De Vries JE (1988) IgE production by normal human B cells induced by alloreactive T cell clones is mediated by IL-4 and suppressed by IFN-gamma. J Immunol 141(4):1218–1224
9. Vercelli D, Jabara HH, Arai K, Yokota T, Geha RS (1989) Endogenous interleukin 6 plays an obligatory role in interleukin 4-dependent human IgE synthesis. Eur J Immunol 19 (8):1419–1424. https://doi.org/10.1002/eji.1830190811
10. Zhang K, Clark EA, Saxon A (1991) CD40 stimulation provides an IFN-gamma-independent and IL-4-dependent differentiation signal directly to human B cells for IgE production. J Immunol 146(6):1836–1842
11. Tran TH, Nakata M, Suzuki K, Begum NA, Shinkura R, Fagarasan S, Honjo T, Nagaoka H (2010) B cell-specific and stimulation-responsive enhancers derepress Aicda by overcoming the effects of silencers. Nat Immunol 11(2):148–154. https://doi.org/10.1038/ni.1829
12. Crouch EE, Li Z, Takizawa M, Fichtner-Feigl-S, Gourzi P, Montano C, Feigenbaum L, Wilson P, Janz S, Papavasiliou FN, Casellas R (2007) Regulation of AID expression in the immune response. J Exp Med 204 (5):1145–1156. https://doi.org/10.1084/jem.20061952
13. Dedeoglu F, Horwitz B, Chaudhuri J, Alt FW, Geha RS (2004) Induction of activation-induced cytidine deaminase gene expression by IL-4 and CD40 ligation is dependent on STAT6 and NFkappaB. Int Immunol 16 (3):395–404
14. Huong le T, Kobayashi M, Nakata M, Shioi G, Miyachi H, Honjo T, Nagaoka H (2013) In vivo analysis of Aicda gene regulation: a critical balance between upstream enhancers and intronic silencers governs appropriate expression. PLoS One 8(4):e61433. https://doi.org/10.1371/journal.pone.0061433
15. Poltoratsky V, Goodman MF, Scharff MD (2000) Error-prone candidates vie for somatic mutation. J Exp Med 192(10):F27–F30

16. Poltoratsky VP, Wilson SH, Kunkel TA, Pavlov YI (2004) Recombinogenic phenotype of human activation-induced cytosine deaminase. J Immunol 172(7):4308–4313
17. Chang TP, Vancurova I (2013) NFkappaB function and regulation in cutaneous T-cell lymphoma. Am J Cancer Res 3(5):433–445
18. DiDonato JA, Mercurio F, Karin M (2012) NF-kappaB and the link between inflammation and cancer. Immunol Rev 246(1):379–400. https://doi.org/10.1111/j.1600-065X.2012.01099.x
19. Li MO, Wan YY, Sanjabi S, Robertson AK, Flavell RA (2006) Transforming growth factor-beta regulation of immune responses. Annu Rev Immunol 24:99–146. https://doi.org/10.1146/annurev.immunol.24.021605.090737
20. Massague J (2012) TGFbeta signalling in context. Nat Rev Mol Cell Biol 13(10):616–630. https://doi.org/10.1038/nrm3434
21. Muramatsu M, Kinoshita K, Fagarasan S, Yamada S, Shinkai Y, Honjo T (2000) Class switch recombination and hypermutation require activation-induced cytidine deaminase (AID), a potential RNA editing enzyme. Cell 102(5):553–563. https://doi.org/10.1016/s0092-8674(00)00078-7
22. Petersen S, Casellas R, Reina-San-Martin B, Chen HT, Difilippantonio MJ, Wilson PC, Hanitsch L, Celeste A, Muramatsu M, Pilch DR, Redon C, Ried T, Bonner WM, Honjo T, Nussenzweig MC, Nussenzweig A (2001) AID is required to initiate Nbs1/gamma-H2AX focus formation and mutations at sites of class switching. Nature 414 (6864):660–665
23. Matthews AJ, Zheng S, DiMenna LJ, Chaudhuri J (2014) Regulation of immunoglobulin class-switch recombination: choreography of noncoding transcription, targeted DNA deamination, and long-range DNA repair. Adv Immunol 122:1–57. https://doi.org/10.1016/b978-0-12-800267-4.00001-8
24. Battey J, Moulding C, Taub R, Murphy W, Stewart T, Potter H, Lenoir G, Leder P (1983) The human c-myc oncogene: structural consequences of translocation into the IgH locus in Burkitt lymphoma. Cell 34 (3):779–787
25. Neri A, Barriga F, Knowles DM, Magrath IT, Dalla-Favera R (1988) Different regions of the immunoglobulin heavy-chain locus are involved in chromosomal translocations in distinct pathogenetic forms of Burkitt lymphoma. Proc Natl Acad Sci U S A 85(8):2748–2752
26. Shiramizu B, Barriga F, Neequaye J, Jafri A, Dalla-Favera R, Neri A, Guttierez M, Levine P, Magrath I (1991) Patterns of chromosomal breakpoint locations in Burkitt's lymphoma: relevance to geography and Epstein-Barr virus association. Blood 77 (7):1516–1526
27. Akasaka H, Akasaka T, Kurata M, Ueda C, Shimizu A, Uchiyama T, Ohno H (2000) Molecular anatomy of BCL6 translocations revealed by long-distance polymerase chain reaction-based assays. Cancer Res 60 (9):2335–2341
28. Offit K, Louie DC, Parsa NZ, Roy P, Leung D, Lo Coco F, Zelenetz A, Dalla-Favera R, Chaganti RS (1995) BCL6 gene rearrangement and other cytogenetic abnormalities in diffuse large cell lymphoma. Leuk Lymphoma 20 (1-2):85–89

Chapter 16

Single-Stranded DNA Aptamers Against TNF and Their Potential Applications

Shao Tao, Pingfang Song, Xiaowei Zhang, Lingshu Zhang, and Cong-Qiu Chu

Abstract

Aptamers are short, single-stranded RNA or DNA sequences, which can bind to protein ligands with high affinity and specificity. Applications of aptamers are broad, ranging from drugs and drug delivery vehicles to biosensors. Tumor necrosis factor (TNF) is an inflammatory cytokine that plays a critical role in the pathogenesis of several autoimmune inflammatory diseases. Blocking TNF activity by monoclonal antibodies or TNF receptor fusion protein has been tremendously successful in treating these diseases. However, manufacturing these biological TNF inhibitors is expensive and a significant proportion of patients do not respond to TNF blockade. Here we describe selection of single-stranded DNA aptamers for TNF blockage, and their bioactivity in blocking TNF-mediated cytotoxicity in vitro. These TNF-binding aptamers have the potential to serve as alternatives to biological TNF inhibitors and to be used as in vivo probes for TNF detection.

Key words Aptamers, ssDNA, SELEX, Tumor necrosis factor, In vivo imaging, Therapeutics

1 Introduction

Tumor necrosis factor (TNF) is a pleiotropic cytokine with both pro-inflammatory and immunoregulatory functions. TNF is the first cytokine that is validated as therapeutic target for rheumatoid arthritis (RA) and other inflammatory diseases. Blocking TNF activity has revolutionized the management of RA and other inflammatory diseases [1, 2]. The benefit of TNF inhibitors (TNFi) to RA patients is well recognized and demonstrated in numerous clinical trials and real-world registries of clinical practice for over 20 years. Specific blockade of TNF activity has categorically proven the critical role of TNF in the pathogenesis of RA and other inflammatory diseases [1, 2]. TNF specifically targeted therapy for these inflammatory conditions has been achieved by using biological TNF inhibitors (TNFi), namely, monoclonal antibodies (mAb) and soluble TNF receptor fusion proteins. However, in spite

Ivana Vancurova and Yan Zhu (eds.), *Immune Mediators in Cancer: Methods and Protocols*, Methods in Molecular Biology, vol. 2108, https://doi.org/10.1007/978-1-0716-0247-8_16,

of the high efficacy and great benefit of TNFi to patients with inflammatory diseases, there are two important issues associated with TNFi therapy. The first is the high cost [3]. This is stemmed from the nature of TNFi, since they are all protein therapeutics, which are produced by costly protein engineering. The second is that a significant proportion of patients do not respond to TNFi treatment. For instance, about 30–40% of RA patients fail to achieve adequate response to TNFi [4, 5]. Current standard practice still applies the trial and error model. This involves administration of full dose of one TNFi in a patient before it is determined whether the patient has an adequate response or not. If the patient fails to respond to one TNFi, another TNFi or other biologics will be tried. This trial process can take up to 3 months. The trial of TNFi is not only expensive, but also has the patient exposed to potentially adverse effects from TNFi. Many pharmacogenetics studies have attempted to identify genotypes to predict RA patients to respond to TNFi but have failed to be replicated in independent cohort of patients (reviewed in ref. [6]). A TNFi response prediction guided personalized medicine is required, but this still remains a challenge. Alternative approaches are required.

TNF is an effector molecule that is required to be present at the site of the tissue to mediate inflammation. For example, TNF is expressed in synovial tissue of RA patients [7] and in the mucosa of patient with Crohn's disease [8]. But the TNF levels in the inflamed tissues vary from zero to high levels of expression [7]. Therefore, in vivo probing and quantifying TNF would represent a practical approach to predict therapeutic response. In small pilot studies, ^{99m}Tc-labeled anti-TNF mAb, infliximab and adalimumab have been used to image TNF in RA joints before and after TNFi treatment. Patients with high pre-therapy uptake of ^{99m}Tc-labeled anti-TNF mAb had more therapeutic benefit than those who showed less uptake in the inflamed joints before therapy [9]. These studies suggest that detection of TNF at arthritic joints may have value for prediction of TNFi response. However, isotope exposure has potential safety concerns. Non-radiative labeled in vivo probing is highly desirable. Recently, Atreya et al. labeled adalimumab with fluorescein isothiocyanate (FITC) and topically applied it to the inflamed mucosa of patients with Crohn's disease [10]. The FITC-adalimumab stained positive cells in the colon were visualized and quantified by laser colonoscopy. The TNF producing cells in the colon positively correlated with treatment response rate [10]. Thus, it is feasible to quantify TNF expression in vivo with non-radiation methods.

To overcome the drawbacks associated with mAb and soluble receptors, we sought alternative agents for specific detection and targeting of TNF activity without compromising the therapeutic effects and reducing the cost. Aptamers fulfill the criteria to substitute for biological agents to block TNF. Aptamers are single-stranded 20–100 nucleotides that bind to molecular targets with high affinity and specificity due to their stable three-dimensional shapes [11, 12]. Aptamers are synthesized random sequences of RNA or DNA which are pooled to serve as a library. Each library of aptamers consists of around 10^{-15} unique nucleotide sequences to bind to a wide array of protein families. In theory, one can find at least one aptamer from a library of aptamers for any given protein. Aptamers bind to protein ligand through conformational tertiary structure with an extremely high affinity and specificity which are comparable to those of mAb, and hence aptamers are referred as "chemical antibodies." In addition, aptamers possess some unique characteristics as therapeutic agents. For instance, using chemical substitutions and other modifications, aptamers elicit minimal immunogenicity in vivo relative to mAb. Their relatively small physical size results in an improved transportation and enhanced tissue penetration. Straightforward chemical synthesis makes them amenable to backbone modification and rapid in vitro selection. Thereby aptamers can be reproducibly and economically synthesized in a large scale for clinical applications [11, 12]. Pegaptanib, an RNA aptamer against vascular endothelial growth factor (VEGF), has been approved by the FDA to treat wet age-related macular degeneration [13] and many other aptamers are being explored for therapeutic purposes. Aptamers have also been extensively investigated for use as probes for in vivo molecular and cellular imaging using non-radioactive bioluminescence dye. Aptamer-based imaging probes can be formulated either by directly linking to fluorescent molecules or by conjugating aptamers to nanoparticle-based optical probes. These aptamer-based molecular imaging probes have been used to image biomarkers and cellular proteins such as integrins, tumor antigens for in vivo tracking tumor progress and therapeutic response [14].

In this chapter, we apply the standard in vitro SELEX (Systematic Evolution of Ligands by Exponential Enrichment) protocol [15] to select single-stranded DNA (ssDNA) aptamers for human TNF using a ssDNA library containing 10^{15} random sequences (Fig. 1). The selected aptamers were then screened for their affinity and bioactivity to neutralize TNF cytotoxicity in vitro. These TNF-binding aptamers can potentially be developed for therapy and in vivo quantification of TNF expression.

2 Materials

2.1 Materials for Systematic Evolution of Ligands by Exponential Enrichment (SELEX)

1. 13 mm Millipore Swinnex filter.
2. Syringes (10 mL).
3. Single-stranded DNA (ssDNA) library (TriLink BioTechnologies, catalog # O-32001-40), store at −20 °C.

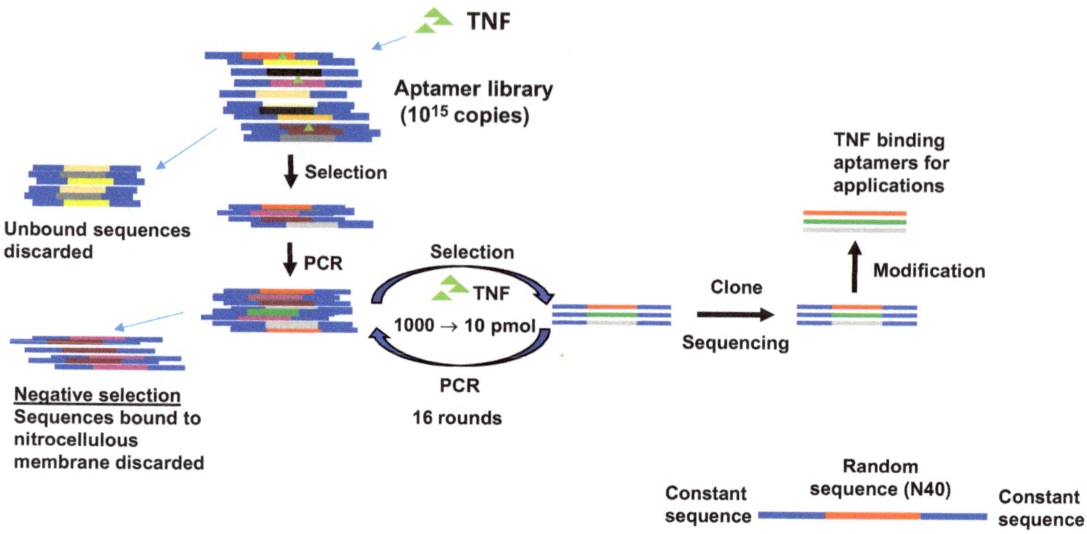

Fig. 1 A schematic SELEX procedure for selection of ssDNA aptamer binding to human TNF. The protocol was based on a published method for ssDNA aptamer selection with modification. (SELEX: systematic evolution of ligands by exponential enrichment)

4. 20 μM Forward primer 5′-TAGGGAAGAGAAGGACATA TGAT-3′ (TriLink BioTechnologies, catalog # O-32001-40), store at −20 °C.
5. 20 μM Reverse primer 5′-TAGGGAAGAGAAGGACATAT GAT-3′ (TriLink BioTechnologies, catalog # O-32001-40), store at −20 °C.
6. Recombinant human TNF (*see* **Note 1**), store at −80 °C.
7. CleanAmp PCR 2× Master Mix (TriLink BioTechnologies, catalog # L-5101-100), store at −20 °C.
8. 3.0% LE agarose gel, store at room temperature.
9. Ethidium bromide (EtBr), store at room temperature.
10. 1.5% Low-melting-point agarose gel, store at room temperature.
11. GelRed (Biotium, catalog # 41002), store at 4 °C.
12. Binding buffer; 20 mM HEPES, 2 mM $CaCl_2$, 50 nM NaCl. Store at room temperature.
13. Nitrocellulose membrane.
14. 7.0 M Urea, store at room temperature.
15. Phenol, store at 4 °C.
16. 25:24:1, v/v UltraPure™ Phenol:Chloroform:Isoamyl Alcohol.
17. 3 M Sodium acetate, pH 5.5, store at room temperature.

18. 100% Ethanol and 70% ethanol, store at −20 °C.
19. DEPC-treated molecular biology grade water, store at room temperature.

2.2 Materials for Aptamer-Based Enzyme-Linked Binding Assay

1. 96-Well flat-bottom EIA/RIA microtiter plates.
2. Coupling buffer: Na_2CO_3–$NaHCO_3$, pH 8.3, store at room temperature.
3. Recombinant human TNF, store at −80 °C.
4. PBS, store at 4 °C.
5. Tween-20, store at room temperature.
6. 2% Bovine serum albumin (BSA) Fraction V, store at 4 °C.
7. Capture purified anti-human TNF, MAb1 (BioLegend, catalog # 502802), store at 4 °C.
8. Biotin anti-human TNF, Mab11 (BioLegend, catalog # 502904), store at 4 °C.
9. Sheared salmon sperm DNA, store at −20 °C.
10. Biotinylated anti-human TNF MAb11, store at 4 °C.
11. Streptavidin-Horseradish peroxidase (HRP), store at 4 °C.
12. 3,3′,5,5′-Tetramethylbenzidine (TMB), store at 4 °C.
13. 2 N H_2SO_4, store at room temperature.
14. 1.5 mL Eppendorf tubes.
15. 10 mM Tris–HCl, pH 10.5, store at room temperature.
16. 1× RPMI 1640, store at 4 °C.

2.3 Materials for Screening ssDNA Aptamers to Block TNF-Alpha Bioactivity

1. Selected ssDNA aptamers for TNF, stored at −20 °C.
2. Recombinant human TNF, store at −80 °C.
3. L929 mouse fibroblast cell line (ATCC), culture at 37 °C.
4. 96-Well flat-bottom microtiter culture plate.
5. 1× RPMI 1640, store at 4 °C.
6. Fetal bovine serum (FBS), store at −20 °C.
7. 1 mM sodium pyruvate, store at 4 °C.
8. 2 mM L-glutamine, store at 4 °C.
9. Penicillin-streptomycin, store at 4 °C.
10. Sulforhodamine B (SRB), store at room temperature.
11. Trichloroacetic acid (TCA), store at room temperature.
12. 1% (vol/vol) acetic acid, store at room temperature.
13. 10 mM Tris–HCl, pH 10.5, store at room temperature.
14. Gyratory shaker.

3 Methods

3.1 PCR Cycle Optimization for SELEX

1. The procedures described below are based on published protocol for selection of ssDNA aptamers with modifications [15].
2. Put ssDNA library, primers, and CleanAmp PCR 2× Master Mix on ice.
3. Reconstitute both forward and reverse primers to 200 μM, and make aliquots of 20 μM stocks.
4. Reconstitute the ssDNA library to 100 μM, and make 2000 pM stocks.
5. Set up a 50-μL regular PCR (R-PCR) amplification reaction volume on ice as shown below (*see* **Note 2**):

CleanAmp PCR 2× Master Mix	25.0 μL
ssDNA library 0.002 μM	7.50 μL
Forward primer 20 μM	2.50 μL
Reverse primer 20 μM	2.50 μL
ddH_2O	12.5 μL

6. Perform R-PCR amplification, using the following amplification conditions (*see* **Note 3**):

Step	Temperature (°C)	Time (min)
Hot start	94.0	2:00
Amplification (20 cycles)		
Denaturation	94.0	0:30
Annealing	49.0	0:30
Extension	72.0	0:30
Final extension	72.0	5:00
Hold	4.0	

7. Take 5 μL of R-PCR samples at the following cycles: 8, 10, 12, 14, 16, 18, and 20.
8. Perform electrophoresis with a 3% regular agarose gel at 84 V at room temperature with the amplified chosen R-PCR samples.
9. Select a cycle number that yields a band without nonspecific amplicons (*see* **Note 4**).
10. Set up a 50 μL asymmetric PCR (A-PCR) amplification reaction volume on ice as shown below (*see* **Note 4**):

CleanAmp PCR 2× Master Mix	25.0 μL
Amplified R-PCR DNA sample	1.00 μL
Forward primer 20 μM	2.50 μL
ddH_2O	21.5 μL

11. Perform A-PCR amplification, using the following amplification conditions (*see* **Note 5**):

Step	Temperature (°C)	Time (min)
Hot start	94.0	2:00
Amplification (30 cycles)		
Denaturation	94.0	0:30
Annealing	49.0	0:30
Extension	72.0	2:00
Final extension	72.0	5:00
Hold	4.0	

12. Take 5 μL of R-PCR samples at the following cycles: 18, 20, 22, 24, 26, 28, and 30.
13. Perform electrophoresis with a 3% regular agarose gel at 84 V at room temperature with the amplified chosen A-PCR samples.
14. Select a cycle number that yields the brightest band without nonspecific amplicons (*see* **Note 6**).
15. The selected R-PCR and A-PCR cycles are to be used for in vitro SELEX amplifications (*see* below).

3.2 In Vitro SELEX for TNF-Specific ssDNA Aptamers

1. Reconstitute 100 μg of lyophilized TNF in 100 μL of binding buffer (*see* **Note 7**) to result in 57 pM stock, or 17.54 μL per 1000 pmol.
2. Add 1000 pmol ssDNA (10 μL from the 100 μM ssDNA library) and 72.5 μL of binding buffer, and mix.
3. Incubate the ssDNA-binding buffer mixture at 95 °C for 5 min and then allow to cool down at room temperature for 10 min.
4. Add 1000 pmol TNF (17.5 μL from 57 pM stock) and the ssDNA-binding buffer mixture, mix, and incubate at room temperature for 25 min (*see* **Note 8**).
5. Allow the mixture to immobilize onto nitrocellulose membrane (*see* **Note 9**).
6. Wash the nitrocellulose membrane five times with 150 μL of binding buffer to wash off unbound ssDNAs.

7. Transfer the washed nitrocellulose membrane into a 1.5 mL Eppendorf tube.
8. Pipette 500 μL of 7 M urea into the nitrocellulose membrane-containing Eppendorf tube.
9. Heat the Eppendorf tube on a heat block at 95 °C for 5 min to elute the TNF-ssDNA aptamer complexes.
10. Transfer the ssDNA aptamers-containing urea into another 1.5 mL Eppendorf tube, and discard the nitrocellulose membrane.
11. Pipette 500 μL of phenol into the ssDNA aptamers-containing urea under chemical hood.
12. Vortex and centrifuge the phenol-ssDNA mixture at 13.2 rpm for 20 min with a tabletop centrifuge at room temperature.
13. Pipette the ssDNA-containing aqueous phase into a new 1.5 mL Eppendorf tube. Discard the phenol portion.
14. Measure the volume of the ssDNA-containing liquid.
15. Pipette the same volume of Phenol:Chloroform:Isoamyl Alcohol into the new 1.5 mL Eppendorf tube to clean up potential phenol contamination in the ssDNA aptamers.
16. Vortex and centrifuge the mixture at 13.2 rpm for 15 min with a tabletop centrifuge. Pipette the aqueous-phase layer into a new 1.5 mL Eppendorf tube.
17. Add 1/10 volume of 3 M sodium acetate, pH 5.2, of the aqueous-phase ssDNA and 2.5× volume 100% ethanol of sodium acetate and ssDNA mixture and vortex.
18. Incubate the mixture at −20 °C overnight. Centrifuge at 16.1 × *g* for 30 min at 4 °C with a tabletop centrifuge.
19. Discard the supernatant with care.
20. Wash the ssDNA pellet with 500 μL of ice-cold 70% ethanol at 16.1 × *g* for 20 min with a tabletop centrifuge.
21. Air-dry the washed ssDNA product and reconstitute with molecular biology grade (DEPC-treated) water.
22. Measure the purified ssDNA concentration with Spectrophotometer ND-1000 using ssDNA-33 setting. Record the measurement.
23. Amplify 300 pM of the ssDNA with the optimized R-PCR.
24. Perform electrophoresis with a 3% regular agarose gel at 84 V at room temperature to confirm one single band without nonspecific amplicons.
25. Set up and perform the optimized 50 μL asymmetric PCR (A-PCR) amplification reaction.

26. Perform electrophoresis with a 1.5% low-melting-point agarose gel at 92 V at 4 °C.
27. Excise out the ssDNA bands from the low-melting agarose gel under UV.
28. Transfer the ssDNA-containing gel fragment into a 1.5 mL Eppendorf tube.
29. Submerge the gel fragment with 1× TE buffer.
30. Incubate the TE buffer submerged gel fragment at 65 °C for 5 min or until completely melted.
31. Add equal volume of phenol to the 1.5 mL Eppendorf tube for purification.
32. Repeat **steps 12–22**.
33. Verify the purified ssDNA for the correct size on a 1.5% LE agarose gel.
34. Subject the purified ssDNA to the second round of SELEX with a decreased concentration of TNF.
    (a) The ssDNA:TNF ratio for each round (a total of 16 rounds) of SELEX as follows:
    - 1000 pmol ssDNA and 1000 pmol TNF (1:1)
    - 1000 pmol ssDNA and 500 pmol TNF (2:1)
    - 1000 pmol ssDNA and 500 pmol TNF (2:1)
    - 1000 pmol ssDNA and 100 pmol TNF (10:1)
    - 1000 pmol ssDNA and 100 pmol TNF (10:1)
    - 1000 pmol ssDNA and 100 pmol TNF (10:1)
    - 1000 pmol ssDNA and 20 pmol TNF (50:1)
    - 1000 pmol ssDNA and 20 pmol TNF (50:1)
    - 1000 pmol ssDNA and 20 pmol TNF (50:1)
    - 1000 pmol ssDNA and 20 pmol TNF (50:1)
    - 1000 pmol ssDNA and 10 pmol TNF (100:1)
    - 1000 pmol ssDNA and 10 pmol TNF (100:1)
    - 1000 pmol ssDNA and 10 pmol TNF (100:1)
    - 1000 pmol ssDNA and 10 pmol TNF (100:1)
    - 1000 pmol ssDNA and 10 pmol TNF (100:1)
    - 1000 pmol ssDNA and 10 pmol TNF (100:1).
35. Perform negative selection to eliminate nitrocellulose membrane-specific ssDNA every four rounds of SELEX (*see* **Note 10**).
36. Perform Next Generation Sequencing (NGS) for selected aptamers (*see* **Note 11**).

37. Select the top 225 most frequent ssDNA sequences post NGS.
38. Synthesize the 225 ssDNA sequences for Aptamer-Based Enzyme-Linked Binding Assay.

3.3 Liquid Phase Capture Aptamer-Linked OligoNucleotide Assay

1. Coat each well of a 96-well flat-bottom EIA/RIA microtiter plate with 25 μL of 8 μg/mL of capture purified anti-human TNF (MAb1) (*see* **Note 12**) in PBS at 4 °C overnight.
2. Wash the plate three times with 1× PBS containing 0.05% (v/v) Tween-20.
3. Block the plate with 150 μL of 2% BSA and 150 μL of 100 μg/mL sheared salmon sperm DNA in 1× PBS for TNF-selected 5′ biotinylated aptamer wells for 2 h at room temperature.
4. Incubate 150 ng/mL of TNF with either 20 ng/mL of biotinylated anti-human TNF (MAb11) (*see* **Note 13**) in 1× PBS containing 0.5% BSA and 0.005% Tween-20 or 800 nM of 5′biotinylated aptamers in 1× PBS containing 10 μg/mL sheared salmon sperm DNA and 0.005% Tween-20 in 1.5 mL Eppendorf tubes for 2 h at room temperature.
5. Wash the plate four times with 1× PBS containing 0.05% (v/v) Tween-20.
6. Add 25 μL of streptavidin-HRP at a ratio of 1:1000 diluted in 1× PBS containing 0.05% (v/v) Tween-20 for 30 min at room temperature.
7. Wash the plate five times with 1× PBS containing 0.05% (v/v) Tween-20.
8. Develop with 25 μL of TMB.
9. Stop the development by adding 25 μL of 2 N H_2SO_4.
10. Read the absorbance at 450 nm on a plate reader, and record the data.

3.4 Screening ssDNA Aptamers by Inhibiting TNF Bioactivity

1. The method described here is modified based on published methods to assay TNF bioactivity and monoclonal antibodies in blocking TNF activity [16, 17].
2. Seed and culture 2 × 10^4 L929 mouse fibroblast cells/well in RPMI 1640 medium supplemented with 10% FBS, 2 mM L-glutamine, 1 mM sodium pyruvate, 100 μg/mL penicillin G, and 100 μg/mL streptomycin, at 37 °C and 5% CO_2 in a flat-bottom 96-well microtiter culture plate overnight.
3. Incubate each synthesized ssDNA aptamer with TNF at different ratios (aptamer:TNF):
   (a) 100 (0.05725 μM or 11.45 pmol):1 (0.0005725 μM or 0.1145 pmol).
   (b) 50:1.

(c) 25:1.

(d) 12.5:1.

(e) 6.25:1.

(f) 3.125:1.

4. Incubate these mixtures and a positive IC_{50} control (10 ng/mL TNF only) in supplemented RPMI1640 medium for 2 h at room temperature prior to incubation with the seeded L929 cells.
5. Incubate the plate (wells containing aptamer, TNF and L929 cells; wells containing TNF and L929 cells; and wells containing L929 cells) for 20 h at 37 °C and 5% CO_2 (*see* **Note 14**).
6. Add 100 μL of cold 20% (wt/vol) trichloroacetic acid to the cell-seeded wells without removing the supernatant.
7. Incubate at 4 °C for 1 h to fix the cells.
8. Wash and air-dry the wells (*see* **Note 15**).
9. Add 100 μL/well of 0.057% SRB and incubate at room temperature for 30 min.
10. Wash the wells immediately with 1% (vol/vol) acetic acid to remove unbound dye. Air-dry the wells (*see* **Note 16**).
11. Add 200 μL of 10 mM Tris–HCl, pH 10.5, to the wells.
12. Shake the plate for 5 min on a Gyratory shaker at room temperature.
13. Measure absorbance of the plate at OD_{510}.
14. Calculate L929 cytotoxicity with the equation: % of cells killed = 100 − mean $OD_{sample}/OD_{negative\ control} \times 100$.

4 Notes

1. It is important that TNF is carrier-free for aptamer selection to avoid selection of carrier protein-binding aptamers.
2. The established R-PCR amplification reaction (molar concentrations and volumes of the primers and the ssDNA library) may need to be adjusted. Such adjustment is to be determined by evaluating the dsDNA bands on an agarose gel.
3. The established R-PCR amplification conditions may need to be adjusted. Such adjustment is to be determined by evaluating the dsDNA bands on an agarose gel.
4. Run a 3% agarose gel with the amplified R-PCR samples. The dsDNA is 86-nucleotide base pairs. The correct dsDNA band should correspond to the same location as the same size dsDNA ladder band.

5. The established A-PCR amplification reaction (molar concentrations and volumes of the primers and the ssDNA library) may need to be adjusted. Such adjustment is to be determined by evaluating the dsDNA bands on an agarose gel.
6. Run a 3% agarose gel with the amplified A-PCR samples. The ssDNA is 86-nucleotide bases, which is equivalent to 43-nucloetide base pairs. The correct ssDNA band should correspond to the same location as the same size 43-nucleotide base pair dsDNA ladder band. It is potentially possible to also see dsDNA on the gel as well. Make sure there are no nonspecific ssDNA amplicons to prevent any potential contamination while doing gel-exercising.
7. Reconstitute the TNF under the culture hood. Let it sit at room temperature for 30 min with several pulse vortexes. Spin down the reconstitute at 0.2 × *g* for 30 s at 4 °C with a tabletop centrifuge. Make aliquots and store them at −80 °C.
8. The mixture is incubated at RT on a rotator.
9. After incubation, vortex and spin down the mixture at 0.2 × *g* for 30 s with a tabletop centrifuge. Assemble a 13 mm Millipore Swinnex filter mount with a piece of nitrocellulose membrane pre-wet with binding buffer in place. Use a p200 pipette to pipette the 100 μL volume onto the membrane through the syringe filter holder. Wash the membrane five times with 150 μL of binding buffer using a 1 mL syringe. Remove the nitrocellulose membrane with a tweezer and place it in a 1.5 mL Eppendorf tube.
10. Negative selections eliminate ssDNAs specific to nitrocellulose membranes that are used to immobilize ssDNA-TNF complexes. Assemble a 13 mm Millipore Swinnex filter mount with a piece of nitrocellulose membrane pre-wet with binding buffer in place. Use a p200 pipette to pipette a mixture of only 10 μL ssDNA (1000 pmol) and 190 μL binding buffer onto an in-place nitrocellulose membrane. Use a 1 mL syringe to pressure out the mixture from the membrane. Collect the mixture in a 1.5 mL Eppendorf tube. Discard the membrane. Measure the ssDNA concentration in the collected mixture. Use this ssDNA for the next round of SELEX.
11. Sequences of selected aptamers can be verified by molecular cloning and Sanger sequencing. However, next generation sequencing is more efficient for a large number of aptamers to be sequenced though the cost is high.
12. (*see* also **Note 13**) The two clones of monoclonal antibodies to human TNF, MAb1 and MAb11 are paired antibodies for quantitative ELISA to measure TNF. We have used either purified MAb1 or MAb11 as the capture antibody and generated similar results.

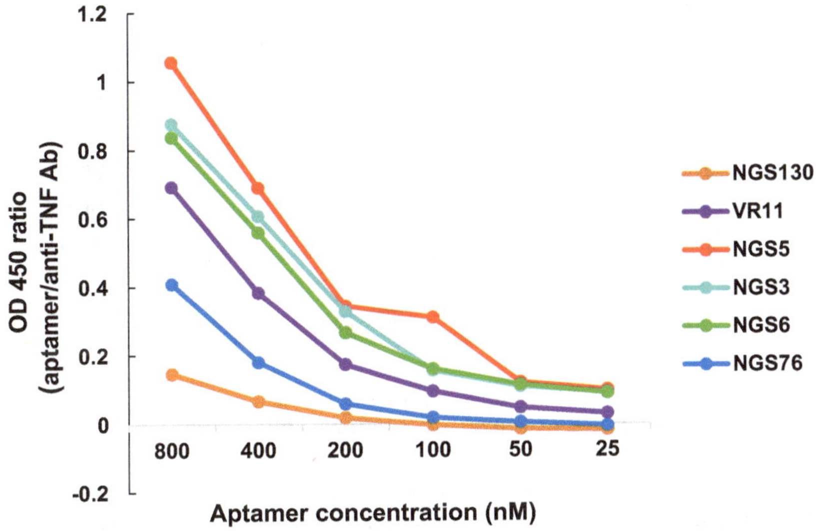

Fig. 2 Binding of ssDNA aptamers selected by SELEX to TNF. Aptamers were biotinylated and incubated with recombinant TNF in liquid phase, and detected by modified ELONA assay. The binding of aptamer to TNF was quantified in reference to the binding of a monoclonal anti-TNF antibody

13. Biotinylated aptamers were custom manufactured by Integrated DNA Technology. Here biotinylated MAb11 antibody is incubated with TNF to serve as a positive control for verifying biotinylated aptamers in binding to TNF in liquid phase. As mentioned in **Note 12**, when purified MAb11 antibody was used as capture antibody, biotinylated MAb1 is used to incubate with TNF as a positive control. As shown in Fig. 2, in each batch of the binding assay, the reading of biotinylated anti-TNF (MAb1 or MAb11) to TNF in the same batch is used as a reference and the ratio of OD_{450} (aptamer/anti-TNF Ab) is expressed. The ratio of OD_{450} (aptamer/anti-TNF Ab) can be compared between batches. In Fig. 2, we also included a short ssDNA (25 nucleotides) aptamer, VR11 [18] as a comparison in measuring the selected ssDNA aptamers.
14. In the bioassay (Fig. 3), the therapeutic anti-TNF monoclonal antibody, infliximab is included as a positive control to compare the bioactivity of TNF-binding aptamers. Infliximab is a chimeric monoclonal antibody used to treat a variety of inflammatory diseases. Infliximab has the high affinity in binding to human TNF [19].
15. Wash each plate four times by submerging the plate slowly in a container filled with tap water. Remove excess residual water in the wells by gently tapping the plate on paper towels. Air-dry each plate either at room temperature or expose the plate to the air nozzle at a slow-flowing rate on a lab bench.
16. Wash the wells four times. Air-dry each plate either at room temperature or expose the plate to the air nozzle at a slow-flowing rate on a lab bench.

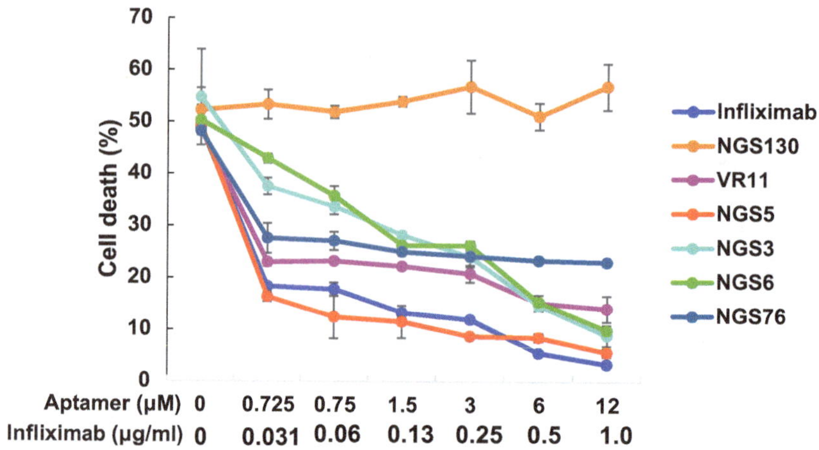

Fig. 3 Bioassay of TNF-binding aptamers. The bioactivity of TNF-binding aptamers was determined by blockade of TNF in a cytotoxicity assay. L929 cells are sensitive to TNF-induced death. 2×10^4 of L929 cells/well were seeded on a flat-bottom 96-well microtiter plate and incubated at 37 °C and 5% CO_2 overnight. Each aptamer was incubated with TNF at different ratios (aptamer:TNF): 100 (0.05725 μM or 11.45 pmol):1 (0.0005725 μM or 0.1145 pmol), 50:1, 25:1, 12.5:1, 6.25:1, and 3.125:1. These mixtures and a positive IC_{50} control (10 ng/mL TNF only) were incubated in supplemented RPMI 1640 medium for 2 h prior to incubation with the seeded cells. After an additional 20-h incubation, the cells were fixed with TCA, dyed with SRB, and absorbance at OD_{450} was measured to determine the cytotoxicity. Data represent an average of two to three tests. NGS 130 is the negative control and Infliximab is the positive control

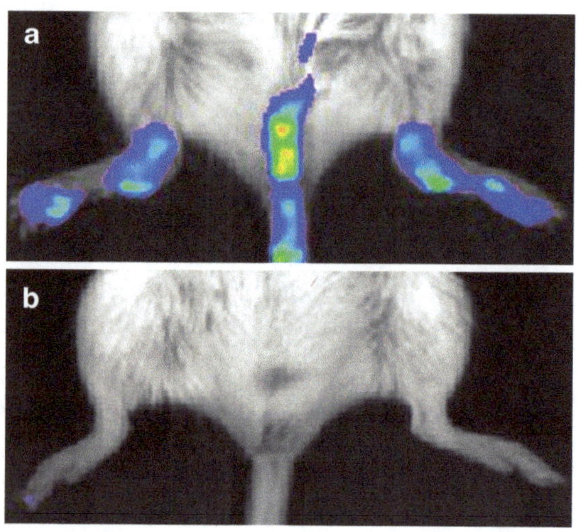

Fig. 4 Detection of TNF in vivo by TNF binding an aptamer. An SKG mouse with arthritis induced by intraperitoneal injection of zymosan was injected with IRDye800CW, and was scanned by IVIS Spectrum CT. (**a**) Arthritic SKG mouse showing TNF expression in hinder paws. (**b**) Normal SKG mouse showing no TNF expression (*see* **Note 17**)

17. In Fig. 4, we show an example of potential application of TNF-binding aptamers. A near-infrared fluorescent dye, IRDye800CW-labeled one selected aptamer (NGS5) (custom labeled by Integrated DNA Technology) was injected

intravenously in an SKG mouse with arthritis induced by intraperitoneally injected zymosan [20]. Expression of TNF was detected by NGS5 and visualized by an IVIS Spectrum CT scanner (Perkin-Elmer). Ongoing work with these aptamers is to determine whether they could serve as therapeutic agents to treat TNF-mediated inflammatory diseases.

Acknowledgement

This work was supported by an Innovative Grant and a Pilot Grant of Rheumatology Research Foundation (CQC). ST was supported by a Graduate Student Proctorship of Rheumatology Research Foundation. LSZ was supported by a scholarship of China Scholarship Council.

References

1. Feldmann M, Maini RN (2010) Anti-TNF therapy, from rationale to standard of care: what lessons has it taught us? J Immunol 185 (2):791–794
2. Taylor PC, Feldmann M (2009) Anti-TNF biologic agents: still the therapy of choice for rheumatoid arthritis. Nat Rev Rheumatol 5 (10):578–582
3. Schabert VF, Watson C, Joseph GJ, Iversen P, Burudpakdee C, Harrison DJ (2013) Costs of tumor necrosis factor blockers per treated patient using real-world drug data in a managed care population. J Manag Care Pharm 19 (8):621–630
4. Klareskog L, van der Heijde D, de Jager JP, Gough A, Kalden J, Malaise M et al (2004) Therapeutic effect of the combination of etanercept and methotrexate compared with each treatment alone in patients with rheumatoid arthritis: double-blind randomised controlled trial. Lancet 363(9410):675–681
5. Maini RN, Breedveld FC, Kalden JR, Smolen JS, Davis D, Macfarlane JD et al (1998) Therapeutic efficacy of multiple intravenous infusions of anti-tumor necrosis factor alpha monoclonal antibody combined with low-dose weekly methotrexate in rheumatoid arthritis. Arthritis Rheum 41(9):1552–1563
6. Umicevic Mirkov M, Cui J, Vermeulen SH, Stahl EA, Toonen EJ, Makkinje RR et al (2013) Genome-wide association analysis of anti-TNF drug response in patients with rheumatoid arthritis. Ann Rheum Dis 72 (8):1375–1381
7. Chu CQ, Field M, Feldmann M, Maini RN (1991) Localization of tumor necrosis factor alpha in synovial tissues and at the cartilage-pannus junction in patients with rheumatoid arthritis. Arthritis Rheum 34(9):1125–1132
8. Murch SH, Braegger CP, Walker-Smith JA, MacDonald TT (1993) Location of tumour necrosis factor alpha by immunohistochemistry in chronic inflammatory bowel disease. Gut 34 (12):1705–1709
9. Malviya G, Conti F, Chianelli M, Scopinaro F, Dierckx RA, Signore A (2010) Molecular imaging of rheumatoid arthritis by radiolabelled monoclonal antibodies: new imaging strategies to guide molecular therapies. Eur J Nucl Med Mol Imaging 37(2):386–398
10. Atreya R, Neumann H, Neufert C, Waldner MJ, Billmeier U, Zopf Y et al (2014) In vivo imaging using fluorescent antibodies to tumor necrosis factor predicts therapeutic response in Crohn's disease. Nat Med 20(3):313–318
11. Bouchard PR, Hutabarat RM, Thompson KM (2010) Discovery and development of therapeutic aptamers. Annu Rev Pharmacol Toxicol 50:237–257
12. Keefe AD, Pai S, Ellington A (2010) Aptamers as therapeutics. Nat Rev Drug Discov 9 (7):537–550
13. Campa C, Harding SP (2011) Anti-VEGF compounds in the treatment of neovascular age related macular degeneration. Curr Drug Targets 12(2):173–181
14. Wang AZ, Farokhzad OC (2014) Current progress of aptamer-based molecular imaging. J Nucl Med 55(3):353–356
15. Marimuthu C, Tang TH, Tominaga J, Tan SC, Gopinath SC (2012) Single-stranded DNA

(ssDNA) production in DNA aptamer generation. Analyst 137(6):1307–1315

16. Galloway CJ, Madanat MS, Mitra G (1991) Monoclonal anti-tumor necrosis factor (TNF) antibodies protect mouse and human cells from TNF cytotoxicity. J Immunol Methods 140 (1):37–43
17. Shiau MY, Chiou HL, Lee YL, Kuo TM, Chang YH (2001) Establishment of a consistent L929 bioassay system for TNF-alpha quantitation to evaluate the effect of lipopolysaccharide, phytomitogens and cytodifferentiation agents on cytotoxicity of TNF-alpha secreted by adherent human mononuclear cells. Mediat Inflamm 10(4):199–208
18. Orava EW, Jarvik N, Shek YL, Sidhu SS, Gariepy J (2013) A short DNA aptamer that recognizes TNFalpha and blocks its activity in vitro. ACS Chem Biol 8(1):170–178
19. Mitoma H, Horiuchi T, Tsukamoto H, Ueda N (2018) Molecular mechanisms of action of anti-TNF-alpha agents—comparison among therapeutic TNF-alpha antagonists. Cytokine 101:56–63
20. Yomogida K, Wu S, Baravati B, Avendano C, Caldwell T, Maniaci B et al (2013) Cell penetrating recombinant Foxp3 protein enhances Treg function and ameliorates arthritis. Biochem Biophys Res Commun 434 (2):263–267

Chapter 17

Probing Metabolic Changes in IFNγ-Treated Ovarian Cancer Cells

Pritpal Kaur, Shreya Nagar, Madhura Bhagwat, Mohammad M. Uddin, Yan Zhu, and Ales Vancura

Abstract

Interferon-γ (IFNγ) is a pleiotropic cytokine that signals to many different cell types. IFNγ has both antitumor functions and pro-tumorigenic effects and regulates different aspects of cell physiology, including metabolism. Cancer cells undergo a complex rearrangement of metabolic pathways that allows them to satisfy the needs of increased proliferation, and many cancer cells redirect glucose metabolism from oxidative phosphorylation to aerobic glycolysis. In this chapter, we describe a protocol that utilizes the Agilent Seahorse XFp Analyzer to assess mitochondrial respiration and glycolysis in ovarian cancer cells treated with IFNγ.

Key words Oxygen consumption rate, Extracellular acidification, Mitochondrial respiration, Glycolysis, Interferon-γ, Ovarian cancer

1 Introduction

Interferon-γ (IFNγ) is a pleiotropic cytokine predominantly produced by cells of the immune system [1]. Since IFNγ receptor is expressed by most, if not all, cell types, IFNγ affects many different tissues, including adipose tissue, neurons, and tumors [1]. IFNγ signaling through JAK kinase and STAT1 transcription factor regulates different aspects of cell physiology, including transcription, epigenetic modifications of chromatin, and metabolism. IFNγ affects mTORC1 (mammalian target of rapamycin complex 1), AMPK (AMP-activated protein kinase), and GSK3 (glycogen synthase kinase 3) [1, 2]; however, systematic analyses of the effect of IFNγ on metabolism of nonimmune cells have not been performed. In this study, we present a general approach for investigating IFNγ's effect on oxidative phosphorylation and glycolysis in cancer cells.

Cancer cells undergo a complex rearrangement of metabolic pathways that allows them to satisfy the needs of increased

Ivana Vancurova and Yan Zhu (eds.), *Immune Mediators in Cancer: Methods and Protocols*, Methods in Molecular Biology, vol. 2108, https://doi.org/10.1007/978-1-0716-0247-8_17,

proliferation [3]. Tumors contain functional mitochondria that support proliferation by providing precursors for anabolic pathways [4]. On the other hand, many cancer cells redirect glucose metabolism from the tricarboxylic acid cycle and oxidative phosphorylation to aerobic glycolysis [5]. Better understanding of the regulatory links between metabolism, mitochondrial function, and growth control will lead to improved treatment strategies for cancer.

In this chapter, we describe a protocol that utilizes the Agilent Seahorse XFp Analyzer to assess mitochondrial respiration and glycolysis in ovarian cancer cells treated with IFNγ. The XFp (extracellular flux) analyzer measures changes in oxygen concentration (oxygen consumption rate, OCR) and pH (extracellular acid release, ECAR) in medium surrounding monolayer of cells in cell culture plate [6]. The XFp Analyzer utilizes cell culture plates and sensor cartridges. The sensor cartridges feature solid-state sensors at the tips of probes that measure oxygen and proton concentrations in the media. The sensor cartridge is periodically lowered into the cell culture plate just above the cell monolayer, creating a transient micro chamber in which OCR and ECAR are measured. In Seahorse XFp Cell Mito Stress Test assay, three different modulators are injected through ports in the sensor cartridge to analyze different parameters of mitochondrial function. Oligomycin, an ATP synthase inhibitor, is injected first to reveal oxygen consumption due to ATP synthesis. Uncoupler FCCP (carbonyl cyanide-4 trifluoromethoxy phenylhydrazone) is injected second to dissipate proton gradient across the mitochondrial inner membrane. FCCP allows proton transport through the membrane, bypassing ATP synthase, and reveals maximal respiration. Lastly, a mixture of rotenone and antimycin A (Rot/AA) is injected to the wells. Rot/AA inhibit mitochondrial respiration, and the oxygen consumption recorded in the presence of Rot/AA corresponds to non-mitochondrial oxygen consumption.

2 Materials

2.1 Cell Culture

1. SKOV3 cells (American Type Culture Collection).
2. RPMI complete medium: RPMI medium supplemented with 10% fetal bovine serum (FBS), 2 mM glutamine, 1 mM sodium pyruvate, 10 mM HEPES, and 1% penicillin-streptomycin solution.
3. IFNγ stock solution: Dissolve IFNγ in sterile water to a final concentration of 50 μg/mL. Store at −80 °C (*see* **Note 1**).
4. 0.25% Trypsin-EDTA.
5. 15 mL Centrifuge tubes.

6. 1.5 mL Micro-centrifuge tubes.
7. Trypan Blue solution.
8. Hemocytometer.
9. Seahorse XFp cell culture miniplate.
10. Seahorse XFp sensor cartridges.
11. Seahorse XF RPMI medium, pH 7.4. Store at 4 °C.
12. Seahorse XF 1 M glucose solution. Store at 4 °C.
13. Seahorse XF 100 mM sodium pyruvate solution. Store at 4 °C.
14. Seahorse XF 200 mM L-glutamine solution. Store at 4 °C.
15. 5% Humdified CO_2 incubator.

2.2 Agilent Seahorse XFp Mito Stress Assay

1. Seahorse XF Calibrant buffer.
2. Seahorse XF Cell Mito Stress Test kit.
3. Sterile distilled water.
4. Microscope.
5. Seahorse XFp Analyzer.
6. Non-CO_2 incubator.

2.3 Result Analysis

1. Seahorse Wave desktop software.
2. Seahorse XFp Cell Mito Stress Test Report Generator.
3. Microsoft Excel.

3 Methods

In this section, we describe the XFp Cell Mito Stress Test assay procedure to measure OCR and ECAR in living cells using Seahorse XFp Analyzer. This assay provides in-depth understanding of mitochondrial pathways and the cause of their dysregulation under stress conditions. It includes several modulator of mitochondrial respiration such as oligomycin, FCCP, and Rot/AA. They target complexes involved in the electron transport chain and reveal basal respiration, ATP-linked respiration, maximal respiration, and spare capacity. The XFp Analyzer measures oxygen and proton concentrations in the media above the cell monolayer through a solid-state probes in the cartridges. During the assay, the sensor probes are periodically lowered into the wells of the cell culture miniplate, where they measure both OCR and ECAR. The results are analyzed in the Wave software and in the Seahorse XFp Report Generators.

3.1 Determination of the Optimal Cell Density for the OCR and ECAR Assays

To determine OCR and ECAR, it is important that cells are in monolayer. Thus, it is important to determine the optimal cell density for all cell types. Cell seeding number depends on the well surface area and cell type. Seahorse XFp Analyzer is compatible with 8-well XFp cell culture miniplate. The surface area of wells is about 11.40 mm^2. Estimate the number of the cells based on previous experiments or using Seahorse bioscience cell line reference database (https://www.agilent.com/cell-reference-database/). If it is a new cell line, then do optimal cell density assay as follows. This procedure is to find optimal cell seeding number, so no need to repeat it for same cell line.

Day 1

1. Add 80 μL of RPMI complete medium in wells A and H (background wells; the first and last wells of the Seahorse XFp cell culture miniplate).
2. Seed 10,000, 20,000, and 40,000 cells/well in duplicates into wells B, C, D, E, F, and G of the cell culture miniplate by plating 80 μL of appropriately diluted cell suspension (*see* **Note 2**).
3. Add 400 μL water in moats around the wells and incubate the cell culture miniplate at 37 °C in 5% CO_2 humidified atmosphere for 16–24 h.
4. Hydrate sensor cartridges:
   (a) Open the pack of cartridges and carefully separate the utility plate and sensor cartridge. Put the cartridge upside down on the bench (*see* **Note 3**).
   (b) Add 200 μL of sterile distilled water in each well and 400 μL of sterile distilled water to the moats around the wells.
   (c) Carefully put the cartridge back on the utility plate and incubate it in a non-CO_2 incubator at 37 °C overnight (*see* **Note 4**).

Day 2

5. Turn on the XFp Analyzer at least 2 h before the assay to make sure that the machine is stable at 37 °C (*see* **Note 5**).
6. Warm 10 mL XF calibrant buffer to 37 °C.
7. Take out the sensor cartridge from non-CO_2 incubator and discard the water from all wells and moats by pipetting.
8. Add 200 μL of XF calibrant buffer in each well and 400 μL of XF calibrant buffer to the moats around the wells of the sensor cartridge.
9. Incubate the sensor cartridge at 37 °C for an hour.

10. Prepare 10 mL XF RPMI complete medium (assay medium) and keep it warm at 37 °C (*see* **Note 6**).
11. Wash the cells with assay media:
    (a) Remove 60 μL of growth medium from each well of cell culture miniplate (*see* **Note 7**).
    (b) Add 180 μL assay medium to each well carefully without disturbing cell layer and then remove 180 μL medium from the wells (*see* **Note 8**).
    (c) Repeat **step b** twice.
12. Add 180 μL of the assay medium to make the final volume 200 μL in all wells.
13. Incubate the cell culture miniplate in non-CO_2 incubator at 37 °C for an hour (*see* **Note 9**).
14. Prepare a new assay template in the Wave software, save it on the USB flash drive, and transfer it to the XFp Analyzer before starting the assay (*see* **Note 10**).
15. Press "START" button and carefully load the sensor cartridge with utility plate (*see* **Note 11**).
16. After calibration, replace the utility plate with cell culture miniplate and press "CONTINUE" to start the sample analysis (*see* **Note 12**).
17. When the reading of the OCR and ECAR is completed, transfer the result to USB flash drive in Excel format.
18. Trypsinize the cells from each well and count the cell number for normalization of the results.
19. Analyze the result using the Wave software on a desktop computer. Plot the OCR against the cell number to determine optimal cell density for further Seahorse XFp assays (Fig. 1).

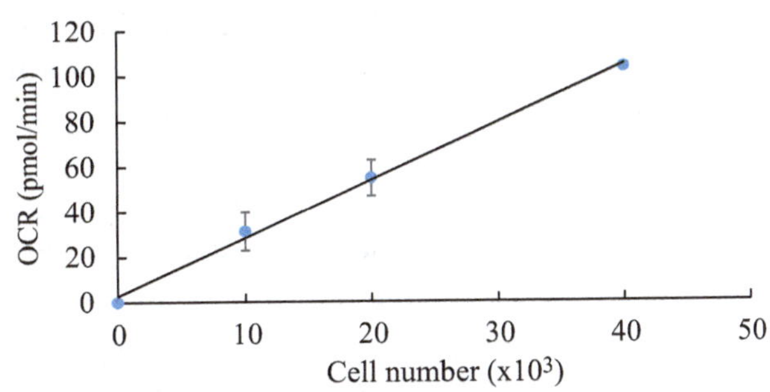

Fig. 1 Optimization of cell seeding number for OCR measurement in SKOV3 cells. SKOV3 cells were seeded at 10,000, 20,000 and 40,000 cells/well and incubated for 24 h. OCR was measured using protocol described in **Note 10**

3.2 Mitochondria Stress Assay

Day 1

1. Add 80 μL of RPMI complete medium in wells A and H (background wells) of the Seahorse XF cell culture miniplate.
2. Seed 20,000 cells/well by plating suspension of SKOV3 cells (2.5×10^5 cells/mL) in RPMI complete medium to wells B-G. Add 400 μL water in moats around the wells and incubate the plate in a humidified 5% CO_2 atmosphere at 37 °C for 16–24 h.

Day 2

3. Take out the Seahorse XFp cell culture miniplate from the incubator and observe under microscope to make sure that the cells are healthy and in monolayer.
4. Carefully remove the medium and cell debris from the well without disturbing the adhered cells.
5. Add 80 μL of complete RPMI medium supplemented with IFNγ to achieve 0, 10, and 50 ng/mL IFNγ (each concentration in duplicate) in wells B-G (*see* **Note 13**).
6. Incubate the miniplate in a humidified 5% CO_2 atmosphere at 37 °C for 24 h.
7. Hydrate sensor cartridges as described under Subheading 3.1, **step 4**.

Day 3

8. Prepare the XFp Analyzer, sensor cartridges, and cell culture miniplates as described under Subheading 3.1, **steps 5–14** (*see* **Note 5**).
9. Prepare the compounds of the Seahorse XFp Cell Mito Stress Test kit by reconstituting the content of the individual vials in the assay medium as follows (*see* **Note 14**):
   (a) Add 280 μL of the assay medium into the oligomycin vial to prepare stock solution of 45 μM.
   (b) Add 288 μL of the assay medium into the FCCP vial to prepare stock solution of 50 μM.
   (c) Add 216 μL of the assay medium into the Rot/AA vial to prepare stock solution of 25 μM.

   The stock solutions should be prepared fresh on the day of the assay and should not be refrozen.
10. Dilute the stock solutions into working solutions as follows:
   (a) To prepare 15 μM working solution of oligomycin, add 100 μL of stock solution into 200 μL assay medium.
   (b) To prepare 5 μM working solution of FCCP, add 30 μL of stock solution into 270 μL assay medium.
   (c) To prepare 5 μM working solution of Rot/AA, add 60 μL of stock solution into 240 μL assay medium.

11. Load the working solutions of the individual compounds in ports of all the wells, including background wells:
    (a) Add 20 μL of 15 μM oligomycin in all ports A to get 1.5 μM as final concentration.
    (b) Add 22 μL of 5 μM FCCP in all ports B to get 0.5 μM as final concentration.
    (c) Add 25 μL of 5 μM Rot/AA in all ports C to get 0.5 μM as final concentration.
12. Create assay template in the Wave software (*see* **Note 15**).
13. Press "START" button and carefully load the sensor cartridge with utility plate (*see* **Note 11**).
14. After calibration, replace the utility plate with cell culture miniplate and press "CONTINUE" to start the sample analysis (*see* **Note 12**).
15. When the reading of the OCR and ECAR is completed, transfer the result to USB flash drive in Excel format.
16. Trypsinize the cells from each well and count the cell number for normalization of the results.

3.3 Analysis of Results

1. Transfer the result from the USB flash drive to a computer and save the files.
2. Open the result in the Wave software and click on export and select "Seahorse XF Cell Mito Stress Test Report Generator" and save the file (*see* **Note 16**).
3. Download the Seahorse XFp Cell Mito Stress Test Report Generator from this link (https://www.agilent.com/en/products/cell-analysis/xf-cell-mito-stress-test-report-generator).
4. Open the result in Report Generator and analyze the result (Figs. 2 and 3).

4 Notes

1. Aliquot IFNγ in sterile microcentrifuge tubes and store at −80 °C to avoid repeated freeze-thaw cycles that might decrease IFNγ biological activity.
2. Cell density could vary depending on the cell type. Generally, it ranges from 10,000 to 40,000 cells/well.
3. Do not touch the bottom tip of sensor cartridges because it is labeled with a solid-state sensor material that detects change in both pH and CO_2.

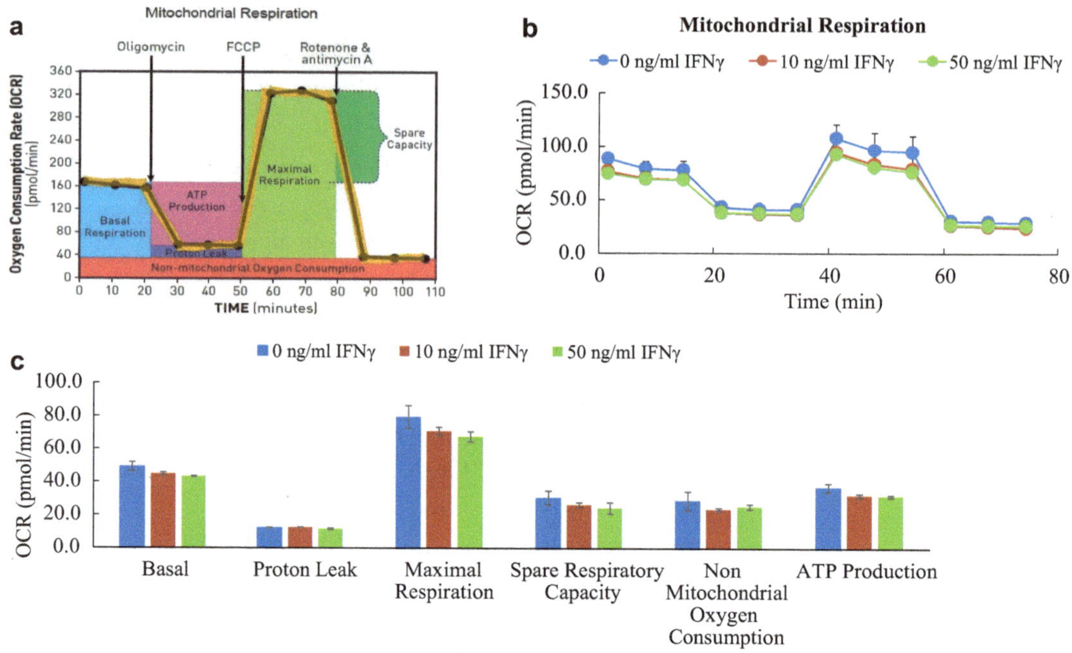

Fig. 2 Mitochondrial stress test of IFNγ-treated SKOV3 cells. (**a**) A schematic diagram of mitochondrial stress test (Agilent Seahorse). (**b**) Oxygen consumption rate was measured in SKOV3 cells seeded at 20,000 cells/well, incubated for 24 h, and treated with 0 (control), 10, and 50 ng/mL of IFNγ. OCR was measured under basal conditions followed by the sequential addition of oligomycin (1.5 μM), FCCP (0.5 μM), and rotenone & antimycin A (0.5 μM) as indicated. Each data point represents an OCR measurement. (**c**) Respiratory parameters derived from (**b**) are basal respiration, proton leak, maximal respiration, spare respiratory capacity, non-mitochondrial respiration, and ATP production (*see* (**a**) for explanation)

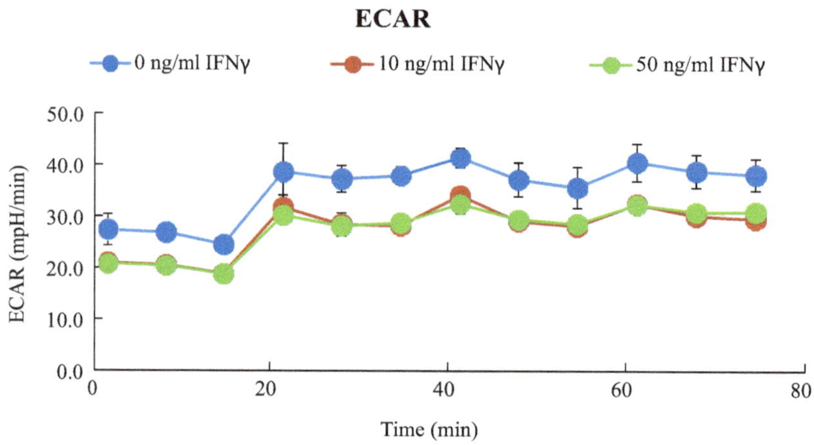

Fig. 3 ECAR of IFNγ-treated SKOV3 cells. ECAR was measured in SKOV3 cells seeded at 20,000 cells/well, incubated for 24 h, and treated with 0 (control), 10, and 50 ng/mL of IFNγ

4. Cartridges are incubated in non-CO_2 incubator because it has no cells. Incubator should be humidified to prevent evaporation.
5. In the last step of washing the cells, add only 160 μL of the assay medium to make the total volume 180 μL in each well. Assay should be performed at 37 °C, therefore turn "ON" XFp Analyzer at least 2 h before assay.
6. Preparation of XF RPMI complete assay medium for SKOV3 cells. All the chemicals like medium and calibrant buffer should be at pH-7.4.
   (a) Aliquot 10 mL XF RPMI medium, pH-7.4.
   (b) Add 100 μL of XF 1.0 M glucose to get final concentration (10 mM).
   (c) Add 100 μL of XF 100 mM sodium pyruvate to get final concentration (1 mM).
   (d) Add 100 μL of XF 200 mM L-glutamine to get final concentration (2 mM).
   (e) Warm the media to 37 °C.
7. The cells must be attached to the wells. Do not remove all media from the wells to prevent cells from drying out.
8. Do not mix or disrupt cell layer.
9. Cell culture miniplate is incubated in non-CO_2 incubator before the assay to remove CO_2 from the plate. It improves the accuracy of the ECAR measurement.
10. Prepare a new assay template in the Wave software. Include experimental details such as cell type, media, and passage of the cells. Assign wells: A and H, background; B and C, 10,000 cells/well; D and E, 20,000 cells/well; F and G, 40,000 cells/well. After assigning of the wells, enter the protocol command. Determination of the basal respiration does not require injection of any chemicals and the protocol command includes only several cycles of OCR and ECAR measurement (each cycle is 3 min) alternating with mixing of the media in the wells that is accomplished by repeated lowering and raising of the probes into the wells (each mixing cycle is also 3 min). The example of protocol command below has 8 cycles of mixing and measuring:

Command	Time (min)
Calibrate	
Equilibrate	
Cycles	8×
Mix	3.00
Wait	0.00
Measure	3.00
End	

11. Remove the cover of cartridge plate before keeping it in the XFp Analyzer. DO NOT shake the cartridge to prevent leakage from the ports.
12. Remove the cover of cell culture miniplate before keeping it in XFp Analyzer.
13. Sterile distilled water is used as a control. Drug treatment preparation was done as follows:
    (a) For 50 ng/mL IFNγ, 80 μL of 0.5 μg/mL was added in 720 μL growth media.
    (b) For 10 ng/mL IFNγ, 16 μL of 0.5 μg/mL was added in 784 μL growth media.
    (c) Control, 10 ng/mL IFNγ and 50 ng/mL IFNγ were performed in duplicates. Well A and H are supplemented with growth media (background).
14. Reconstitute the compounds on the day of assay. Do not refreeze.
15. Review the "XFp Cell Mito Stress Test" template in the Wave software. Fill in all experimental details in the template such as cell type, medium, passage and assign well as a control and experimental well. Protocol commands will remain same as in "XFp Cell Mito Stress Test" template. Export the template from the Wave software to the XFp Analyzer using USB flash drive.
16. The Wave software is required for data analysis. Download the Seahorse Wave software from this link (https://www.agilent.com/en/products/cell-analysis/software-download-for-wave-desktop).

Acknowledgment

This work was supported by NIH grant GM120710 to A. Vancura.

References

1. Ivashkiv LB (2018) IFNγ: signaling, epigenetics and roles in immunity, metabolism, disease and cancer immunotherapy. Nat Rev Immunol 18:545–558
2. Su X, Yu Y, Zhong Y, Giannopoulou EG, Hu X, Liu H, Cross JR, Ratsch G, Rice CM, Ivashkiv LB (2015) Interferon-γ regulates cellular metabolism and mRNA translation to potentiate macrophage activation. Nat Immunol 16:838–849
3. Sciacovelli M, Gaude E, Hilvo M et al (2014) The metabolic alterations of cancer cells. Methods Enzymol 542:1–23
4. Vyas S, Zaganjor E, Haigis MC (2016) Mitochondria and cancer. Cell 166:555–566
5. Vander Heiden MG, Cantley LC, Thompson CB (2009) Understanding the Warburg effect: the metabolic requirements of cell proliferation. Science 324:1029–1033
6. Ferrick DA, Neilson A, Beeson C (2008) Advances in measuring cellular bioenergetics using extracellular flux. Drug Discov Today 13:268–274

Part III

Expression and Regulation of Immune Mediators in Cancer Cells

Chapter 18

Immunoblotting Analysis of Intracellular PD-L1 Levels in Interferon-γ-Treated Ovarian Cancer Cells Stably Transfected with Bcl3 shRNA

Sveta Padmanabhan, Yue Zou, and Ivana Vancurova

Abstract

Expression of the immune checkpoint programmed death ligand 1 (PD-L1, CD274) is increased in many types of cancer, including ovarian cancer (OC), but the mechanisms that regulate the PD-L1 expression are not fully understood. In addition to binding to PD-1 on T cells, thus inhibiting T cell-mediated antitumor responses, PD-L1 has also tumor-intrinsic effects that include increased cancer cell survival and proliferation, and that might be in part mediated by the intracellular PD-L1. In this chapter, we describe a protocol for the analysis of the intracellular PD-L1 protein levels in OC cells by immunoblotting. Our results show that interferon-γ (IFNγ) induces the intracellular levels of PD-L1 and the proto-oncogene Bcl3 in OC cells. However, the PD-L1 expression is significantly decreased in OC cells stably transfected with Bcl3 shRNA, demonstrating that the IFNγ-induced PD-L1 expression in OC cells is mediated by Bcl3. These data identify the IFNγ-Bcl3-PD-L1 axis as a novel therapeutic target in OC, and suggest that targeting Bcl3 may provide a novel strategy to regulate the PD-L1 expression, and especially the tumor-intrinsic PD-L1 effects mediated by the intracellular PD-L1 in OC cells.

Key words Bcl3, Interferon-γ, Immune escape, Intracellular protein levels, Oncoprotein, Ovarian cancer, PD-L1

1 Introduction

Programmed death ligand-1 (PD-L1, CD274) is an immune checkpoint protein expressed on the surface of cancer cells. By binding to PD-1 on T cells, PD-L1 inhibits T cell-mediated antitumor responses, resulting in immune escape [1–3]. However, PD-L1 has also tumor-intrinsic effects, which might be in part mediated by the intracellular PD-L1, and that include increased cancer cell proliferation, survival, and mTOR signaling [4–6].

PD-L1 expression is increased in many types of cancers, including ovarian cancer (OC), and is stimulated by interferon-γ (IFNγ) [7–10]. However, the mechanisms of how IFNγ induces the PD-L1 expression in OC cells are poorly understood. We have

Ivana Vancurova and Yan Zhu (eds.), *Immune Mediators in Cancer: Methods and Protocols*, Methods in Molecular Biology, vol. 2108, https://doi.org/10.1007/978-1-0716-0247-8_18, © Springer Science+Business Media, LLC, part of Springer Nature 2020

recently shown that the IFNγ-induced PD-L1 expression in OC cells is mediated by the proto-oncogene Bcl3, which is overexpressed in OC tissues, and is also induced by IFNγ [11]. In this chapter, we describe a protocol to analyze the intracellular PD-L1 protein levels in IFNγ-stimulated OC cells stably transfected with Bcl3 shRNA, by using immunoblotting. Using this approach, our data show that the intracellular PD-L1 and Bcl3 levels in OC cells are increased by IFNγ; however, the IFNγ-induced PD-L1 expression is significantly decreased in cells stably transfected with Bcl3 shRNA (Fig. 1). Targeting the Bcl3 expression may provide a novel strategy to regulate the PD-L1 expression, and especially the tumor-intrinsic PD-L1 effects mediated by the intracellular PD-L1, in OC cells. The protocol described below includes a preparation of whole cell extracts (WCE) from IFNγ-treated OC cells, followed by SDS electrophoresis, immunoblotting, and densitometric evaluation of the intracellular PD-L1 and Bcl3 levels.

2 Materials

2.1 Cell Culture

1. SKOV3 cells (American Type Culture Collection).
2. RPMI complete medium (CM): RPMI 1640 medium supplemented with 10% fetal bovine serum (FBS), 2 mM glutamine, 1 mM sodium pyruvate, and 1% penicillin-streptomycin solution.
3. 75 cm^2 Culture flasks.
4. 0.25% Trypsin-EDTA.
5. 15 mL Centrifuge tubes.
6. Phosphate-buffered saline, pH 7.4 (PBS).
7. Trypan Blue solution.
8. 1.5 mL Micro centrifuge tubes.
9. Standard 6-well plates with clear flat bottom.
10. Interferon-γ stock solution: Dissolve IFNγ in 1×PBS to a final concentration of 50 μg/mL. Store at −80 °C (*see* **Note 1**).

2.2 Preparation of Whole Cell Extracts

1. 0.25% Trypsin EDTA.
2. RPMI complete medium.
3. 1.5 mL Micro centrifuge tubes.
4. Phosphate-buffered saline, pH 7.4 (PBS).
5. 5× Sample buffer (5×SB): To 3 mL of distilled water, add 1 mL of 0.5 M Tris–HCl, pH 6.8, 1.6 mL of 50% glycerol, 1.6 mL of 10% SDS, 0.4 mL of 1% (w/v) bromophenol blue,

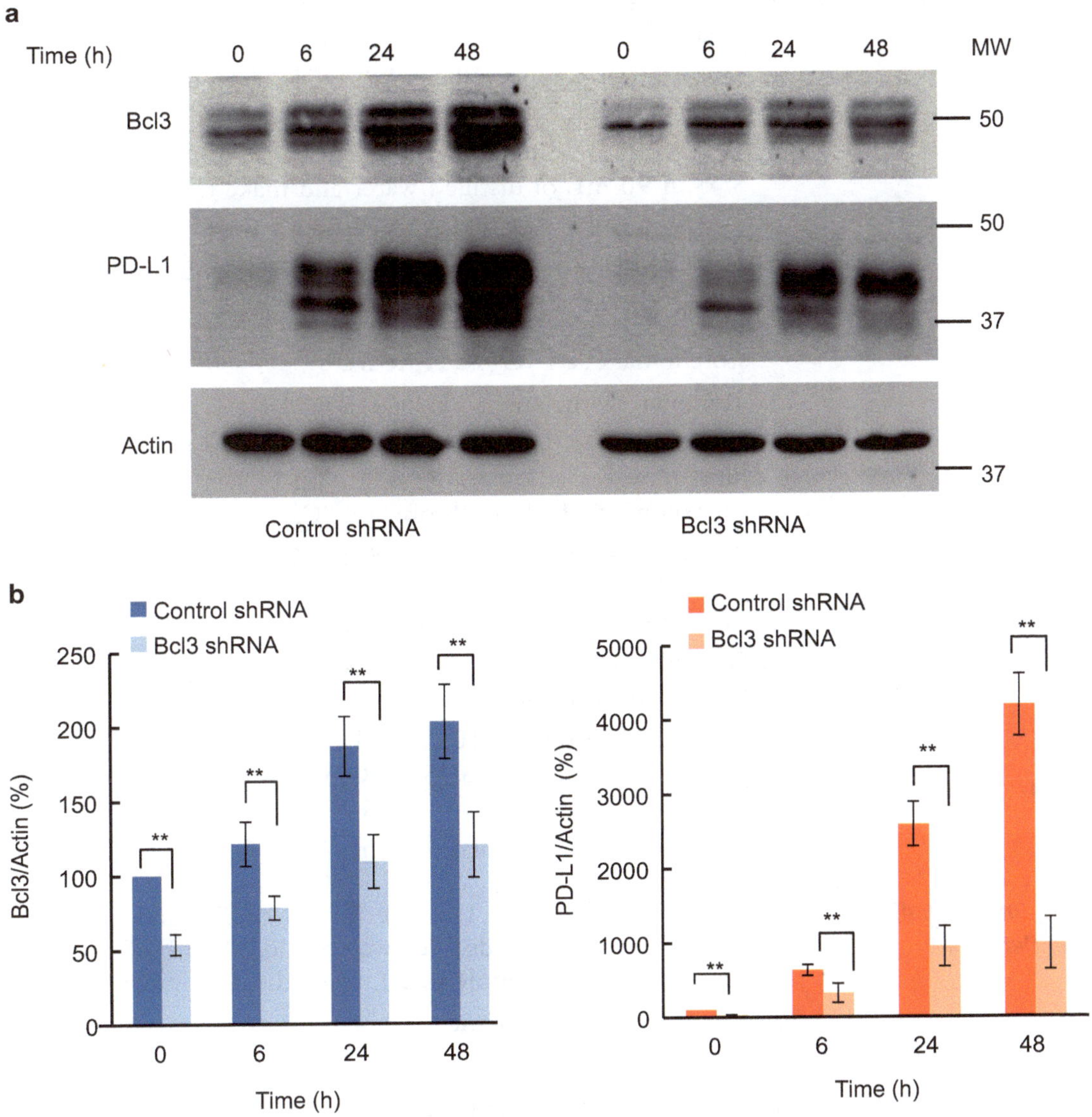

Fig. 1 Immunoblotting analysis of Bcl3 and PD-L1 intracellular levels in IFNγ-stimulated OC cells stably transfected with Bcl3 shRNA. (**a**) Immunoblotting of WCE prepared from IFNγ-treated (50 ng/mL) SKOV3 cells stably transfected with Bcl3 or control shRNA, and analyzed by using Bcl3 and PD-L1 antibodies. To confirm equal protein loading, the membrane was stripped and re-probed with actin antibody. Each lane corresponds to approximately 5×10^4 cells. (**b**) The Bcl3 and PD-L1 bands were scanned and their densities were normalized to the densities of actin used as a loading control. The values for untreated cells were arbitrarily set to 100%, and the other values are presented relative to these values. The data represent the means of three experiments ± SE (Mann-Whitney U test)

and 0.4 mL of 2-mercaptoehanol. Add 2-mercaptoethanol just before use and store at room temperature (*see* **Note 2**).

6. 2× Sample buffer (*see* **Note 3**).

2.3 SDS-PAGE

1. 70% Ethanol: Add 300 mL of distilled water to 700 mL of ethanol.
2. 10% Ammonium persulfate (APS): Dissolve 100 mg of APS in 1 mL of distilled water (*see* **Note 4**).
3. 10% (w/v) Sodium dodecyl sulfate (SDS): Dissolve 10 g of SDS in 90 mL of distilled water and make up the volume to 100 mL. Store at room temperature.
4. 30% Acrylamide/*bis* solution: Dissolve 29.2 g of acrylamide and 0.8 g of *N′N′*-bis-methylene-acrylamide in 50 mL of distilled water, and make up the volume to 100 mL. Filter and store in dark at 4 °C (*see* **Note 5**).
5. Tetramethylethylenediamine (TEMED).
6. 1.5 M Tris–HCl, pH 8.8: Dissolve 18.15 g of Tris in 50 mL of distilled water, adjust to pH 8.8 using 1 M HCl, and make up the volume to 100 mL. Store at 4 °C.
7. 0.5 M Tris–HCl, pH 6.8: Dissolve 6 g of Tris in 50 mL of distilled water, adjust to pH 6.8 using 1 M HCl, and make up the volume to 100 mL. Store at 4 °C.
8. Glass plates, casting frames, and stand, plastic combs, clamping frame and electrode assembly.
9. 10× Running buffer (10×RB): Dissolve 30.3 g of Tris, 144 g of glycine, and 10 g of SDS in 600 mL of distilled water. Make up the volume to 1 L. Store at 4 °C.
10. Kaleidoscope pre-stained markers.

2.4 Immunoblotting and Detection

1. Transfer Buffer (TB): Dissolve 3.03 g of Tris and 14.4 g of glycine in 500 mL of distilled water. Add 200 mL of methanol and make up the volume to 1 L using distilled water.
2. Nitrocellulose membrane.
3. Extra thick filter paper.
4. Semidry transfer apparatus.
5. 10×TBS: Dissolve 81.8 g of NaCl and 3.04 g of $MgCl_2$ in 500 mL of distilled water, and add 100 mL of 1 M Tris–HCl, pH 7.5. Make up the volume to 1 L using distilled water and store at 4 °C.
6. TBST: Add 2.5 mL of 20% Tween-20 to 100 mL of 10×TBS, and adjust the volume to 1 L with distilled water. Store at 4 °C.
7. TBSTM blocking solution: Dissolve 5 g of nonfat dry milk in 100 mL of TBST and store at 4 °C. Filter. Prepare fresh each day.
8. Small containers for incubating the membranes with antibodies.
9. Bcl3, PD-L1, and actin antibodies.

10. Horseradish peroxidase (HRP)-labeled secondary IgG antibodies.
11. ECL western blotting detection reagents and chemiluminescence imaging system.
12. Stripping buffer: Dissolve 7.5 g of glycine, 0.5 g of SDS, and 5 mL of Tween-20 in 400 mL of distilled water, adjust the pH to 2.2 with 1 M HCl, and make up the volume to 500 mL. Prepare fresh just before use.

3 Methods

In this section, we describe the protocol for analysis of intracellular Bcl3 and PD-L1 protein levels in IFNγ-treated OC cells. The main steps of the protocol are: (1) SKOV3 cell culture and incubation with IFNγ; (2) preparation of whole cell extracts (WCE); (3) SDS-PAGE, and (4) immunoblotting, detection, and analysis (Fig. 1). This protocol can be easily modified and used for analysis of different intracellular proteins in different cell types. On average, it can be accomplished within 3–4 days.

3.1 Cell Culture

1. Grow SKOV3 cells in CM medium until they reach about 80% confluency (*see* **Note 6**).
2. Discard the media, and wash the cells with 7 mL of PBS. Detach the cells by adding 4 mL of pre-warmed (37 °C) 0.25% trypsin-EDTA, followed by 15-min incubation at 37 °C in a 5% CO_2 humidified atmosphere (*see* **Note 7**).
3. Neutralize the trypsin by adding 8 mL of CM, transfer the cell suspension to a 15 mL centrifuge tube, and centrifuge at 130 × *g* for 5 min at room temperature.
4. Discard the supernatants and resuspend the cell pellets in 5 mL of CM.
5. To count the cells, transfer 50 μL of the above cell suspension into a 1.5 mL micro-centrifuge tube, and add 50 μL of 1×PBS and 100 μL of Trypan Blue solution. Mix well by pipetting (*see* **Note 8**).
6. Add 10 μL of the Trypan Blue-cell suspension obtained from **step 5** to each chamber of the hemocytometer.
7. Count the number of viable cells, and calculate the cell concentration using the following formula: Cell concentration = average cell count in four squares × 4 × 10^4 cells/mL.
8. Dilute the cells suspension obtained from **step 4** to a final concentration of 0.5 × 10^6 cells/mL using CM.
9. Mix well, and plate 2 mL of the above cell suspension into each well of a 6-well plate, so that each well has 1 × 10^6 cells.

10. Incubate the plate 24 h at 37 °C in a 5% CO_2 humidified atmosphere tissue culture incubator, to allow cell attachment.
11. After 24 h, discard the medium, and add 2 mL of new CM containing IFNγ of the required concentration into each well.
12. Incubate cells for 24 h at 37 °C in 5% CO_2 humidified atmosphere.

3.2 Preparation of Whole Cell Extracts

All the following steps are performed on ice or at 4 °C, unless otherwise stated.

1. Following cell incubation, collect 2 mL of unattached cell suspension from each well, and transfer it into two labeled 1.5 mL micro-centrifuge tubes; each tube will get 1 mL of the cell suspension. Centrifuge at 1700 × *g* for 5 min (*see* **Note 9**).
2. Detach the adherent cells still in the wells by adding 800 μL of 0.25% trypsin-EDTA, followed by 10 min incubation at 37 °C in 5% CO_2 humidified atmosphere.
3. After 10 min, neutralize trypsin by adding 700 μL of CM into each well.
4. Carefully discard supernatants from the centrifuged 1.5 mL micro-centrifuge tubes (from **step 1**), and resuspend the cell pellets in 1.5 mL of the trypsinized cell solution from **step 3**. Centrifuge at 1700 × *g* for 5 min.
5. Discard supernatants, and wash the cells using 1 mL of ice-cold 1×PBS. Centrifuge at 1700 × *g* for 5 min.
6. Carefully discard supernatants, resuspend the pellets in 200 μL of 2×SB, and boil the samples immediately for 7 min in a boiling water bath (*see* **Note 10**).
7. After boiling, centrifuge tubes at 1700 × *g* for 5 min at room temperature.
8. Transfer supernatants into new 1.5 mL tubes, and store at −80 °C.

3.3 SDS-PAGE

1. Clean electrophoresis glass plates and combs using 70% ethanol.
2. Place the plates in the casting frame and fasten it to the casting stand (*see* **Note 11**).
3. To prepare two 12% resolving gels, mix in a beaker: 3.4 mL of distilled water, 4 mL of 30% acrylamide/*bis*, 2.5 mL of 1.5 M Tris–HCl, pH 8.8, and 0.1 mL of 10% SDS.
4. Swirl the ingredients, and just before casting the gels, add 5 μL of TEMED and 50 μL of 10% APS to induce polymerization. Mix well again.

5. Immediately after adding TEMED and APS, pour the gels using a micropipette. Carefully overlay the gels with distilled water to even the gel tops and remove air bubbles.
6. Allow the resolving gels to polymerize for 45 min.
7. Once the gels are polymerized, remove water on the top by inverting the casting stand and using Kim wipes.
8. Prepare stacking gels (4%) by mixing 6.1 mL of distilled water, 1.3 mL of 30% acrylamide/*bis*, 2.5 mL of 0.5 M Tris–HCl, pH 6.8, and 0.1 mL of 10% SDS.
9. Swirl the ingredients, and add 10 μL of TEMED and 50 μL of 10% APS.
10. Add combs to gels in the casting frame, and fill the remaining spaces by adding the stacking gel solution using a micropipette (*see* **Note 12**).
11. Allow stacking gels to polymerize for 1 h.
12. Meanwhile, thaw the frozen protein samples by boiling them for 7 min.
13. Place the plates in the running module and assemble them in the gel tank.
14. Fill the inner chamber with 1×RB, and gently remove the combs.
15. Clean the wells with 1×RB using a syringe.
16. Using gel loading tips, load the samples, as well as pre-stained markers, into the wells (*see* **Note 13**).
17. Fill the tank with 1×RB.
18. Run gels at 120 V until the blue dye reaches the bottom of the gel (*see* **Note 14**).

3.4 Immunoblotting and Detection

1. Dissemble plates, discard the stacking gels, and soak the resolving gels each in 400 mL of TB for 10 min.
2. Soak two filter papers and one nitrocellulose membrane per gel in TB for 10 min.
3. Clean the anode platform of semidry transfer apparatus with 70% ethanol and assemble the sandwich in the order from bottom to top (*see* **Note 15**):
   - (a) Filter paper (top).
   - (b) Gel.
   - (c) Nitrocellulose membrane.
   - (d) Filter paper (bottom).
4. Place lid on top, and run the transfer according to the parameters below:
   - (a) One 12% gel: 18 V, 3 A, 35 min.
   - (b) Two 12% gels: 20 V, 3 A, 50 min.

5. After transfer, disassemble the sandwich, and cut the nitrocellulose membrane with transferred proteins to the size of the blocking container, to minimize the amount of needed antibody (*see* **Note 16**).
6. Transfer membranes to containers for incubation with antibodies, and add blocking solution (TBSTM) to each container (*see* **Notes 17** and **18**).
7. Incubate membranes in the blocking solution TBSTM for 2 h at room temperature, with gentle rocking (*see* **Note 19**).
8. After 2 h, remove the blocking solution, and add primary antibody diluted in TBSTM solution. Each primary antibody requires different dilution; follow the protocol recommended by the manufacturer.
9. Incubate membranes with primary antibodies for 2 h at room temperature, followed by overnight incubation at 4 °C, with gentle rocking.
10. After incubation with primary antibody, remove the antibody solution, and wash the membranes six times in 50 mL of TBST, 5 min each wash.
11. Transfer membranes into new blocking containers, and add secondary HRP-labeled antibody diluted 1:2000 in TBSTM (*see* **Note 20**).
12. Incubate on a rocking platform for 1 h at room temperature.
13. Remove the secondary antibody solution, and wash the membranes six times with TBST buffer, 5 min each wash.
14. Mix required amounts of ECL solution A and solution B in a 15 mL centrifuge tube as shown below (*see* **Note 21**):
    (a) 1 membrane: 2 mL of solution A and 50 μL of solution B.
    (b) 2 membranes: 3 mL of solution A and 75 μL of solution B.
15. Carefully blot the membranes to remove any remaining TBST, place them on parafilm, and add enough ECL solution A + B to cover the surface of the membranes. Incubate at room temperature for 5 min.
16. Cover the membranes with plastic wrap and visualize proteins using chemiluminescence imaging system.
17. To probe the membranes with other antibodies, incubate them twice in 50 mL of stripping buffer (10 min each wash), followed by two 5 min washes in TBST.
18. Block the membranes for 2 h in 5% TBSTM at room temperature with gentle rocking.
19. Incubate the membranes with primary and secondary antibodies as described above.

4 Notes

1. Aliquot IFNγ in sterile microcentrifuge tubes and store at −80 °C to avoid repeated freezing-thawing cycles that might decrease IFNγ biological activity.
2. 5×SB (without 2-mercaptoethanol) can be prepared and stored at room temperature in dark. Before each experiment, use the required amount of 5×SB, and add 2-mercaptoethanol.
3. Prepare required volumes of 2×SB by diluting 5×SB with distilled water just before use.
4. Always prepare fresh APS. Old APS results in incomplete catalysis and long polymerization time.
5. Unpolymerized acrylamide is toxic and can be easily absorbed by skin. Proper gloves should be worn while handling the gels.
6. It is optimum to grow the cells until they reach about 80% confluence.
7. Do not "over-thaw" the trypsin-EDTA solution; remove it from water bath right after it melts. Increasing temperature of trypsin decreases its activity.
8. Make sure to mix the cells evenly by pipetting up and down. Uneven mixing results in incorrect cell counts.
9. It is advisable to centrifuge all tubes in one position—hinges either up or down, so that the pellets can be easily seen.
10. Boiling the protein samples in 2×SB sample buffer denatures proteins, so the samples can be stored for longer periods. It is better to aliquot the samples in smaller volumes, so that they are not repeatedly thawed.
11. Make sure that the plates are leak-proof by aligning them correctly. Otherwise, the gel solution might leak.
12. Avoid air bubbles, which could result in improper well formation.
13. Load markers in different positions in the two gels, so that they can be used to differentiate the gels.
14. Keep checking the gel run. Fall in the level of the running buffer halts the run.
15. Avoid air bubbles, especially between the gel and the membrane. Bubbles result in improper transfer of proteins.
16. To avoid cutting out an important piece of membrane with transferred proteins, cut along the outer borders of the markers and the blue dye on the bottom of the gel.
17. For blocking, use either TBSTM, or 5% BSA in TBST, which works better for most phospho-proteins.

18. The membrane has to be completely covered with the blocking solution. Typically, 6 mL of blocking solution will be sufficient for one membrane in a small container.
19. Western blotting can be interrupted at this point, by blocking overnight at 4 °C.
20. Always use the secondary antibody raised against animal species in which the primary antibody was raised.
21. Since ECL solutions are light sensitive, keep the solution mixture in dark.

Acknowledgment

This work was supported by National Institutes of Health Grant CA202775 (to I.V.).

References

1. Freeman GJ, Long AJ, Iwai Y et al (2000) Engagement of the PD-1 immunoinhibitory receptor by a novel B7 family member leads to negative regulation of lymphocyte activation. J Exp Med 192:1027–1034
2. Iwai Y, Ishida M, Tanaka Y et al (2002) Involvement of PD-L1 on tumor cells in the escape from host immune system and tumor immunotherapy by PD-L1 blockade. Proc Natl Acad Sci U S A 99:12293–12297
3. Loke P, Allison JP (2003) PD-L1 and PD-L2 are differentially regulated by Th1 and Th2 cells. Proc Natl Acad Sci U S A 100:5336–5341
4. Azuma T, Yao S, Zhu G et al (2008) B7-H1 is a ubiquitous antiapoptotic receptor on cancer cells. Blood 111:3635–3643
5. Chang CH, Qiu J, O'Sullivan D et al (2015) Metabolic competition in the tumor microenvironment is a driver of cancer progression. Cell 162:1229–1241
6. Clark CA, Gupta HB, Sareddy G et al (2016) Tumor-intrinsic PD-L1 signals regulate cell growth, pathogenesis, and autophagy in ovarian cancer and melanoma. Cancer Res 76:6964–6974
7. Sanmamed MF, Chen L (2018) A paradigm shift in cancer immunotherapy: from enhancement to normalization. Cell 175:313–326
8. Ribas A, Wolchok JD (2018) Cancer immunotherapy using checkpoint blockade. Science 359:1350–1355
9. Lin H, Wei S, Hurt EM et al (2018) Host expression of PD-L1 determines efficacy of PD-L1 pathway blockade-mediated tumor regression. J Clin Invest 128:805–815
10. Abiko K, Matsumura N, Hamanishi J et al (2015) IFN-gamma from lymphocytes induces PD-L1 expression and promotes progression of ovarian cancer. Br J Cancer 112:1501–1509
11. Zou Y, Uddin MM, Padmanabhan S et al (2018) The proto-oncogene Bcl3 induces immune checkpoint PD-L1 expression, mediating proliferation of ovarian cancer cells. J Biol Chem 293:15483–15496

Chapter 19

Flow Cytometry Analysis of Surface PD-L1 Expression Induced by IFNγ and Romidepsin in Ovarian Cancer Cells

Sveta Padmanabhan, Yue Zou, and Ivana Vancurova

Abstract

Expression of programmed death ligand-1 (PD-L1, CD274) on cancer cells is regulated by interferon-γ (IFNγ) signaling as well as by epigenetic mechanisms. By binding to PD-1 on cytotoxic T cells, PD-L1 inhibits T cell-mediated antitumor responses, resulting in immune escape. This chapter describes analysis of the surface PD-L1 expression in ovarian cancer (OC) cells using flow cytometry (FC). Our data demonstrate that the surface PD-L1 expression in OC cells is induced by IFNγ as well as by the class I histone deacetylase (HDAC) inhibition by romidepsin, suggesting that class I HDAC inhibition might provide a useful strategy to modulate the PD-L1 levels on OC cells.

Key words HDAC, HDAC inhibition, Interferon-γ, Immune escape, Flow cytometry, Ovarian cancer, PD-L1, Romidepsin

1 Introduction

Programmed death ligand-1 (PD-L1, B7-H1, or CD274) is a glycoprotein expressed on the surface of antigen-presenting cells, as well as different types of cancer cells. The tumor-expressed PD-L1 binds to PD-1 on cytotoxic T cells, resulting in the inhibition of T cell-mediated antitumor responses and immune escape [1–3]. In addition, the tumor-expressed PD-L1 has tumor intrinsic effects that include increased cancer cell proliferation, survival, and mTOR signaling [4–7]. While the inhibition of T cell-mediated antitumor responses is mediated by the surface PD-L1, the intrinsic functions of PD-L1 might be partly mediated by the intracellular PD-L1.

The PD-L1 expression in cancer cells is induced by interferon-γ (IFNγ) through the JAK-STAT-IRF signaling [8, 9]. In addition, recent studies have shown that the PD-L1 expression is regulated by epigenetic mechanisms, and that inhibition of histone deacetylases (HDAC) increases PD-L1 expression in cancer cells, suggesting that HDAC inhibition might increase effectiveness of immune

Ivana Vancurova and Yan Zhu (eds.), *Immune Mediators in Cancer: Methods and Protocols*, Methods in Molecular Biology, vol. 2108, https://doi.org/10.1007/978-1-0716-0247-8_19,

checkpoint inhibitors in cancer treatment [10–17]. This is particularly important in solid tumors, such as ovarian cancer (OC), where HDAC inhibitors and immune checkpoint inhibitors, as single agents, have produced disappointing results.

Ovarian cancer is the leading cause of death from gynecologic cancer in the United States, with a high morbidity and low survival rates [18–20]. Recent studies have shown that IFNγ induces PD-L1 expression in OC cells, resulting in their increased proliferation and tumor growth [21–23]. Here, we analyzed whether the surface PD-L1 expression is induced also by the FDA-approved class I HDAC inhibitor romidepsin. Using flow cytometry (FC) analysis of the surface PD-L1 expression in SKOV3 cells, our data show that romidepsin increases the PD-L1 surface expression in OC cells by about 100%. These results suggest that HDAC inhibition might provide a useful strategy to modulate the PD-L1 levels on OC cells. The protocol below describes an FC analysis of the surface PD-L1 expression in IFNγ- and romidepsin-treated OC cells. However, it can also be modified for the analysis of PD-L1 in other types of cancer cells.

2 Materials

2.1 Cell Culture

1. SKOV3 cells (American Type Culture Collection).
2. RPMI complete medium: RPMI 1640 medium supplemented with 10% fetal bovine serum (FBS), 1% penicillin-streptomycin, 2 mM L-glutamine, 10 mM HEPES, and 1 mM sodium pyruvate.
3. Phosphate-buffered saline (PBS), pH 7.4.
4. Interferon gamma (IFNγ) stock solution: Dissolve IFNγ in sterile PBS to a final concentration of 50 μg/mL. Aliquot, and store at −80 °C (*see* **Note 1**).
5. Romidepsin stock solution: Dissolve romidepsin in sterile DMSO to a final concentration of 10 μM. Aliquot, and store at −80 °C (*see* **Note 1**).
6. 0.25% Trypsin-EDTA solution.
7. T-75 flasks.
8. T-25 flasks.
9. Trypan Blue solution.
10. Hemocytometer.
11. 1.5 mL Microcentrifuge tubes.
12. 15 mL Centrifuge tubes.

2.2 Cell Preparation for Flow Cytometry

1. HBSS (Hank's Balanced Salt Solution), without calcium, magnesium, or phenol red.
2. Accutase™ cell detachment solution.
3. RPMI complete medium: RPMI 1640 medium supplemented with 10% FBS, 1% penicillin-streptomycin, 2 mM L-glutamine, 10 mM HEPES, and 1 mM sodium pyruvate.
4. Incubation buffer: Dissolve 0.5% bovine serum albumin (BSA) in 100 mL of HBSS and filter. Prepare fresh and store at 4 °C.
5. Human-specific rabbit monoclonal PD-L1 IgG antibody for FC (*see* **Note 2**).
6. Control IgG.
7. Anti-rabbit IgG Alexa 488 conjugate secondary antibody for FC.
8. 1.5 mL Microcentrifuge tubes.
9. 15 mL Centrifuge tubes.
10. Slides and coverslips.

3 Methods

The protocol below describes FC analysis of PD-L1 expressed on the surface of OC cells, using antibody that specifically recognizes the extracellular domain of PD-L1. Using this approach, our data show that IFNγ induces the surface PD-L1 expression in SKOV3 cells approximately 28-fold (Fig. 1), and HDAC class 1 inhibition by romidepsin approximately two-fold (Fig. 2). The protocol can be easily modified and used for analysis of surface PD-L1 in other cells.

3.1 Cell Culture

1. Grow SKOV3 cells in a T-75 flask containing RPMI complete medium until they reach about 80% confluence.
2. Discard the medium and wash cells with 7 mL of PBS. Add 4 mL of pre-warmed 0.25% trypsin-EDTA solution to the flask, and incubate at 37 °C till the cells detach (*see* **Note 3**).
3. Add an equal volume of RPMI medium to neutralize the trypsin.
4. Collect cells in a 15 mL centrifuge tube and centrifuge at 300 × *g* at 4 °C for 5 min. Discard supernatant, and resuspend cells in 5 mL of RPMI medium (*see* **Note 4**).
5. For cell counting, transfer 50 μL of the above cell suspension into a 1.5 mL centrifuge tube, add 50 μL of PBS, and 100 μL of trypan blue solution. Mix thoroughly by pipetting.
6. Add 10 μL of the above cell mixture into each chamber of the hemocytometer.

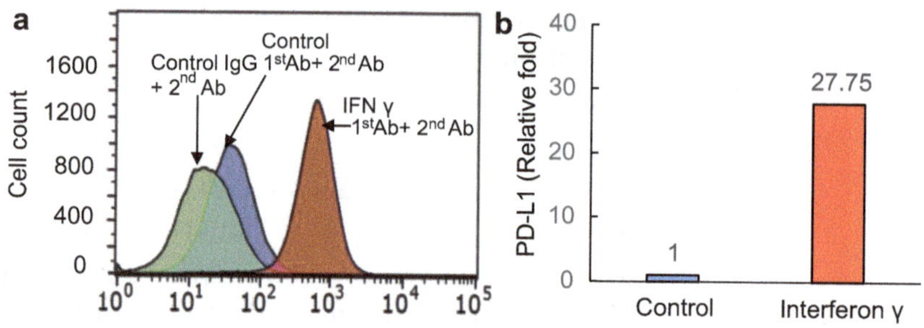

Fig. 1 Flow cytometry analysis of surface PD-L1 expression in IFNγ-treated OC cells. (**a**) Histogram of PD-L1 surface expression in IFNγ-treated SKOV3 cells, illustrating the fluorescence intensity (horizontal axis) against the number of events detected (vertical axis). Cells incubated with isotype-matched control IgG are plotted in green; untreated cells are plotted in blue, and IFNγ (50 ng/mL, 48 h)-treated cells are plotted in red. (**b**) Relative fold surface expression of PD-L1 in untreated cells vs. IFNγ-treated cells

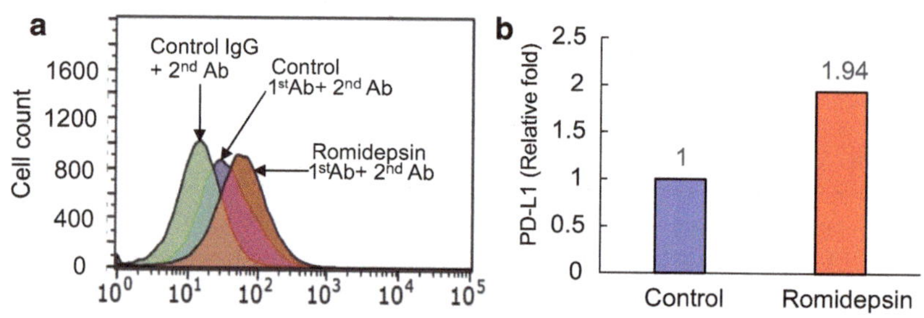

Fig. 2 Flow cytometry analysis of surface PD-L1 expression in romidepsin-treated OC cells. (**a**) Histogram of PD-L1 surface expression in romidepsin-treated SKOV3 cells, illustrating the fluorescence intensity (horizontal axis) against the number of events detected (vertical axis). Cells incubated with isotype-matched control IgG are plotted in green; untreated cells are plotted in blue, and romidepsin (10 nM, 48 h)-treated cells are plotted in red. (**b**) Relative fold surface expression of PD-L1 in untreated cells vs. romidepsin-treated cells

7. Count the number of viable cells and calculate the total cell concentration using the formula: Cell concentration = average cell count in four squares × 4 × 10^4 cells/mL.
8. Dilute the cell suspension from **step 4** to a final concentration of 0.5 × 10^6 cells/mL using fresh RPMI medium.
9. Add 800 μL of the cell suspension to a T-25 flask containing 5 mL of RPMI complete medium, so that each flask contains about 4 × 10^5 cells (*see* **Note 5**).
10. Allow cells to attach to the flask for 24 h, aspirate the medium, and add 5 mL of fresh RPMI complete medium to each flask.
11. Set up the experimental protocol for cell-surface PD-L1 detection in IFNγ- and romidepsin-treated cells as follows:
    (a) No Antibody.
    (b) Control IgG and secondary antibody.

(c) PD-L1 primary antibody and secondary antibody in untreated cells.

(d) PD-L1 primary antibody and secondary antibody in IFN-γ-treated cells.

(e) PD-L1 primary antibody and secondary antibody in romidepsin-treated cells.

12. Incubate cells for 48 h with IFNγ (final concentration 50 ng/mL), romidepsin (10 nM), or with an equal volume of sterile vehicle solution at 37 °C in a 5% humidified CO_2 incubator (*see* **Note 6**).

3.2 Cell Preparation for Flow Cytometry

1. Discard tissue culture medium and wash cells with sterile, room-temperature HBSS. Remove liquid by aspiration (*see* **Note 7**).
2. Add 3 mL of pre-warmed Accutase™ Cell Detachment Solution into each T-25 flask to cover the cells (*see* **Note 8**).
3. Incubate at 37 °C for 5 min, monitor cells under microscope every 2–3 min until more than 80% cells are detached (*see* **Note 9**).
4. Add 4 mL of RPMI complete medium to neutralize Accutase, and pipette gently up and down multiple times to disperse any cell clumps (*see* **Note 10**).
5. Transfer the entire content to a new pre-labeled 15 mL centrifuge tube.
6. Confirm the presence of single cells by removing 10 μL of the above cell suspension, placing it on a slide, and observing under microscope (*see* **Note 11**).
7. Centrifuge the cell suspension from **step 5** at 300 × *g* for 5 min. Discard supernatant and collect the cell pellets. Gently resuspend the cell pellets in 8 mL of HBSS, and centrifuge again at 300 × *g* for 5 min. Discard the supernatant.
8. Wash the cell pellets in 5 mL of Incubation buffer. Resuspend the washed cell pellet in 1 mL of Incubation buffer, and transfer the cell suspension to a pre-labeled dark-colored Eppendorf tube (*see* **Note 12**).
9. Centrifuge again at 300 × *g* for 5 min, collect the cell pellet, and add primary PD-L1 antibody diluted in the Incubation buffer; incubate on ice for 60 min (*see* **Note 13**).
10. Centrifuge at 300 × *g* for 5 min, remove the supernatant, and collect the cell pellet. Wash the cell pellet twice in 1.5 mL of Incubation buffer. During each wash, gently resuspend the cell pellet, mix by inverting, and incubate on ice for 10 min. Centrifuge each time at 300 × *g* for 5 min (*see* **Note 14**).

11. Resuspend the cell pellets in 100 μL of Incubation buffer containing secondary antibody, and incubate on ice for 60 min (*see* **Note 15**).
12. Wash the cell pellets twice with 1.5 mL of Incubation buffer as in **step 10**. Centrifuge each time at 300 × *g* for 5 min.
13. Resuspend cells in Incubation buffer to a concentration of 7×10^5 to 1×10^6 cells/mL, and analyze samples by flow cytometry (*see* **Note 16**).

3.3 Data Analysis

1. Acquire at least 40,000 events during sample acquisition. Here, guavaSoft 3.3 (Millipore) was used for data analysis (*see* **Note 17**).
2. PD-L1 expression can be quantified by measuring the increase in fluorescence intensity in treated samples compared with untreated cells (Figs. 1 and 2).

4 Notes

1. Aliquot IFNγ and romidepsin stock solutions in sterile microcentrifuge tubes and store at −80 °C to avoid repeated freeze thaw cycles that may decrease the biological activity.
2. For FC analysis of surface antigens, it is important to use antibody that recognizes the extracellular domain of the particular protein. Here, we used the Cell Signaling rabbit monoclonal antibody #86744 that recognizes the extracellular domain of PD-L1.
3. Thaw aliquots of 0.25% trypsin-EDTA solution by placing them in the incubator at 37 °C in a 5% CO_2 humidified atmosphere. If trypsin is not pre-warmed at 37 °C, cells may not detach completely.
4. Resuspend cells by pipetting up and down, and by gently inverting the tube; avoid vortexing.
5. Cells must be plated so that each flask yields about 1 million cells after 48 h incubation. Plate one T-25 flask per condition. The cells must not be over-confluent since the surface PD-L1 expression might be reduced due to contact inhibition.
6. After adding IFN or romidepsin, gently rotate the plate in a circular motion to assure an equal distribution of the drug in the medium.
7. Wash with HBSS thoroughly 5–6 times to remove dead cells, and any leftover medium and serum.
8. Thaw aliquots of Accutase by placing them in the 37 °C incubator in a 5% CO_2 humidified atmosphere.

9. If most cells are still attached after 5-min incubation, remove the original Accutase solution, add a fresh Accutase solution, and continue the incubation with periodical microscopic observation. The detachment times may vary for different cell types.
10. Pipette gently 6–7 times to disperse any cell clumps.
11. Approximately 80–90% of the cells must be single, and not clumped. The flow cytometry instrument will detect PD-L1 expressed only on single cells. Clumped cells will produce inaccurate results.
12. Use dark-colored Eppendorf tubes so that after addition of secondary antibody, the loss of fluorescence is minimized.
13. Pre-dilute the primary antibody with Incubation buffer to avoid a pipetting error. After addition of primary antibody, resuspend the cells gently to ensure that all the cells are exposed to the antibody and there are no clumps. Here we used PD-L1 antibody obtained from Cell Signaling # 86744 (1:100 dilution).
14. Incubation on ice between the washes ensures that the cells are thoroughly washed.
15. Minimize exposure of the secondary antibody to light. Pre-dilute the secondary antibody with Incubation buffer to avoid a pipetting error. Pipette gently and ensure that all cells are exposed to secondary antibody. The tubes must be kept on ice and in dark. Exposure to light would lead to loss of fluorescence. Here we used anti-rabbit IgG Alexa 488 conjugate obtained from Cell Signaling (# 4412) in a 1:750 dilution.
16. The cells must have a minimum concentration of 5×10^5 cells/mL, and a volume of 500 μL for appropriate detection. Analyze immediately after incubation. Vortex samples for 30 s just before FC detection to disperse any cell clumps.
17. Before acquiring the data, ensure that the capillary in the flow cytometer is clean and ready for sample analysis; follow the manufacturer's instructions. If analyzing more than one sample, run a quick clean between the samples so that any debris deposited in the capillary do not interfere with the sample analysis.

Acknowledgment

This work was supported by National Institutes of Health Grant CA202775 (to I.V.).

References

1. Freeman GJ, Long AJ, Iwai Y et al (2000) Engagement of the PD-1 immuno-inhibitory receptor by a novel B7 family member leads to negative regulation of lymphocyte activation. J Exp Med 192:1027–1034
2. Iwai Y, Ishida M, Tanaka Y et al (2002) Involvement of PD-L1 on tumor cells in the escape from host immune system and tumor immunotherapy by PD-L1 blockade. Proc Natl Acad Sci U S A 99:12293–12297
3. Loke P, Allison JP (2003) PD-L1 and PD-L2 are differentially regulated by Th1 and Th2 cells. Proc Natl Acad Sci U S A 100:5336–5341
4. Azuma T, Yao S, Zhu G et al (2008) B7-H1 is a ubiquitous antiapoptotic receptor on cancer cells. Blood 111:3635–3643
5. Chang CH, Qiu J, O'Sullivan D et al (2015) Metabolic competition in the tumor microenvironment is a driver of cancer progression. Cell 162:1229–1241
6. Clark CA, Gupta HB, Sareddy G et al (2016) Tumor-intrinsic PD-L1 signals regulate cell growth, pathogenesis, and autophagy in ovarian cancer and melanoma. Cancer Res 76:6964–6974
7. Clark CA, Gupta HB, Curiel TJ (2017) Tumor cell-intrinsic CD274/PD-L1: a novel metabolic balancing act with clinical potential. Autophagy 13:987–988
8. Garcia-Diaz A, Shin DS, Moreno BH et al (2017) Interferon receptor signaling pathways regulating PD-L1 and PD-L2 expression. Cell Rep 19:1189–1201
9. Ivashkiv LB (2018) IFNγ: signalling, epigenetics and roles in immunity, metabolism, disease and cancer immunotherapy. Nat Rev Immunol 18:545–558
10. Woods DM, Sodré AL, Villagra A et al (2015) HDAC inhibition upregulates PD-1 ligands in melanoma and augments immunotherapy with PD-1 blockade. Cancer Immunol Res 3:1375–1385
11. Cacan E (2017) Epigenetic-mediated immune suppression of positive co-stimulatory molecules in chemoresistant ovarian cancer cells. Cell Biol Int 41:328–339
12. Briere D, Sudhakar N, Woods DM et al (2018) The class I/IV HDAC inhibitor mocetinostat increases tumor antigen presentation, decreases immune suppressive cell types and augments checkpoint inhibitor therapy. Cancer Immunol Immunother 67:381–392
13. Iwasa M, Harada T, Oda A et al (2019) PD-L1 upregulation in myeloma cells by panobinostat in combination with interferon-γ. Oncotarget 10:1903–1917
14. Llopiz D, Ruiz M, Villanueva L et al (2019) Enhanced anti-tumor efficacy of checkpoint inhibitors in combination with the histone deacetylase inhibitor Belinostat in a murine hepatocellular carcinoma model. Cancer Immunol Immunother 68:379–393
15. Terranova-Barberio M, Thomas S, Ali N et al (2017) HDAC inhibition potentiates immunotherapy in triple negative breast cancer. Oncotarget 8:114156–114172
16. Bae J, Hideshima T, Tai YT et al (2018) Histone deacetylase (HDAC) inhibitor ACY241 enhances anti-tumor activities of antigen-specific central memory cytotoxic T lymphocytes against multiple myeloma and solid tumors. Leukemia 32:1932–1947
17. Knox T, Sahakian E, Banik D et al (2019) Selective HDAC6 inhibitors improve anti-PD-1 immune checkpoint blockade therapy by decreasing the anti-inflammatory phenotype of macrophages and down-regulation of immunosuppressive proteins in tumor cells. Sci Rep 9(1):6136
18. Armbruster S, Coleman RL, Rauh-Hain JA (2018) Management and treatment of recurrent epithelial ovarian cancer. Hematol Oncol Clin North Am 32:965–982
19. Chodon T, Lugade AA, Battaglia S, Odunsi K (2018) Emerging role and future directions of immunotherapy in advanced ovarian cancer. Hematol Oncol Clin North Am 32:1025–1039
20. Vaughan S, Coward JI, Bast RC Jr et al (2011) Rethinking ovarian cancer: recommendations for improving outcomes. Nat Rev Cancer 11:719–725
21. Abiko K, Matsumura N, Hamanishi J et al (2015) IFN-γ from lymphocytes induces PD-L1 expression and promotes progression of ovarian cancer. Br J Cancer 112:1501–1509
22. Mandai M, Hamanishi J, Abiko K et al (2016) Dual faces of IFNγ in cancer progression: a role of PD-L1 induction in the determination of pro- and antitumor immunity. Clin Cancer Res 22:2329–2334
23. Zou Y, Uddin MM, Padmanabhan S et al (2018) The proto-oncogene Bcl3 induces immune checkpoint PD-L1 expression, mediating proliferation of ovarian cancer cells. J Biol Chem 293:15483–15496

Chapter 20

Analysis of PD-L1 Transcriptional Regulation in Ovarian Cancer Cells by Chromatin Immunoprecipitation

Yue Zou, Sveta Padmanabhan, and Ivana Vancurova

Abstract

The immune checkpoint molecule, programmed death ligand 1 (PD-L1; B7-H1, CD274), induces T cell apoptosis and tolerance, thus inhibiting the antitumor immunity. PD-L1 expression is increased in many types of cancer, including ovarian cancer (OC), and correlates with poor prognosis. However, the mechanisms that regulate the PD-L1 expression in cancer cells are incompletely understood. The transcriptional regulation of *PD-L1* expression is orchestrated by several transcription factors, including NFκB. The human *PD-L1* promoter contains five NFκB-binding sites. Interferon-γ (IFNγ) stimulation of OC cells induces p65, and particularly K314/315 acetylated p65 recruitment to all five NFκB-binding sites in *PD-L1* promoter, resulting in increased *PD-L1* expression. In this chapter, we describe a protocol that uses chromatin immunoprecipitation (ChIP) to analyze the transcriptional regulation of *PD-L1* by measuring recruitment of NFκB p65 and K314/315 acetylated p65 to *PD-L1* promoter in human OC cells.

Key words Chromatin immunoprecipitation, Interferon-γ, NFκB, Ovarian cancer, p65, PD-L1, Promoter recruitment, Transcriptional regulation

1 Introduction

Programmed death ligand 1 (PD-L1; B7-H1, CD274) is expressed by hematopoietic cells, but also by many cancer cells. PD-L1 interacts with PD-1 that is expressed on T cells, resulting in the suppression of T cell activity. In the context of hematopoietic cells, binding of PD-L1 to PD-1 prevents autoimmunity by suppressing autoreactive T cells. However, in tumor microenvironment, the PD-L1 interaction with PD-1 inhibits the tumor-killing activity of cytotoxic T cells, resulting in immune escape. Expression of PD-L1 is increased in many types of cancer, including ovarian cancer (OC), and correlates with poor prognosis. However, the mechanisms that regulate the *PD-L1* expression in cancer cells are poorly understood.

Recent studies have shown that *PD-L1* transcription is regulated by the transcription factor NFκB, particularly by p65 NFκB

Ivana Vancurova and Yan Zhu (eds.), *Immune Mediators in Cancer: Methods and Protocols*, Methods in Molecular Biology, vol. 2108, https://doi.org/10.1007/978-1-0716-0247-8_20,

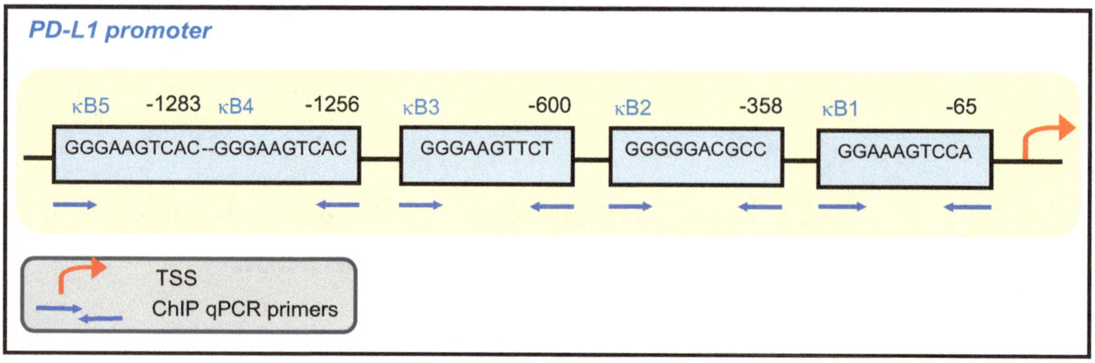

Fig. 1 Schematic illustration of NFκB-binding sites in human *PD-L1* promoter. Human *PD-L1* promoter contains five putative NFκB-binding sites: κB1 (−65), κB2 (−358), κB3 (−600), κB4 (−1256), and κB5 (−1283). Four specific ChIP primers were designed to analyze the NFκB recruitment to *PD-L1* promoter

[1–6]. The human *PD-L1* promoter contains five NFκB-binding sites: κB1 site (GGAAAGTCCA) located at position −65 upstream from the transcription start site (TSS), κB2 site (GGGGGACGCC) located −358 from TSS, κB3 site (GGGAAGTTCT) located −600 from TSS, and κB4/κB5 sites containing an identical putative NFκB-binding sequence (GGGAAGTCAC) located −1256 and −1283 from TSS (Fig. 1).

Expression of PD-L1 in OC cells is induced by interferon-γ (IFNγ) [7, 8]. Recent studies from our laboratory have shown that IFNγ induces recruitment of p65, and especially K314/315 acetylated (ac)-p65 to all five NFκB-binding sites in *PD-L1* promoter in OC cells [8]. In this chapter, we describe a protocol that uses chromatin immunoprecipitation (ChIP) to analyze the regulation of *PD-L1* expression by NFκB in ovarian cancer SKOV3 cells. The main points of this protocol are: (1) ChIP analysis of NFκB recruitment to *PD-L1* promoter using p65, K314/315 ac-p65, and control IgG antibodies; and (2) quantitative real-time PCR analysis using primers for human *PD-L1* promoter. Even though in this chapter we use IFNγ-stimulated ovarian cancer SKOV3 cells, this protocol should be easily modifiable to analyze the *PD-L1* regulation by NFκB in other cell types as well.

2 Materials

2.1 Cell Culture

1. SKOV3 cells (American Type Culture Collection).
2. RPMI complete medium: RPMI supplemented with 10% fetal bovine serum (FBS), 2 mM glutamine, 1 mM sodium pyruvate, and 1% penicillin-streptomycin solution.
3. 75 cm^2 Culture flasks.
4. 6-Well plates with clear flat bottom.

2.2 Chromatin Immunoprecipitation

1. 37% Formaldehyde solution: Aliquot in sterile 15 mL tubes in the laminar flow cabinet, and store at room temperature.
2. 2.5 M Glycine solution: Dissolve 3.75 g of glycine in 20 mL of deionized water, and store at room temperature.
3. Phosphate-buffered saline (PBS, pH 7.4).
4. 100 mM Phenylmethylsulfonyl fluoride (PMSF): Dissolve 17 mg of PMSF in 1 mL of absolute ethanol. Store at −20 °C (*see* **Note 1**).
5. Protease inhibitor cocktail for mammalian cell extracts containing pepstatin A, bestatin, leupeptin, aprotinin, 4-[2-aminoethyl]-benzenesulfonyl fluoride [AEBSF], and trans-epoxysuccinyl-L-leucylamido [4-guanidino] butane (E-64) (*see* **Note 2**).
6. Lysis buffer: 50 mM HEPES, pH 7.4, 1% (v/v) Triton X-100, 1 mM EDTA, 150 mM NaCl. Store at 4 °C. Add protease inhibitors (1 mM PMSF and 1% (v/v) protease inhibitor cocktail) and 0.1% (w/v) deoxycholic acid (Na salt) just before use.
7. Protein A/G PLUS-Agarose.
8. Immunoprecipitating antibodies: Antibodies recognizing human p65, K314/315 ac-p65, and control human IgG.
9. Low salt immune complex wash buffer: 50 mM HEPES, pH 7.4, 1% (v/v) Triton X-100, 1 mM EDTA, 100 mM NaCl. Adjust pH to 8.1. Store at 4 °C. Add protease inhibitors (1 mM PMSF and 1% (v/v) protease inhibitor cocktail) and 0.1% (w/v) deoxycholic acid (Na salt) just before use.
10. High salt immune complex wash buffer: 50 mM HEPES, pH 7.4, 1% (v/v) Triton X-100, 1 mM EDTA, 150 mM NaCl. Adjust pH to 8.1. Store at 4 °C. Add protease inhibitors (1 mM PMSF and 1% (v/v) protease inhibitor cocktail) and 0.1% (w/v) deoxycholic acid (Na salt) just before use.
11. LiCl immune complex wash buffer: 0.25 M LiCl, 0.5% (v/v) IGEPAL CA-630, 0.5% (w/v) deoxycholic acid (Na salt), 1 mM EDTA, 10 mM Tris–HCl, pH 8.1. Adjust pH to 8.1. Store at 4 °C. Add protease inhibitors (1 mM PMSF and 1% (v/v) protease inhibitor cocktail) just before use.
12. 1× Tris-EDTA (TE) buffer: 1 mM EDTA, 10 mM Tris–HCl, pH 8.1. Adjust pH to 8.1. Store at 4 °C.
13. Elution buffer: 1% SDS, 0.1 M $NaHCO_3$. Add 100 μL of 10% SDS and 100 μL of 1 M $NaHCO_3$ to 800 μL of deionized water to make 1 mL of elution buffer. Prepare fresh before each reaction; each sample requires 300 μL of elution buffer (*see* **Note 3**).
14. 5 M NaCl: Dissolve 29.2 g of NaCl in 100 mL of deionized water. Store at 4 °C.

15. 0.5 M EDTA: Dissolve 14.6 g of ethylenediaminetetraacetic acid (EDTA) disodium salt dihydrate in 100 mL of deionized water. Adjust pH to 8.0. Store at 4 °C.
16. 1 M Tris–HCl, pH 6.5: Dissolve 12.1 g of Tris base in 80 mL of deionized water. Adjust pH to 6.5. Bring the total volume to 100 mL, filter, and store at 4 °C.
17. 1 M Tris–HCl, pH 8.0: Dissolve 12.1 g of Tris base in 80 mL of deionized water. Adjust pH to 8.0. Bring the total volume to 100 mL, filter, and store at 4 °C.
18. Proteinase K solution, 20 mg/mL.
19. Phenol:chloroform:isoamyl alcohol mixture, 25:24:1, pH 8.0.
20. Ethanol, absolute.
21. 70% Ethanol: Add 70 mL of absolute ethanol to deionized water to make up a volume of 100 mL. Store at 4 °C.
22. Linear polyacrylamide (LPA), 25 mg/mL.
23. 3 M sodium acetate (NaOAc): Dissolve 6.15 g of anhydrous NaOAc in 25 mL of deionized water. Adjust pH to 5.2 using glacial acetic acid. This stock solution can be stored at room temperature.
24. Nuclease-free water.

2.3 Real-Time Polymerase Chain Reaction

1. SYBR Green Supermix.
2. Real-Time PCR Plates, 96 well.
3. Optical tape.
4. Specific primers (10 μM working stock solutions) for different promoter regions.
5. Nuclease-free water.

3 Methods

In this section, we describe the protocol for analysis of NFκB recruitment to *PD-L1* promoter using chromatin immunoprecipitation (ChIP) in ovarian cancer SKOV3 cells. However, this protocol can be easily modified for other cells as well. The recruitment is quantified by real-time PCR. On average, this protocol can be accomplished within 3–5 days. Figure 1 illustrates the NFκB-binding sites in human *PD-L1* promoter. Figure 2 illustrates the recruitment of p65, K314/315 ac-p65, and control IgG to the NFκB-binding sites in *PD-L1* promoter in IFNγ-treated SKOV3 cells.

3.1 Cell Culture and Chromatin Immunoprecipitation (ChIP)

1. Grow SKOV3 cells in RPMI complete medium to 0.5×10^6 cells/mL concentration. Incubate in a humidified 5% CO_2 atmosphere at 37 °C overnight. At desired times, cross-link proteins to DNA by adding 54 μL of 37% formaldehyde stock

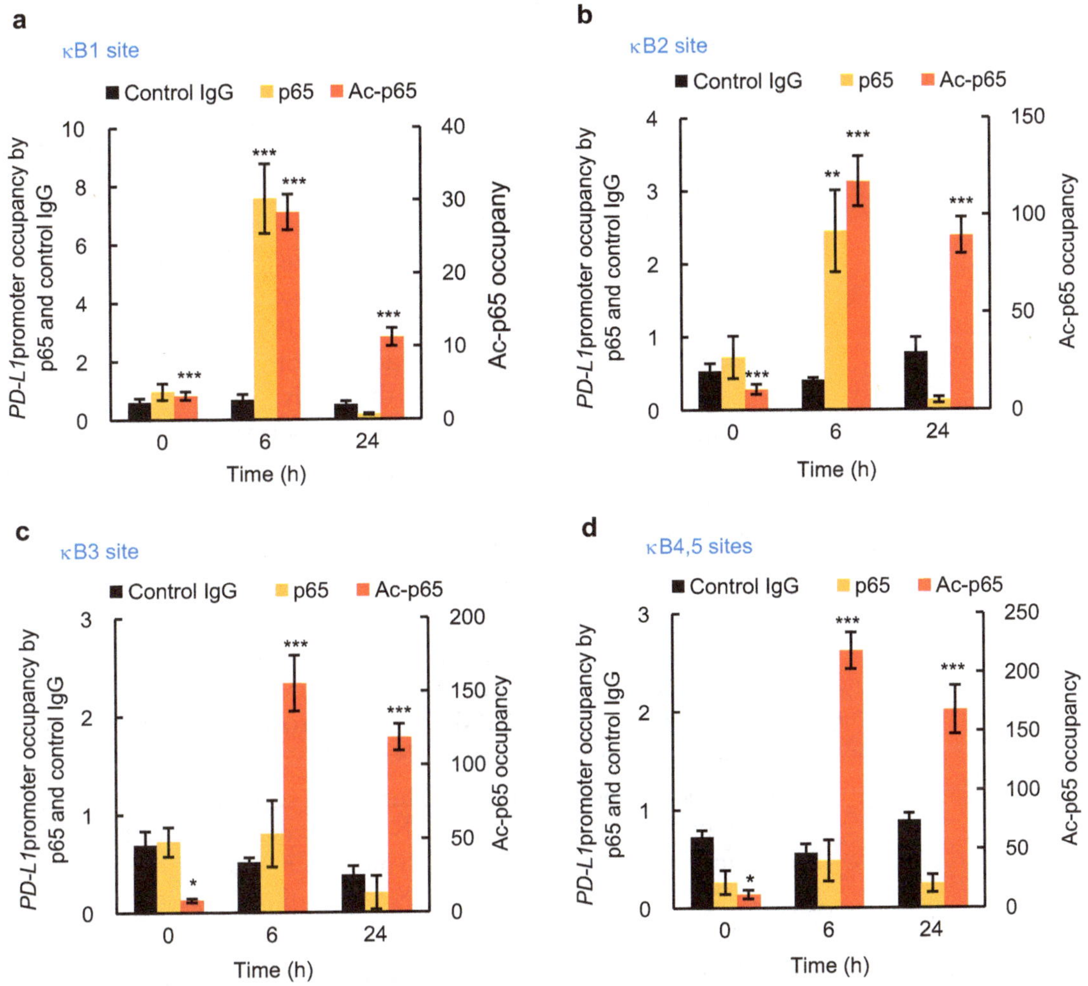

Fig. 2 ChIP analysis of p65, K314/315 ac-p65, and control IgG recruitment to κB1 **(a)**, κB2 **(b)**, κB3 **(c)**, and κB4,5 **(d)** sites in *PD-L1* promoter in SKOV3 cells. Recruitment of p65, K314/315 ac-p65, and control IgG to human *PD-L1* promoter in IFN-treated SKOV3 cells was analyzed by ChIP and quantified by real-time PCR. The data are presented as fold difference in occupancy of the particular protein at the particular locus in comparison with the human IGX1A locus, and represent the mean ± SE of three experiments. Asterisks denote a statistically significant ($^{*}p < 0.05$; $^{**}p < 0.01$; $^{***}p < 0.001$) change compared to ChIP using control IgG at the corresponding time (Mann-Whitney U test)

solution to 2 mL of cell culture, so that the final concentration of formaldehyde is 1%. Perform this step in the laminar flow cabinet.

2. Incubate cells with formaldehyde for 15 min in culture incubator (37 °C, 5% CO_2). Be consistent with the fixation condition for all time points (*see* **Note 4**).
3. Neutralize the formaldehyde-induced cross-linking by adding 100 μL of 2.5 M glycine solution into each well so that the final concentration of glycine is 0.125 M.

4. Collect cells into 15 mL centrifuge tubes and then centrifuge at 1700 × *g* for 5 min in a refrigerated centrifuge (*see* **Note 5**).
5. Carefully remove the supernatant as much as possible. Resuspend the cell pellets in 2 mL of ice-cold PBS containing the protease inhibitors (1 mM PMSF and 1% protease inhibitor cocktail) and centrifuge at 1700 × *g* for 5 min in a refrigerated centrifuge. Repeat this wash step one more time.
6. Carefully remove the supernatant as much as possible. Resuspend the cell pellets in 500 μL of ice-cold lysis buffer containing the protease inhibitors (1 mM PMSF and 1% protease inhibitor cocktail) and 0.1% deoxycholic acid (Na salt). Incubate on ice for 10 min to aid the cell lysis.
7. Sonicate the cell lysates on ice to shear DNA into 400–500 bp fragments. Sonication conditions: four 10-s pulses at output 40 (*see* **Note 6**).
8. Centrifuge the sonicated samples for 15 min at 14,000 × *g* at 4 °C. Transfer the supernatants to new prechilled 2 mL microcentrifuge tubes and discard the pellets.
9. Dilute the sonicated cell supernatants to a final volume of 2 mL by adding 1.5 mL of ice-cold lysis buffer containing the protease inhibitors (1 mM PMSF and 1% protease inhibitor cocktail) and 0.1% deoxycholic acid (Na salt).
10. Set aside a portion of the diluted cell supernatant (100 μL) to quantify the amount of DNA present in the sample. This sample is considered to be your input/starting material and needs to have the protein-DNA cross-links reversed by heating at 65 °C for 6 h (*see* **step 26**).
11. To reduce the nonspecific background, add 80 μL of protein A/G PLUS-agarose slurry to 1.9 mL of the diluted cell supernatant (from **step 9**, above) and incubate for 1 h at 4 °C while rotating the tubes in a rotator (*see* **Note 7**).
12. Pellet the agarose beads by a brief centrifugation at 150 × *g* at 4 °C, and carefully divide the 1.9 mL supernatant in two prechilled 1.5 mL microcentrifuge tubes. Each tube (with ~1 mL cell lysate) can be used to set up individual immunoprecipitation.
13. Add 4 μg of specific immunoprecipitating antibody per reaction and incubate overnight at 4 °C with constant rotation in a rotator (*see* **Note 8**).
14. The next day, add 100 μL of protein A/G PLUS-agarose slurry to each sample and incubate for 2 h at 4 °C with rotation to collect the specific antibody-protein-DNA complexes (*see* **Note 9**).

15. Pellet the agarose beads with bound protein complexes by gentle centrifugation (150 × *g* at 4 °C for 1 min). Carefully discard the supernatants containing unbound, nonspecific protein-DNA complexes. The A/G PLUS-agarose pellets should now contain only the specific antibody-protein-DNA complexes.
16. Add 1 mL of ice-cold low salt immune complex wash buffer containing protease inhibitors (1 mM PMSF and 1% protease inhibitor cocktail) and 0.1% deoxycholic acid (Na salt) to the tubes containing the protein A/G agarose-antibody-protein complexes. Incubate the complexes at 4 °C for 5 min with constant rotation.
17. Pellet agarose beads by centrifugation (150 × *g* at 4 °C for 1 min). Carefully discard the supernatants and keep the pellets on ice.
18. Add 1 mL of ice-cold high salt immune complex wash buffer containing the protease inhibitors and 0.1% deoxycholic acid (Na salt) to protein A/G agarose-antibody-protein complexes and incubate at 4 °C for 5 min with constant rotation.
19. Pellet the agarose beads by centrifugation (150 × *g* at 4 °C for 1 min). Carefully discard the supernatants and keep the pellets on ice.
20. Add 1 mL of ice-cold LiCl wash buffer containing the protease inhibitors to the bead pellets. Incubate the beads at 4 °C for 5 min with constant rotation.
21. Centrifuge the beads at 150 × *g* at 4 °C for 1 min. Carefully discard the supernatants.
22. Add 1 mL of ice-cold 1× TE buffer and incubate the beads at 4 °C for 5 min with constant rotation. Centrifuge as described above and carefully remove the supernatant as much as possible. Repeat this step twice.
23. Add 150 μL of freshly prepared elution buffer to the pelleted A/G agarose-antibody-protein complexes. Vortex briefly (5–10 s) and incubate at room temperature for 15 min with constant rotation.
24. Pellet down the agarose beads by centrifuging at 150 × *g* for 1 min at room temperature. Carefully transfer the supernatant (eluate) to a new, labeled 1.5 mL microcentrifuge tube.
25. Add 150 μL of freshly prepared elution buffer to the pellets. Repeat **step 23** as described above to elute the remaining proteins from the agarose beads. Centrifuge at 150 × *g* for 1 min at room temperature and transfer the supernatant (eluate) to the 1.5 mL microcentrifuge tube already containing 150 μL of supernatant from the **step 24**. You should now have 300 μL of the eluate per reaction.

26. Add 15 μL of 5 M NaCl to the combined eluates (300 μL) and 5 μL of 1 M NaCl to the input/starting material (100 μL, from **step 10**) to reverse the protein-DNA crosslinks. Incubate the complexes for 6 h in a 65 °C water bath.
27. After 6 h, add 6 μL of 0.5 M EDTA, 12 μL of 1 M Tris–HCl, pH 6.5, and 1 μL of 20 mg/mL proteinase K to the combined eluates and incubate for 1 h at 42 °C.
28. For the input sample, add 10 μL of 10% SDS, 2 μL of 0.5 M EDTA, 10 μL of 1 M Tris–HCl, pH 8.0, and 2 μL of 20 mg/mL proteinase K and incubate for 1 h at 45 °C.
29. Add equal volume of phenol:chloroform:isoamyl alcohol (25:24:1, pH 8.0) to the microcentrifuge tubes containing the eluate and the input sample. Vortex vigorously for 5 s. Centrifuge at 12,000 × *g* for 3 min at room temperature. Collect the top (aqueous) layers into new microcentrifuge tubes.
30. Repeat **step 29** (above) and collect again the top (aqueous) layers into new microcentrifuge tubes.
31. Add 1/10th volume of 3 M NaOAc, pH 5.2, 2 μL of LPA, and twice the volume of 100% (absolute) ethanol to the aqueous layers from **step 30** (above). Mix by inverting the tubes. Keep the microcentrifuge tubes at −20 °C overnight to allow DNA precipitation (*see* **Note 10**).
32. The next day, centrifuge the microcentrifuge tubes at 12,000 × *g* for 30 min at 4 °C. Collect the DNA containing pellets.
33. Wash the pellets with 1 mL of ice-cold 70% ethanol. Centrifuge at 12,000 × *g* for 15 min at 4 °C. Collect the pellets. Try to remove as much ethanol as possible. Allow to air-dry until the white pellets become invisible.
34. Dissolve the DNA pellets in 50 μL of nuclease-free water and store the samples at −80 °C. Perform real-time PCR as described below.

3.2 Real-Time Polymerase Chain Reaction

1. Prepare a 100 μM stock of each primer using nuclease-free water, for both the forward and reverse primers. From the 100 μM primer stocks, prepare 10 μM working stock solutions for PCR reaction using the nuclease-free water (*see* **Note 11**).
2. Each PCR reaction has a volume of 25 μL and will use 1 μL of each 10 μM primer, so that the final concentration of each primer in PCR reaction is 0.4 μM.
3. The input DNA should be diluted two times in nuclease-free water before performing PCR reaction. Each PCR reaction (25 μL volume) for the input sample will use 3 μL of two times diluted input DNA.

4. Set up the PCR reactions on ice.
5. Each reaction using immunoprecipitated DNA has a total volume of 25 μL, and is set up as follows (*see* **Note 12**):
   (a) SYBR® Green Supermix: 12.5 μL.
   (b) Nuclease-free water: 7.5 μL.
   (c) Forward primer (10 μM): 1.0 μL.
   (d) Reverse primer (10 μM): 1.0 μL.
   (e) Immunoprecipitated DNA sample: 3.0 μL.
6. Each reaction using input DNA has a total volume of 25 μL, and is set up as follows (*see* **Note 13**)
   (a) SYBR® Green Supermix: 12.5 μL.
   (b) Nuclease-free water: 7.5 μL.
   (c) Forward primer (10 μM): 1.0 μL.
   (d) Reverse primer (10 μM): 1.0 μL.
   (e) Input DNA sample (two times diluted): 3.0 μL.
7. After loading the master-mix and the DNA into the wells of the PCR plate, seal the plate carefully using an optical tape and continue with the real-time PCR reaction in the thermal cycler.
8. Each reaction for both the immunoprecipitated and input samples should include a positive and negative control (*see* **Note 14**).

4 Notes

1. PMSF is unstable in aqueous environment. It is essential that it is dissolved in absolute alcohol (ethanol, methanol, or isopropanol); it will not freeze at −20 °C. Add PMSF to buffers in the final working concentration of 1 mM just before use.
2. This protease inhibitor cocktail contains protease inhibitors with a broad specificity for the inhibition of serine, cysteine and aspartic proteases, and aminopeptidases. It should be stored at −20 °C, and added to buffers just before use.
3. Prepare stock solutions of 10% SDS and 1 M $NaHCO_3$ by dissolving 5 g of SDS in 50 mL of deionized water, and 4.2 g of $NaHCO_3$ in 50 mL deionized water, respectively. These stock solutions can be stored at room temperature.
4. Formaldehyde is a reversible protein-DNA cross-linking agent that preserves protein-DNA interactions in cells.
5. It is helpful always to centrifuge the tubes in one position (for example, when using 1.5 mL microcentrifuge tubes, position

them with cap snaps facing toward the center of the rotor). This way you can always expect the pellets to be at the same place.

6. Make sure to keep the samples on ice at all times in between the shearing. In addition, it is also helpful to place the tip of the sonicator in a beaker filled with ice for 30 s in between successive 10-s pulses to ensure that the tip is not overheated. When using a new sonicator, it is important to calibrate it so that the sheared DNA fragments are between 400 and 500 bp in size.
7. Make sure protein A/G PLUS-agarose slurry is completely resuspended before adding.
8. In this protocol, we used p65 NFκB antibody, K314/315 ac-p65 antibody, and control IgG in the final amounts of 4 μg of antibody per each immunoprecipitation reaction.
9. At this point, the agarose beads bind the antibody-protein-DNA complexes.
10. The presence of LPA during ethanol precipitation results in complete recovery of fragments larger than 20 base pairs. The nucleic acid-LPA co-precipitate is visible upon addition of ethanol.
11. The primers for amplifying the NFκB-binding sites in *PD-L1* promoter were designed to anneal optimally at 55 °C. Prepare a 10 μM working stock solution of each primer, and store at −20 °C.
12. It is convenient to prepare a master-mix by mixing all components (for desired amount of reactions) except for the DNA. Prepare the master-mix in a 1.5 mL microcentrifuge tube. Aliquot 22 μL of the master-mix into each well of the PCR plate. Add 3 μL of immunoprecipitated DNA sample into each well.
13. Prepare a master-mix containing all of the above except the input DNA in a 1.5 mL microcentrifuge tube. Aliquot 22 μL of the master-mix into each well of the PCR plate. Add 3 μL of input DNA sample (two times diluted) into each well.
14. The positive control primers provide a control for successful chromatin immunoprecipitation and gene transcription. In this protocol, we used the ChIP-qPCR human positive control primer GAPDH-1. The negative primer provides a reference of the amount of nonspecific genomic DNA that co-immunoprecipitates during the procedure. In this protocol, we used ChIP-qPCR human IGX1A negative control primer (GPH 100001C(-)01A).

Acknowledgment

This work was supported by NIH grant CA202775 to I. Vancurova.

References

1. Huang G, Wen Q, Zhao Y et al (2013) NF-κB plays a key role in inducing CD274 expression in human monocytes after lipopolysaccharide treatment. PLoS One 8:e61602
2. Peng J, Hamanishi J, Matsumura N et al (2015) Chemotherapy induces programmed cell death-ligand 1 overexpression via the nuclear factor-κB to Foster an immunosuppressive tumor microenvironment in ovarian cancer. Cancer Res 75:5034–5045
3. Gowrishankar K, Gunatilake D, Gallagher SJ et al (2015) Inducible but not constitutive expression of PD-L1 in human melanoma cells is dependent on activation of NF-κB. PLoS One 10:e0123410
4. Lim SO, Li CW, Xia W et al (2016) Deubiquitination and stabilization of PD-L1 by CSN5. Cancer Cell 30:925–939
5. Bouillez A, Rajabi H, Jin C et al (2017) MUC1-C integrates PD-L1 induction with repression of immune effectors in non-small-cell lung cancer. Oncogene 36:4037–4046
6. Maeda T, Hiraki M, Jin C et al (2018) MUC1-C induces PD-L1 and immune evasion in triple-negative breast cancer. Cancer Res 78:205–215
7. Abiko K, Matsumura N, Hamanishi J et al (2015) IFN-gamma from lymphocytes induces PD-L1 expression and promotes progression of ovarian cancer. Br J Cancer 112:1501–1509
8. Zou Y, Uddin MM, Padmanabhan S et al (2018) The proto-oncogene Bcl3 induces immune checkpoint PD-L1 expression, mediating proliferation of ovarian cancer cells. J Biol Chem 293:15483–15496

Chapter 21

Real-Time PCR Assay for the Analysis of Alternative Splicing of Immune Mediators in Cancer

Ruizhi Wang, Md. Faruk Hossain, Jovan Mirkovic, Samuel Sabzanov, and Matteo Ruggiu

Abstract

Alternative splicing evolved as a very efficient way to generate proteome diversity and to regulate cell homeostasis from a limited number of genes. Moreover, changes in the relative amounts of different splice variants derived from the same pre-mRNA are a hallmark in cancer, and aberrant expression of alternatively spliced mRNAs has been linked to cancer initiation and progression. Therefore, splice variants are critical tools to assess disease progression and clinical prognosis, and hold great promise as potential targets for therapeutic intervention. In order to understand the role that such splice variants play in cancer, it is vital to be able to accurately quantify their expression levels in different cell types and organs, both in normal conditions and in disease. In this chapter we describe a protocol to efficiently detect, analyze, and quantify alternative splicing patterns of immune mediators such as chemokines, cytokine and their receptors and ligands in cancer by quantitative PCR.

Key words RNA, Alternative splicing, Splice variant, Reverse transcription, qPCR, Cancer

1 Introduction

Sequencing of the human genome revealed that we have a surprisingly low number of genes, with coding sequences being only ~1–1.5% of our genome for ~26,000 genes [1–3]. Therefore, the great variation in gene expression in higher eukaryotes and metazoans cannot be explained simply by a larger number of genes and alleles. Pre-mRNA alternative splicing (AS) arose during evolution as a rapid, efficient, and highly regulated way to increase proteome diversity from a limited number of genes. ~95% of human genes undergo AS [4, 5], enabling the number of mRNAs—and thus proteins—arising from genes to be amplified ~10-fold [6], resulting in multiple protein isoforms (or splice variants) being produced from a single gene [7, 8]. The importance of AS is underlined by the discovery that ~50% of genetic mutations that result in disease affect pre-mRNA splicing [9–11].

Ivana Vancurova and Yan Zhu (eds.), *Immune Mediators in Cancer: Methods and Protocols*, Methods in Molecular Biology, vol. 2108, https://doi.org/10.1007/978-1-0716-0247-8_21,

The importance of AS in generating proteome diversity and in regulating homeostasis in the immune system has been discussed elsewhere [12–16]. Moreover, alterations in the ratio of different splice variants derived from the same pre-mRNA are a hallmark in cancer, with cancer tissues often producing aberrant splice forms that are not present in normal tissues [17–19]. This suggests that dysregulation of cancer-associated splice variants may play a crucial role in cancer initiation and progression [20]. As such, splice variants are important biomarkers for disease progression and clinical prognosis and, alongside their regulatory mechanisms, are potential targets for therapeutic intervention [21–24].

Interestingly, splicing isoforms of several cell membrane receptors and intracellular immune mediators often display opposite functions in cancer cells (Fig. 1). Fas (CD95/Apo-1) is a cell

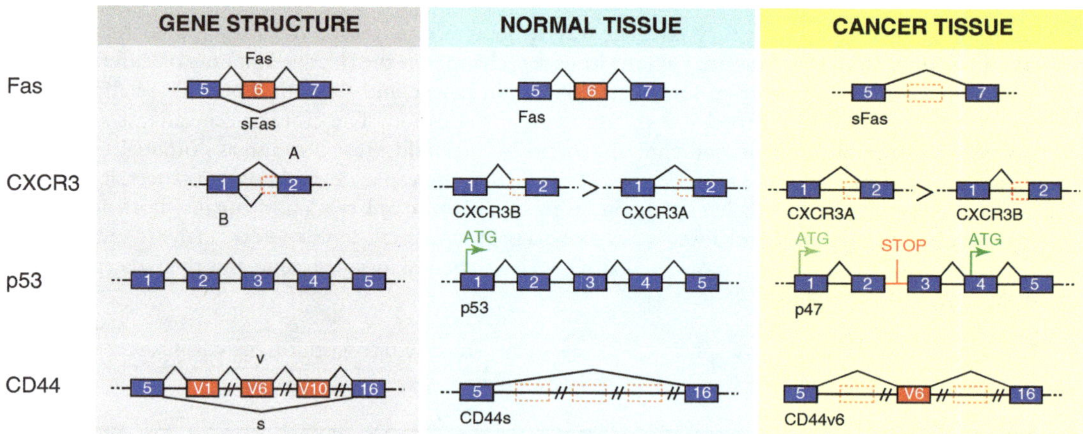

Fig. 1 Alternative splicing of immune mediators in normal tissue and in cancer tissue. Schematic representation of four genes that encode for immune mediators (Fas, CXCR3, p53, and CD44), showing the gene structure and splicing patterns, and how their AS changes between normal tissue and cancer tissue. Constitutive exons are shown in blue, while alternative regions are shown in red. The transmembrane domain of the cell surface receptor Fas is encoded by exon 6; skipping of this exon, therefore, gives rise to a soluble form of the receptor termed sFas, which cannot trigger intracellular Fas-mediated apoptosis. Circulating sFas levels are significantly higher in breast cancer patients compared to controls. The gene encoding the G protein-coupled receptor chemokine CXCR3 contains only two exons and one intron, but through usage of two competing 3′ SS can give rise to two different receptors: CXCR3B by using the proximal 3′ SS, and CXCR3A by using the distal 3′ SS. CXCR3B is the dominant splice variant in normal human prostate tissue, while the ratio of the two splice variants is flipped in prostate cancer tissue. The tumor suppressor p53 can generate a second, shorter form by inclusion of intron 2. As this intron contains an in-frame stop codon, translation for the intron-retaining isoform starts from the next downstream in-frame ATG located in exon 4, giving rise to a shorter protein termed p47 which lacks the N-terminal first transactivation domain. p47 is normally present at much lower levels in cells that express p53, but high expression of p47 in cancer cells leads to p53 loss of function by sequestration of p53 in the cytoplasm via p47–p53 heterodimers. The transmembrane glycoprotein CD44 contains 10 alternative, variable exons and undergoes complex AS, resulting in standard isoform (CD44s) and many distinct variant isoforms (CD44v). Among the various CD44v isoforms, expression of CD44v6 is positively correlated with cell metastasis and invasion

surface membrane receptor that belongs to the tumor necrosis factor (TNF) family. Fas binds to Fas ligand (FasL) as an upstream regulator to activate a signaling cascade resulting in apoptotic cell death during cancer progression [25]. Fas has 9 exons and encodes for two main splicing isoforms termed Fas and FasΔE6, with the latter variant skipping exon 6. This AS event is controlled by the splicing factors SPF45 and SRSF7, and by the long noncoding RNA Saf [26–28]. Since Fas exon 6 encodes for the transmembrane domain, splicing of this exon dictates whether Fas protein is anchored to the cell membrane or is released by the cell as a soluble product. The two splice variants, therefore, have opposing biological activities: Inclusion of exon 6 results in a membrane-bound form of Fas which can bind to FasL and activate caspases to promote apoptosis, while exclusion of exon 6 results in a soluble form of Fas (sFas), which lacks the transmembrane domain and cannot trigger intracellular Fas-mediated apoptosis [29–32]. Soluble sFas protects cells against FasL-induced apoptosis [29], and sFas overexpression tilts the normal Fas-to-sFas ratio contributing to tumor progression. Circulating sFas levels are significantly higher in breast cancer patients compared to controls, and circulating sFas levels may reflect the severity of invasive breast cancer and are, therefore, of prognostic value [33, 34]. Moreover, sFas is believed to be one of the mechanisms for tumor immune evasion [35, 36]. Interestingly, a recent paper describes how a novel, soluble splice variant of the cell-surface adhesion molecule L1CAM that lacks the transmembrane domain is expressed in endothelial cells, stimulates angiogenesis, and is upregulated in blood vessels in ovarian cancers [23]. This suggests that splicing-dependent solubilization of cell membrane receptors may be a general mechanism for tumor cells to gain novel functions that may confer a growth advantage.

CXCR3 is a chemokine, G protein-coupled receptor highly expressed on activated T cells. CXCR3 and its ligands CXCL4/PF4, CXCL9/MIG, CXCL10/IP10, and CXCL11/IP9/I-TAC mediate various cellular responses, including cell proliferation, cell migration, or inhibition of migration and apoptosis of endothelial cells [37, 38]. These different cell behaviors are explained, at least in part, by the fact that AS of the CXCR3 gene—which contains only two exons and one intron—generates two distinct receptors: CXCR3A and CXCR3B. CXCR3A mediates interactions and migratory behavior of effector T cells and natural killer cells [39, 40]. CXCR3B is primarily expressed on fibroblasts, endothelial and epithelial cells, and it inhibits cell migration and promotes apoptosis of endothelial cells [37, 41]. CXCR3B is largely identical to CXCR3A in sequence, but it has a different 5′ end. This variant results from an AS event between the same 5′ splice site (SS; donor, GU) used by CXCR3A and a novel 3′ SS (acceptor, AG) 233 nt upstream of the known 3′ SS. As a result of this alternative SS selection, CXCR3B utilizes an alternate in-frame ATG start codon located within the intron sequence 151 nt upstream of the known 3′ SS, giving rise to a form of the receptor that differs from CXCR3A in the first 52 amino acid residues in the NH_2-terminal extracellular domain, while the rest of the protein sequence is identical [37]. The ratio between CXCR3A and CXCR3B is important for the metastatic potential of human prostate cancer cells. Interestingly, while CXCR3B appears to be the dominant splice variant in normal human prostate tissues and cells, CXCR3A mRNA levels are upregulated while CXCR3B mRNA levels are downregulated in prostate cancer samples compared to normal controls. High levels of CXCR3B override the pro-migration ability of CXCR3A to inhibit cell migration [42]. Interestingly, a recent report shows that CXCR3 splice variants are able to selectively activate specific signaling pathways in response to different chemokine ligands. For example, CXCL11-dependent ERK1/2 phosphorylation through CXCR3A is stronger and lasts longer than the one mediated through CXCR3B [43]. Moreover, CXCR3B, which binds to the chemokine ligands CXCL4/PF4 and CXCL10/IP10, can trigger signaling for the cAMP-dependent protein kinase PKA, and subsequently inhibit m-calpain activity, which results in inhibition of cell migration and invasiveness [37, 41, 44–48]. Such nonredundant signaling responses mediated by different CXCR3 splice variants are likely due to chemokines stabilizing distinct receptor splice variant conformations, which in turn could lead to the activation of different intracellular signaling pathways [43].

p53 is a master tumor suppressor with a key role in regulating and maintaining genome integrity and normal cell function [49]. Activation of p53 leads to a series of posttranslational modification resulting in the formation of p53-p53 homodimers; such homodimers, in turn, work to maintain cell homeostasis as well as to reverse the effects of oncogene activation. A second p53 mRNA termed p53 (EII) is generated by retention of intron 2. Since intron 2 contains an in-frame stop codon, translation of the EII mRNA splice variant begins at the next in-frame start codon, which is located in exon 4. The result is a shorter protein termed p47 which lacks the N-terminal first transactivation domain and is therefore also called DeltaN-p53. Interestingly, p47 binds to p53 more strongly than p53 itself, giving rise to p47-p53 heterodimers [50, 51]. p47 is naturally produced in p53-expressing cells but it is expressed at much lower levels than p53. p53 performs its tumor suppressor functions in the nucleus. However, when p47 is expressed in equal or greater amounts than p53, p47-p53 heterodimers sequester p53 in the cytosol where these heterodimers are localized [51, 52]. As a result, p53 is unable to perform its tumor suppressive functions in the nucleus, expression of p53-induced gene products is altered, and the cell is subjected to unchecked growth [53]. Therefore, regulation of p53 pre-mRNA splicing controls coordinated expression of p53 and p47 and, ultimately, the outcome of p53 function.

CD44 is a non-kinase transmembrane glycoprotein which participates in a wide variety of functions including cell-cell interactions, cell adhesion, growth, migration, differentiation, and tumor metastasis [54]. Overexpression of various CD44 isoforms is often associated with tumor progression and metastasis, and CD44 is a well-established molecular marker for cancer stem cells [55, 56]. CD44 has 19 exons including 10 constant exons (exons 1–5 and 16–20) and several variant exons (exons 6–15 or v1–10; the number of variant exons varies from species to species) [57]. The alternative variant exons lie within the region of the gene encoding the variable membrane proximal extracellular domain, and AS can therefore potentially generate more than 1000 different CD44 isoforms [58]. CD44 undergoes complex AS, resulting in standard isoform (CD44s) and many distinct variant isoforms (CD44v); expression of such splice variants is regulated by multiple splicing factors including epithelial splicing regulatory protein 1 (ESRP1), splicing coactivator SRm160, and nuclear RNA binding protein Sam68 [59–62]. Among the various CD44v isoforms, expression of CD44v6 is positively correlated with cell metastasis and invasion. CD44v6 interacts with hepatocyte growth factor receptor (Met) in the presence of hepatocyte growth factor (HGF), and CD44v6-containing isoforms control HGF-dependent Met signaling [63, 64]. CD44v6 is a valuable prognostic maker to determine the length of survival and risk of relapse in different cancers [65, 66].

Given the importance of AS in regulating immune system functions and the prevalence of splicing dysregulation in cancer, it is critical to be able to not only detect but also accurately measure different AS variants present in immune and cancer tissues and cells. The most widely used approaches involve reverse transcriptase polymerase chain reaction (RT-PCR); in a previous article we described a method to detect, analyze, and quantify AS isoforms of interleukin genes by semiquantitative RT-PCR [67]; in this chapter we describe a protocol to detect, analyze, and quantify AS isoforms of interleukin genes by real-time, quantitative RT-PCR (qPCR).

2 Materials

2.1 Cell Culture

1. Cell lines obtained from the American Type Culture Collection.
2. Dulbecco's Modified Eagle Medium (DMEM) supplemented with high glucose (4.5 g/L) containing 10% fetal bovine serum (FBS), 2 mM L-glutamine, and 0.1 mg/mL gentamicin.
3. Phosphate-buffered saline (PBS), pH 7.4 without calcium and magnesium.

4. 6-Well culture dishes.
5. Fluid aspiration system or vacuum pump.
6. Sterile 1.5 mL microcentrifuge tubes.

2.2 RNA Extraction

1. All procedures are performed under RNase-free conditions, using RNase-free glassware and other equipment, and RNase-free H_2O.
2. RNA is extracted from cells using TRIzol Reagent (Life Technologies; *see* **Note 1**).
3. Sterile 1.5 mL microcentrifuge tubes.
4. Chloroform.
5. Isopropyl alcohol.
6. Glycogen RNA grade 20 mg/mL (Thermo Scientific).
7. 75% Ethanol: Add 75 mL of molecular biology grade absolute ethanol to double distilled, sterile RNase-free H_2O to make up a volume of 100 mL. Store at 4 °C.
8. RNase-free H_2O.
9. TURBO DNA-free DNase treatment and removal kit (Life Technologies).
10. Vortex mixer.
11. Spectrophotometer.

2.3 Reverse Transcription

1. RevertAid First Strand cDNA synthesis kit (Thermo Scientific; *see* **Note 2**), containing RevertAid M-MuLV Reverse Transcriptase 200 U/μL, RiboLock™ RNase Inhibitor 20 U/μL, and oligo $d(T)_{18}$ 0.5 μg/μL.
2. Thermocycler PCR machine.
3. PCR tubes (0.2–0.5 mL, depending on PCR machine).
4. RNase-free H_2O.

2.4 Real-Time Quantitative Polymerase Chain Reaction (qPCR)

1. Forward DNA primer 10 μM.
2. Reverse DNA primer 10 μM.
3. PerfeCTa SYBR Green FastMix for iQ (2×; Quantabio).
4. RNase-free H_2O.
5. Thermocycler qPCR machine.
6. 96-Well PCR plates (0.2 mL; *see* **Note 3**).
7. Optical clear sealing film (*see* **Note 4**).
8. Centrifuge with swinging rotor for 96-well plates.
9. Software for statistical analysis such as Excel (Microsoft) or Prism (GraphPad).

3 Methods

In this section, we describe a protocol for the detection, analysis, and quantification of alternatively spliced mRNA isoforms by quantitative, real-time PCR from total RNA extracted from tissue culture cell lines. However, this protocol can be easily modified and used for other applications, such as RNA analysis from tissue samples.

Sequence information for a specific transcript can be obtained from the NCBI website (http://www.ncbi.nlm.nih.gov/gene/). A search by gene name will provide the gene name and ID number, official full name, description, chromosomal location, and genomic sequence. After selecting a specific name/ID, by clicking on "Nucleotide" under the "Related Information" menu on the right-hand side of the page, it is then possible to access the sequence of single mRNA molecules, including specific splice variants of that gene. After selecting a specific transcript variant to analyze, by selecting the "Pick Primers" option from the "Analyze this sequence" menu on the right-hand side of the page it is possible to access Primer-BLAST: a primer-designing software that allows to find primers specific for this transcript. Alternatively, a specific sequence can be analyzed using a primer design software such as AmplifX or PrimerQuest Tool from Integrated DNA Technologies (IDT). In this case, the specific location of exon-exon junction onto the mRNA sequence has to be known in advance (*see* **Note 5**). Given that we are looking at alternatively spliced molecules, it is important that primers are selected to span exon-exon junctions, so that either the forward or the reverse primer is designed to hybridize on the alternatively spliced exon or region, with the other primer hybridizing on the constitutive upstream or downstream exon. Primers for qPCR, in fact, must be designed so that they will amplify only one molecule; in this case, the exon-including isoform. It is more challenging to design primers that would specifically detect the exon-skipping isoform, as primers designed to hybridize on the exons flanking the junction would amplify both the exon-skipping and exon-including isoforms. In this case, one of the primers can be designed with one end complementary to the 3′ end of one exon and the other end complementary to the 5′ end of the next downstream exon, so that amplification will only occur if this primer binds to cDNA only from a transcript that splices these two exons together, and not from a transcript that includes an alternative exon in between. See also this article from the IDT website: https://www.idtdna.com/pages/education/decoded/article/use-splice-junctions-to-your-advantage-in-qpcr.

The advantages and disadvantages of qPCR versus semiquantitative reverse transcription PCR (RT-PCR) have been previously discussed [67]. Briefly, the major advantages of qPCR over semiquantitative RT-PCR include:

1. qPCR monitors the amount of fluorescence incorporated during the reaction as a direct measurement of amplicon (the product of amplification) production at each PCR cycle (that is, in real time) as opposed to endpoint detection as in a conventional PCR.
2. Melting curve analysis allows to confirm the specificity of amplification.
3. It has a very wide dynamic range, that is, a range over which the reaction is linear.
4. It requires about 1000-fold less template than conventional PCR.
5. It allows to quantify small changes (i.e., 10–20% differences) between samples.
6. It is faster, as there is no need to run PCR products on a gel.

The main disadvantages of qPCR over semiquantitative RT-PCR include the fact that the equipment is expensive, and that setting up the proper conditions can be labor-intensive. For example, while in semiquantitative RT-PCR primers that are flanking a region where multiple alternatively spliced exons are present will allow the detection of all splice products on a gel, for qPCR primer pairs will need to be designed for the specific detection of each splice product. Moreover, qPCR may require more template to obtain the same result, as each sample will have to be amplified with primers specific for the alternatively spliced isoform, primers that will detect all transcripts from that gene (or "total transcripts"), and an internal control such as GAPDH, actin, or tubulin (*see* **Note 6**), and each one of these PCR reactions will have to be done in triplicate (or 3 technical replicates).

On average, the entire protocol can be accomplished in 1 day: RNA extraction, reverse transcription, and qPCR. qPCR data are collected in real time, and are generally quantified and plotted either as percentage of exon inclusion over total, or as fold change normalized to a control sample.

3.1 RNA Extraction from Cells Grown in Culture

3.1.1 Cell Culture and Sample Homogenization

1. Grow cells in appropriate medium, such as DMEM with 4.5 g/L of glucose and sodium pyruvate, without L-glutamine supplemented with FBS, L-glutamine, and antibiotics such as gentamicin sulfate. Incubate in a humidified 5% CO_2 atmosphere at 37 °C until subconfluent (*see* **Note 7**).
2. Vacuum aspirate medium.
3. Homogenize the cells by adding directly 500 μL of TRIzol Reagent per well (*see* **Note 8**).
4. Pass the cell lysate several times through a P1000 pipet.
5. Collect cell lysate in sterile 1.5 mL microcentrifuge tubes.
6. Vortex mix for 15″.

3.1.2 Phase Separation

1. Add 100 μL of chloroform (200 μL of chloroform per 1 mL of TRIzol Reagent). Shake tubes vigorously with a vortex for a few seconds.
2. Centrifuge samples at 12–16,000 × *g* for 15 min at 4 °C to separate the phases. Following centrifugation, the mixture separates into a lower red, phenol-chloroform phase, an interphase (which contains DNA), and a colorless aqueous upper phase; RNA is in the colorless aqueous upper phase which is approximately 50% of the total volume.
3. Without touching the interphase, transfer the aqueous phase into a labeled fresh sterile 1.5 mL microcentrifuge tube.

3.1.3 RNA Precipitation

1. Precipitate the RNA by adding one volume (roughly 250 μL) of isopropyl alcohol.
2. Add 2 μL of glycogen as carrier.
3. Mix by inverting the tubes several times, then vortex mix briefly.
4. Incubate samples for 10 min at room temperature and centrifuge at 12–16,000 × *g* for 10 min at 4 °C.
5. Remove supernatant with fluid aspiration system.

3.1.4 RNA Wash

1. Wash RNA pellet by adding 500 μL of 75% ethanol (1 mL of 75% ethanol per 1 mL of TRIzol reagent used for the initial homogenization).
2. Vortex mix the tubes briefly, and centrifuge them at 12–16,000 × *g* for 5 min at 4 °C.
3. Carefully remove supernatant with fluid aspiration system (*see* **Note 9**), and air-dry the pellet for 10 min at room temperature on the bench (*see* **Note 10**).

3.1.5 RNA Resuspension

1. Add 50–100 μL of RNase-free H_2O to the RNA pellet.
2. Resuspend pellet by pipetting up and down, and with the help of a vortex mixer; incubation at 55–60 °C for 10–15′ will help dissolve the pellet, if necessary.
3. Determine the RNA concentration by reading the optical density at 260 nm with a spectrophotometer (*see* **Note 11**).
4. The RNA is ready for downstream applications, or it can be stored at −80 °C.

3.2 TURBO DNase Digestion

1. Set up the TURBO DNase digestion on ice.
2. Digest 5 μg of RNA with 2 μL of TURBO DNase in a final volume of 50 μL; each reaction is set up as follows:
   (a) 10× TURBO DNase buffer: 5 μL.

(b) TURBO DNase 2 U/μL: 2 μL in total, to be added 1 μL at a time.

(c) RNA: equivalent to 5 μg.

(d) RNase-free H_2O: to 50 μL final volume.

3. Incubate with 1 μL of TURBO DNase at 37 °C for 30 min; add the rest (1 μL) of the TURBO DNase and incubate for a further 30 min.
4. Stop the DNase reaction by adding 0.2 volumes (i.e., 10 μL) of resuspended DNase Inactivation Reagent.
5. Incubate for 5 min at room temperature, flicking the tube 2–3 times during the incubation to redisperse the DNase Inactivation Reagent which will tend to sink to the bottom of the tube.
6. Centrifuge tubes at 10,000 × *g* for 1.5 min to pellet the DNase Inactivation Reagent.
5. Carefully transfer the RNA-containing supernatant to a fresh 1.5 mL tube being careful not to disturb the DNase Inactivation Reagent pellet (*see* **Note 12**).
6. The RNA is ready for downstream applications, or it can be stored at −80 °C (*see* **Note 13**).

3.3 Reverse Transcription

1. Set up the reverse transcription (RT) reaction on ice, using 500 ng of total RNA per sample. This is enough for 25–50 RT-PCR or qPCR reactions, depending on the amount of template used in each reaction.
2. Aliquot the equivalent of 500 ng of total RNA in PCR tubes. Add RNase-free H_2O to 11 μL. To each tube add 1 μL of oligo $d(T)_{18}$ 0.5 μg/μL. Final volume: 12 μL.
3. Denature RNA by incubating samples for 5 min at 65 °C in PCR machine. Chill at 4 °C.
4. Each reaction has a final volume of 20 μL and is set up as follows:

(a) 5× Reaction Buffer: 4 μL.

(b) RiboLock™ RNase Inhibitor 20 U/μL: 1 μL.

(c) 10 mM dNTP mix: 2 μL.

(d) RevertAid Reverse Transcriptase 200 U/μL: 1 μL.

5. Incubate samples at 42 °C for 1 h in PCR machine (*see* **Note 14**).
6. Each reverse transcriptase reaction should include a "no enzyme" negative control for genomic DNA contamination.
7. Bring final volume to 50 μL with H_2O, so that 1 μL of RT reaction is the equivalent of 10 ng of starting total RNA.
8. If not to be used immediately, store RT samples at −20 °C for up to a week, or at −80 °C for long-term storage.

3.4 Real-Time Quantitative Polymerase Chain Reaction (qPCR)

3.4.1 qPCR Reaction Assembly

1. Before starting the reaction, calculate the amount of RNA needed for each sample (*see* **Note 15**).
2. Set up the qPCR on ice. Each reaction has a final volume of 20 μL and is set up as follows:
   (a) 2× PerfeCTa SYBR Green SuperMix for iQ: 10 μL.
   (b) Forward primer 10 μM: 0.6 μL, equivalent to 300 nM (final concentration).
   (c) Reverse primer 10 μM: 0.6 μL, equivalent to 300 nM (final concentration).
   (d) RT reaction (template): 2 μL, equivalent to 20 ng of starting RNA.
   (e) RNase-free H_2O: 6.8 μL.
3. Prepare a primer mix and a template mix separately, keeping into account that each sample should have 3 technical replicates.
   (a) Primer mix (amounts are for one well):
   - 2× PerfeCTa SYBR Green SuperMix for iQ: 10 μL.
   - Forward primer 10 μM: 0.6 μL, equivalent to 300 nM (final concentration).
   - Reverse primer 10 μM: 0.6 μL, equivalent to 300 nM (final concentration).
   - Final volume: 11.2 μL.

   (b) Template mix (amounts are for one well):
   - RT reaction (template): 2 μL.
   - RNase-free H_2O: 6.8 μL.
   - Final volume: 8.8 μL.
4. Aliquot the primer mix first (11.2 μL/well), and then add the template mix (8.8 μL/well) to each well. Final volume: 20 μL/well.
5. Seal the plate with film, vortex it briefly, and centrifuge the plate briefly to collect components at the bottom of each reaction tube.

3.4.2 PCR Cycling Protocol and qPCR Quantification

1. Set SYBR as target when setting up the plate setup in the qPCR machine.
2. Set up the qPCR cycling protocol in the qPCR machine. PerfeCTa SYBR Green FastMix can work as both a 2-step and 3-step cycling (*see* **Note 16**). *See* Fig. 2 for an example of a 3-step qPCR cycling protocol.
3. Data are collected at the end of the extension step.

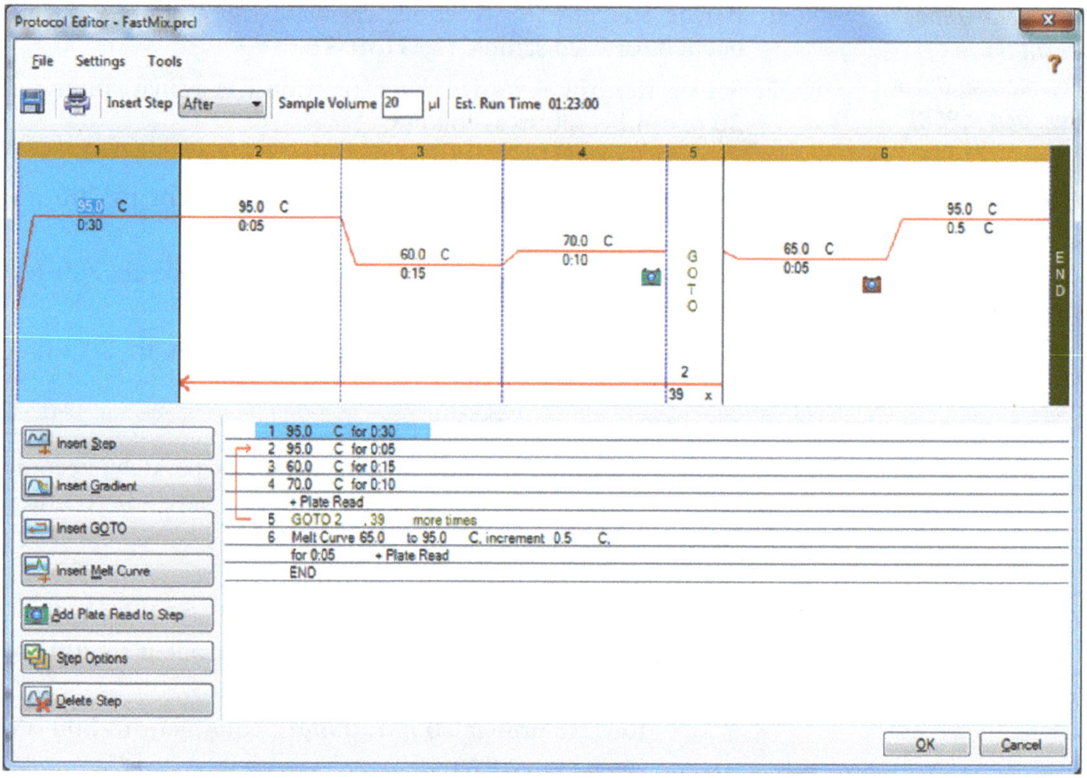

Fig. 2 Example of a 3-step qPCR cycling protocol. This protocol is used with PerfeCTa SYBR Green FastMix for iQ (Quantabio) on a Bio-Rad C1000 Touch Thermal Cycler with CFX96 Real-Time System

4. After the run, when saving and/or exporting the data, include the well, fluorophore, C_T (or C_q) value, and melting temperature. *See* Fig. 3 for examples of qPCR melting curves.
5. Data are quantified using the threshold cycle or C_T value for each single well, where C_T is the intersection between an amplification curve and a threshold line, or the PCR cycle at which a significant difference in normalized reporter signal is first detected. As such, it represents a relative measure of target concentration in a PCR reaction (*see* **Note 17**).
6. Calculate the average C_T value of the 3 technical replicates for each sample, and use that average C_T value for quantification using the $2^{-\Delta\Delta C_T}$ method (*see* **Note 18**).

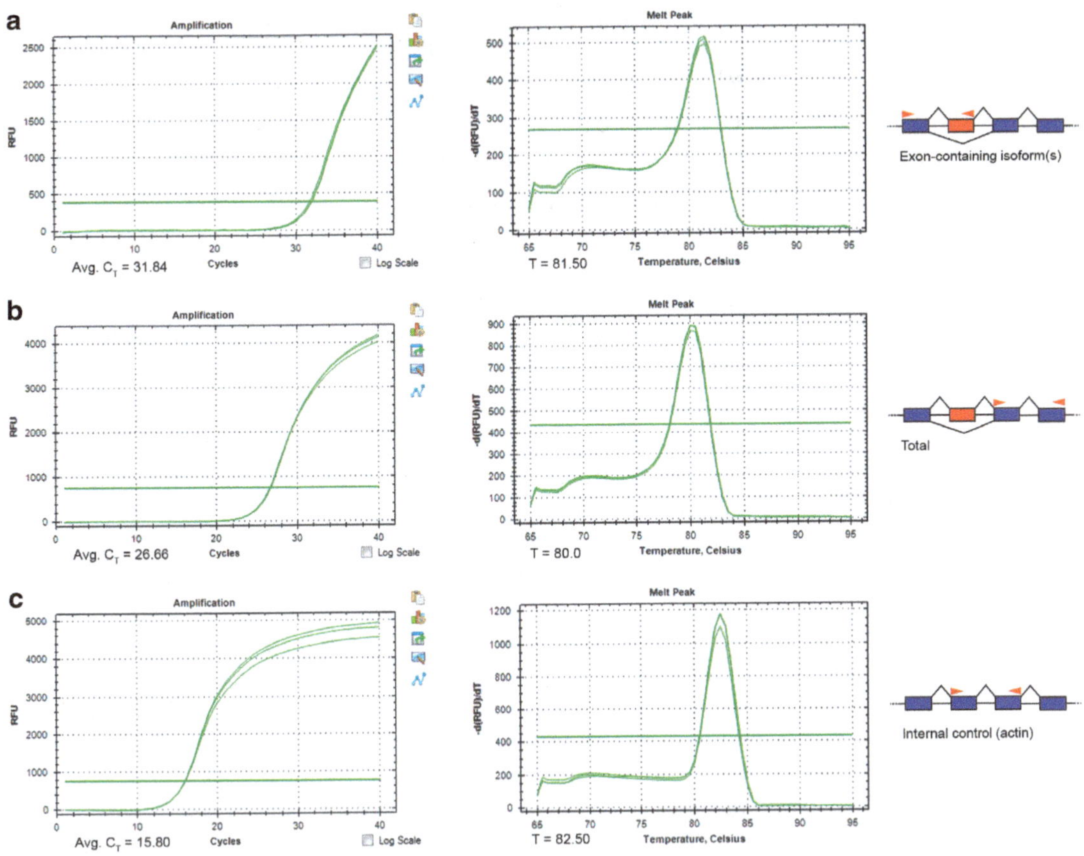

Fig. 3 Examples of qPCR amplification curves and melting curves. Amplification curves (left) and melt peak curves (right) are shown for 3 sets of qPCR primers, with 3 curves for each set of primers corresponding to 3 technical replicates of the same qPCR reaction. qPCR primers and their location on the pre-mRNA are shown as red arrowheads; constitutive exons are shown in blue, while an alternative cassette exon for (**a**, **b**) is shown in red (far right). (**a**) qPCR data obtained with primers designed to detect the exon-containing isoform(s) of a gene that contains an alternatively spliced cassette exon. (**b**) qPCR data obtained with primers designed to amplify all transcripts (total) from the same gene shown in **a**. (**c**) qPCR data obtained with primers designed to amplify transcripts from a control gene (actin). The average C_T value and melting temperatures for the 3 technical replicates are indicated. Note that the melt peak graph shows a single peak for each primer pair used, indicating the presence of a single amplicon in each qPCR reaction. Data were generated using PerfeCTa SYBR Green FastMix for iQ (Quantabio) and a Bio-Rad C1000 Touch Thermal Cycler with CFX96 Real-Time System

4 Notes

1. Other equivalent reagents are RiboZol RNA Extraction Reagent (AMRESCO) and IBI Isolate (IBI).
2. Other reverse transcription enzymes such as SuperScript™ III by Life Technologies work equally well. However, since SuperScript III works at 50 °C instead of 42, this reverse transcriptase is preferable when strong RNA secondary structures are expected.

3. Use a fully skirted 96-well PCR plate, such as Greiner Bio-One cat. #652270 (VWR 75830-566), or USA Scientific cat. #1402-9800.
4. Use an optically clear sealing film, such as Greiner Bio-One cat. #676040, or USA Scientific cat. #2978-2100.
5. Publicly available online resources about genome annotation of AS include the USCS Genome Browser (http://genome.ucsc.edu/), Fast DB and EASANA (both available through https://www.easana.com/), ProSplicer (http://prosplicer.mbc.nctu.edu.tw/), and resources from the Burge Laboratory Web Server (http://hollywood.mit.edu/).
6. Depending on what the goal of the qPCR is, it may not be necessary to include an internal control such as GAPDH, actin, or tubulin. In AS, in fact, what matters is the relative expression of a splice isoform versus the total, or of a splice isoform versus other splice isoforms. An internal control may be useful to look at relative expression levels of the total across samples when, for example, the sample that shows the highest expression levels for a gene that undergoes AS is set to 1 (or 100%). This is assuming that the internal control is expressed at equal levels across all the samples, which may not necessarily be the case. Therefore, when using an internal control to quantify expression it may be better to use more than one control. Otherwise, for each sample the relative expression of a splice isoform is quantified using the total as internal control (the ΔC_T). The sample that shows the highest expression levels of a specific splice variant (exon including, for example) versus the total, could be set to 1, and expression of the same splicing variants in other samples could be shown as fold change versus the sample that shows the highest expression levels of that splice variant.
7. Cells are grown in 6-well plates, such as USA Scientific CytoOne cat. #CC7682-7506. Cells should not be allowed to reach confluency, since that may affect gene expression and AS patterns.
8. 100 μL/cm^2 of culture dish surface area; 1 mL per 50–100 mg of tissue + glass/Teflon homogenizer.
9. Be very gentle in aspirating the supernatant, since at this stage the pellet will detach itself from the minicentrifuge tube very easily.
10. Do not dry the RNA pellet using a vacuum centrifuge and avoid overdrying it; a very dry RNA pellet will be very difficult to resuspend.
11. For a 1-cm pathlength, the optical density at 260 nm (OD_{260}) equals 1.0 for a 40 μg/mL solution of RNA. Calculate the OD_{260}/OD_{280} ratio for an indication of nucleic acid purity.

Pure RNA has an OD_{260}/OD_{280} ratio of ~2.0. Low ratios could be caused by protein or phenol contamination. The expected yield of RNA will vary from cell line to cell line, but a subconfluent 6-well dish should give 10–40 μg of total RNA.

12. The presence of DNase Inactivation Reagent into solutions that may be used for downstream applications can sequester divalent cations and change reaction conditions.

13. The concentration of the RNA, which originally was 5 μg in 50 μL, i.e., 100 ng/μL in the TURBO DNase reaction, has now changed, as the volume has increased after the addition of the DNase Inactivation Reagent. Measure the volume of RNA solution in each tube and calculate its concentration assuming that it contains 5 μg of RNA.

14. For GC-rich RNA templates the reaction temperature can be increased up to 45 °C.

15. For each well the amount of template will be 2 μL of RT reaction, equivalent to 20 ng of starting RNA. Each sample will have to be amplified with various sets of primers: one set to detect each splice isoform, one set to detect the total transcripts, and one set for internal control such as GAPDH, actin, or tubulin (*see* Fig. 3). Each reaction consisting of a set of primers and one template will have to be performed in triplicate (i.e., 3 technical replicates). For example, for a gene that has a cassette exon that can be included or skipped, we will need 1 qPCR reaction to detect the exon including isoform, 1 qPCR reaction to detect total transcripts, 1 qPCR reaction to detect the internal control (GAPDH, actin, or tubulin), i.e., 3 different qPCR reactions, each one in triplicate, for a total of 9 qPCR reactions. Therefore, in this case we will need $9 \times 2 = 18$ μL of RT reaction, equivalent to 180 ng of starting total RNA.

16. Optimal annealing temperature and time or primer concentration may vary from primer set to primer set, and from instrument to instrument. In general, if the qPCR amplicon is large enough to be detected on a gel, we first test the PCR conditions as a semiquantitative RT-PCR; conditions that work for a semiquantitative RT-PCR are a good starting point for a qPCR.

17. The C_T value is called C_q value in certain qPCR machines such as the Bio-Rad C1000 Touch Thermal Cycler with CFX96 Real-Time System.

18. This method has been extensively discussed elsewhere [68, 69]. Briefly, $\Delta C_T = C_T(\text{target gene}) - C_T(\text{reference gene})$, where reference gene is GAPDH, actin, tubulin, etc. $\Delta\Delta C_T = \Delta C_T(\text{target sample}) - \Delta C_T(\text{reference sample})$, where reference sample is the control sample. Please note that this

method of quantification is valid only if the efficiency of amplification for both the target and the reference are approximately equal, and that modified methods that take into account PCR efficiency are available [70]. See also this article from the ThermoFisher Scientific: https://www.thermofisher.com/us/en/home/life-science/pcr/real-time-pcr/real-time-pcr-learning-center/real-time-pcr-basics/real-time-pcr-understanding-ct.html. A variation of this method is to calculate the average $2^{-\Delta C_T}$ for the reference—or control—sample, and to divide all other $2^{-\Delta C_T}$ values by this average $2^{-\Delta C_T}$ value for the reference. This way it is possible to place error bars on the reference sample when graphing the data.

Acknowledgment

This work was supported by NIH grant 1R15GM119099-01 to M. Ruggiu.

References

1. Quackenbush J (2001) The power of public access: the human genome project and the scientific process. Nat Genet 29:4–6
2. Venter JC, Adams MD, Myers EW et al (2001) The sequence of the human genome. Science 291:1304–1351
3. Samuels DC, Han L, Li J et al (2013) Finding the lost treasures in exome sequencing data. Trends Genet 29:593–599
4. Wang ET, Sandberg R, Luo S et al (2008) Alternative isoform regulation in human tissue transcriptomes. Nature 456:470–476
5. Pan Q, Shai O, Lee LJ et al (2008) Deep surveying of alternative splicing complexity in the human transcriptome by high-throughput sequencing. Nat Genet 40:1413–1415
6. Nilsen TW, Graveley BR (2010) Expansion of the eukaryotic proteome by alternative splicing. Nature 463:457–463
7. Modrek B, Resch A, Grasso C et al (2001) Genome-wide detection of alternative splicing in expressed sequences of human genes. Nucleic Acids Res 29:2850–2859
8. Black DL (2003) Mechanisms of alternative pre-messenger RNA splicing. Annu Rev Biochem 72:291–336
9. López-Bigas N, Audit B, Ouzounis C et al (2005) Are splicing mutations the most frequent cause of hereditary disease? FEBS Lett 579:1900–1903
10. Cooper TA, Wan L, Dreyfuss G (2009) RNA and disease. Cell 136:777–793
11. Singh RK, Cooper TA (2012) Pre-mRNA splicing in disease and therapeutics. Trends Mol Med 18:472–482
12. Lynch KW (2004) Consequences of regulated pre-mRNA splicing in the immune system. Nat Rev Immunol 4:931–940
13. Martinez NM, Pan Q, Cole BS et al (2012) Alternative splicing networks regulated by signaling in human T cells. RNA 18:1029–1040
14. Martinez NM, Lynch KW (2013) Control of alternative splicing in immune responses: many regulators, many predictions, much still to learn. Immunol Rev 253:216–236
15. Yabas M, Elliott H, Hoyne GF (2015) The role of alternative splicing in the control of immune homeostasis and cellular differentiation. Int J Mol Sci 17:E3
16. Schaub A, Glasmacher E (2017) Splicing in immune cells-mechanistic insights and emerging topics. Int Immunol 29:173–181
17. Kim E, Goren A, Ast G (2008) Insights into the connection between cancer and alternative splicing. Trends Genet 24:7–10
18. Bruikman CS, Zhang H, Kemper AM et al (2019) Netrin family: role for protein isoforms in cancer. J Nucleic Acids 2019:3947123
19. Li D, Harlan-Williams LM, Kumaraswamy E et al (2019) BRCA1-no matter how you splice it. Cancer Res 79:2091–2098
20. Hagen RM, Ladomery MR (2012) Role of splice variants in the metastatic progression of

prostate cancer. Biochem Soc Trans 40:870–874

21. Wang BD, Lee NH (2018) Aberrant RNA splicing in cancer and drug resistance. Cancers (Basel) 10:E458
22. Coltri PP, Dos Santos MGP, da Silva GHG (2019) Splicing and cancer: challenges and opportunities. Wiley Interdiscip Rev RNA 10: e1527
23. Angiolini F, Belloni E, Giordano M et al (2019) A novel L1CAM isoform with angiogenic activity generated by NOVA2-mediated alternative splicing. Elife 8:e44305
24. Stevens M, Oltean S (2019) Modulation of receptor tyrosine kinase activity through alternative splicing of ligands and receptors in the VEGF-A/VEGFR axis. Cells 8:E288
25. Itoh N, Yonehara S, Ishii A et al (1991) The polypeptide encoded by the cDNA for human cell surface antigen Fas can mediate apoptosis. Cell 66:233–243
26. Cascino I, Papoff G, Eramo A et al (1996) Soluble Fas/Apo-1 splicing variants and apoptosis. Front Biosci 1:d12–d18
27. Villamizar O, Chambers CB, Riberdy JM et al (2016) Long noncoding RNA Saf and splicing factor 45 increase soluble Fas and resistance to apoptosis. Oncotarget 7:13810–13826
28. Fu Y, Wang Y (2018) SRSF7 knockdown promotes apoptosis of colon and lung cancer cells. Oncol Lett 15:5545–5552
29. Cheng J, Zhou T, Liu C et al (1994) Protection from Fas-mediated apoptosis by a soluble form of the Fas molecule. Science 263:1759–1762
30. Cascino I, Fiucci G, Papoff G et al (1995) Three functional soluble forms of the human apoptosis-inducing Fas molecule are produced by alternative splicing. J Immunol 154:2706–2713
31. Kischkel FC, Hellbardt S, Behrmann I et al (1995) Cytotoxicity-dependent APO-1 (Fas/CD95)-associated proteins form a death-inducing signaling complex (DISC) with the receptor. EMBO J 14:5579–5588
32. Ashkenazi A, Dixit VM (1999) Apoptosis control by death and decoy receptors. Curr Opin Cell Biol 11:255–260
33. Ueno T, Toi M, Tominaga T (1999) Circulating soluble Fas concentration in breast cancer patients. Clin Cancer Res 5:3529–3533
34. Sheen-Chen SM, Chen HS, Eng HL et al (2003) Circulating soluble Fas in patients with breast cancer. World J Surg 27:10–13
35. Natoli G, Ianni A, Costanzo A et al (1995) Resistance to Fas-mediated apoptosis in human hepatoma cells. Oncogene 11:1157–1164
36. Owen-Schaub LB, Angelo LS, Radinsky R et al (1995) Soluble Fas/APO-1 in tumor cells: a potential regulator of apoptosis. Cancer Lett 94:1–8
37. Lasagni L, Francalanci M, Annunziato F et al (2003) An alternatively spliced variant of CXCR3 mediates the inhibition of endothelial cell growth induced by IP-10, Mig, and I-TAC, and acts as functional receptor for platelet factor 4. J Exp Med 197:1537–1549
38. Dagan-Berger M, Feniger-Barish R, Avniel S et al (2006) Role of CXCR3 carboxyl terminus and third intracellular loop in receptor-mediated migration, adhesion and internalization in response to CXCL11. Blood 107:3821–3831
39. Romagnani P, Annunziato F, Lazzeri E et al (2001) Interferon-inducible protein 10, monokine induced by interferon gamma, and interferon-inducible T-cell alpha chemoattractant are produced by thymic epithelial cells and attract T-cell receptor (TCR) alphabeta+ CD8+ single-positive T cells, TCRgammadelta+ T cells, and natural killer-type cells in human thymus. Blood 97:601–607
40. Martín-Fontecha A, Thomsen LL, Brett S et al (2004) Induced recruitment of NK cells to lymph nodes provides IFN-gamma for T(H)1 priming. Nat Immunol 5:1260–1265
41. Bodnar RJ, Yates CC, Wells A (2006) IP-10 blocks vascular endothelial growth factor-induced endothelial cell motility and tube formation via inhibition of calpain. Circ Res 98:617–625
42. Wu Q, Dhir R, Wells A (2012) Altered CXCR3 isoform expression regulates prostate cancer cell migration and invasion. Mol Cancer 11:3
43. Berchiche YA, Sakmar TP (2016) CXC chemokine receptor 3 alternative splice variants selectively activate different signaling pathways. Mol Pharmacol 90:483–495
44. Smit MJ, Verdijk P, van der Raaij-Helmer EM et al (2003) CXCR3-mediated chemotaxis of human T cells is regulated by a Gi- and phospholipase C-dependent pathway and not via activation of MEK/p44/p42 MAPK nor Akt/PI-3 kinase. Blood 102:1959–1965
45. Satish L, Blair HC, Glading A et al (2005) Interferon-inducible protein 9 (CXCL11)-induced cell motility in keratinocytes requires calcium flux-dependent activation of mu-calpain. Mol Cell Biol 25:1922–1941
46. Kouroumalis A, Nibbs RJ, Aptel H et al (2005) The chemokines CXCL9, CXCL10, and CXCL11 differentially stimulate G alpha i-independent signaling and actin responses in human intestinal myofibroblasts. J Immunol 175:5403–5411

47. Thompson BD, Jin Y, Wu KH et al (2007) Inhibition of G alpha i2 activation by G alpha i3 in CXCR3-mediated signaling. J Biol Chem 282:9547–9555
48. Petrai I, Rombouts K, Lasagni L et al (2008) Activation of p38(MAPK) mediates the angiostatic effect of the chemokine receptor CXCR3-B. Int J Biochem Cell Biol 40:1764–1774
49. Kruse JP, Gu W (2009) Modes of p53 regulation. Cell 137:609–622
50. Yin Y, Stephen CW, Luciani MG et al (2002) p53 stability and activity is regulated by Mdm2-mediated induction of alternative p53 translation products. Nat Cell Biol 4:462–467
51. Courtois S, Verhaegh G, North S et al (2002) DeltaN-p53, a natural isoform of p53 lacking the first transactivation domain, counteracts growth suppression by wild-type p53. Oncogene 21:6722–6728
52. Maier B, Gluba W, Bernier B et al (2004) Modulation of mammalian life span by the short isoform of p53. Genes Dev 18:306–319
53. Ghosh A, Stewart D, Matlashewski G (2004) Regulation of human p53 activity and cell localization by alternative splicing. Mol Cell Biol 24:7987–7997
54. Ponta H, Sherman L, Herrlich PA (2003) CD44: from adhesion molecules to signalling regulators. Nat Rev Mol Cell Biol 4:33–45
55. Yin T, Wang G, He S et al (2016) Human cancer cells with stem cell-like phenotype exhibit enhanced sensitivity to the cytotoxicity of IL-2 and IL-15 activated natural killer cells. Cell Immunol 300:41–45
56. Chen C, Zhao S, Karnad A et al (2018) The biology and role of CD44 in cancer progression: therapeutic implications. J Hematol Oncol 11:64
57. Tölg C, Hofmann M, Herrlich P et al (1993) Splicing choice from ten variant exons establishes CD44 variability. Nucleic Acids Res 21:1225–1229
58. Screaton GR, Bell MV, Jackson DG et al (1992) Genomic structure of DNA encoding the lymphocyte homing receptor CD44 reveals at least 12 alternatively spliced exons. Proc Natl Acad Sci U S A 89:12160–12164
59. Screaton GR, Bell MV, Bell JI et al (1993) The identification of a new alternative exon with highly restricted tissue expression in transcripts encoding the mouse Pgp-1 (CD44) homing receptor. Comparison of all 10 variable exons between mouse, human, and rat. J Biol Chem 268:12235–12238
60. Cheng C, Sharp PA (2006) Regulation of CD44 alternative splicing by SRm160 and its potential role in tumor cell invasion. Mol Cell Biol 26:362–370
61. Yae T, Tsuchihashi K, Ishimoto T et al (2012) Alternative splicing of CD44 mRNA by ESRP1 enhances lung colonization of metastatic cancer cell. Nat Commun 3:883
62. Prochazka L, Tesarik R, Turanek J (2014) Regulation of alternative splicing of CD44 in cancer. Cell Signal 26:2234–2239
63. Orian-Rousseau V, Chen L, Sleeman JP et al (2002) CD44 is required for two consecutive steps in HGF/c-Met signaling. Genes Dev 16:3074–3086
64. Todaro M, Gaggianesi M, Catalano V et al (2014) CD44v6 is a marker of constitutive and reprogrammed cancer stem cells driving colon cancer metastasis. Cell Stem Cell 14:342–356
65. Kaufmann M, Heider KH, Sinn HP et al (1995) CD44 variant exon epitopes in primary breast cancer and length of survival. Lancet 345:615–619
66. Magyarosy E, Sebestyén A, Timár J (2001) Expression of metastasis associated proteins, CD44v6 and NM23-H1, in pediatric acute lymphoblastic leukemia. Anticancer Res 21:819–823
67. Shakola F, Byrne S, Javed K et al (2014) Radiolabeled semi-quantitative RT-PCR assay for the analysis of alternative splicing of interleukin genes. Methods Mol Biol 1172:343–362
68. Livak KJ, Schmittgen TD (2001) Analysis of relative gene expression data using real-time quantitative PCR and the 2(−Delta Delta C (T)) method. Methods 25:402–408
69. Pfaffl MW (2001) A new mathematical model for relative quantification in real-time RT-PCR. Nucleic Acids Res 29:e45
70. Rao X, Huang X, Zhou Z et al (2013) An improvement of the 2(−delta delta CT) method for quantitative real-time polymerase chain reaction data analysis. Biostat Bioinform Biomath 3:71–85

Chapter 22

Combined Single-Cell Measurement of Cytokine mRNA and Protein in Immune Cells

Julian J. Freen-van Heeren, Benoit P. Nicolet, and Monika C. Wolkers

Abstract

A key feature of immune cells, such as T cells, is their rapid responsiveness to activation. The response rate of T cells depends on the signal strength, and the type of signals they receive. Studying the underlying mechanisms that define responsiveness, however, is confounded by the fact that immune cells do not uniformly respond to activation. Tools that measure gene products on a single-cell level therefore provide additional insights in T cell biology. Here we describe flow cytometry-based fluorescence in situ hybridization (Flow-FISH), a high-throughput assay that allows for the simultaneous measurement of cytokine mRNA and protein levels of the gene(s) of interest by flow cytometry. We present several possible applications of Flow-FISH in human and murine T cells that—with minor adjustments—should also be applicable for other cell types.

Key words Flow-FISH, Immune cells, T cells, mRNA, Protein, Cytokines, Flow cytometry, Single cell

1 Introduction

During our lifetime, we are exposed to a myriad of microbiological threats and malignancies. Our immune system clears infections and protects us from future insults [1–4]. T cells are a critical component of the immune system because they provide life-long immunity. When responding to insults, T cells alter their transcriptional profile and their receptor makeup [5–7]. In addition, they produce copious amounts of effector molecules to clear pathogens or infected cells. This includes the production of pro- and anti-inflammatory cytokines and cytotoxic molecules [8–11]. T cell responses have been studied by flow cytometry, immunohistochemistry, mass spectrometry, ELISA, quantitative PCR, and/or (single cell) RNA sequencing [12–20]. While many insights have been gained by these techniques, they do not measure protein

Julian J. Freen-van Heeren and Benoit P. Nicolet contributed equally to this work.

Ivana Vancurova and Yan Zhu (eds.), *Immune Mediators in Cancer: Methods and Protocols*, Methods in Molecular Biology, vol. 2108, https://doi.org/10.1007/978-1-0716-0247-8_22, © Springer Science+Business Media, LLC, part of Springer Nature 2020

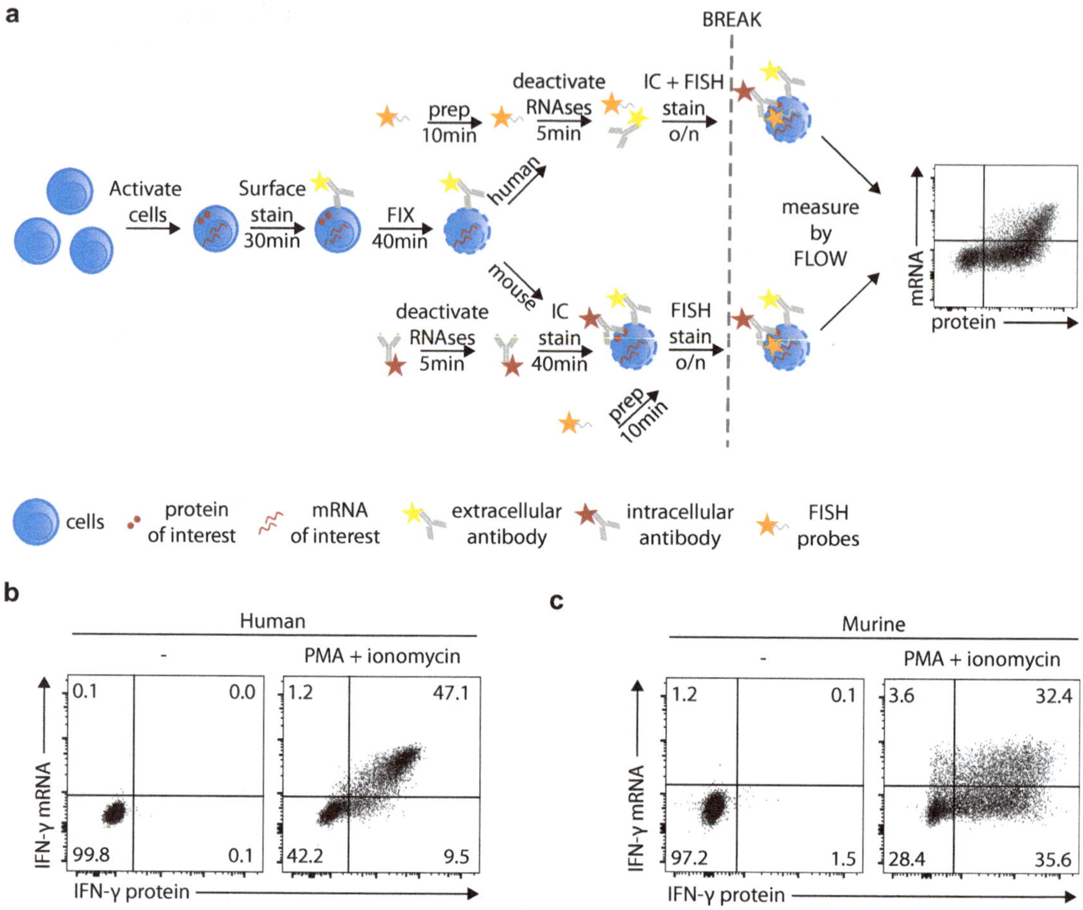

Fig. 1 Flow-FISH allows for the simultaneous measurement of mRNA and protein of one gene with single-cell resolution. (**a**) Schematic representation of the workflow of Flow-FISH. For legend, see bottom of panel. (**b**, **c**) Flow-FISH staining for IFN-γ mRNA and protein from ex vivo human (**b**) and in vitro cultured murine (**c**) CD8$^+$ T cells that were left untreated (−), or that were activated for 4 h with PMA + ionomycin, both in the presence of monensin

production and transcript expression simultaneously on a single-cell level. However, it has recently been appreciated that transcript levels may not reflect the protein output [21–25]. Therefore, to combine the analysis of mRNA and protein levels with single-cell resolution is paramount [26, 27]. One of the methods that allows for this type of simultaneous analysis is flow cytometry-based fluorescence in situ hybridization, or Flow-FISH [28–31]. Flow-FISH utilizes fluorescently labeled probes that anneal specifically to the mRNA of interest in combination with antibody stainings to surface and intracellular proteins. The background of this technique has recently been described elsewhere [27]. Here we describe how Flow-FISH can be used to study human and murine T cell responses (*see* Fig. 1a) and what results should be expected (*see*

Fig. 1b, c). We studied T cell responses, but with minor adjustments this protocol should also be applicable to other cell types.

Flow-FISH can be used to address various types of research questions. Here, we present several examples of such assays.

Flow-FISH can reveal differences in the production kinetics of mRNA and protein of activated T cells in response to activation [29, 31]. For instance, tumor necrosis factor (TNF)-α mRNA is induced within 30 min of 12-*O*-Tetradecanoylphorbol-13-acetate (PMA) + ionomycin stimulation in freshly isolated human T cells, followed by the first measurable protein production at 60 min post activation (*see* Fig. 2a, top panel). Conversely, when T cells were previously activated and subsequently cultured for several days prior to stimulation, both *TNFA* mRNA and the corresponding protein were more rapidly produced upon activation (*see* Fig. 2a, bottom panel). We found that Flow-FISH can also be used to distinguish differential responsiveness in a T cell population when measuring the capacity of $mRNA^{lo}$- and $mRNA^{hi}$-expressing T cells upon activation to produce cytokines [29].

Because Flow-FISH is compatible with the labeling of extracellular markers, it allows for the simultaneous analysis of different T cell populations in one sample. For instance, as reported by literature for human cells [32, 33], only $CD44^{hi}$ memory-like T cells but not $CD44^{lo}$ naïve spleen-derived murine $CD8^{+}$ T cells express mRNA and protein of the pro-inflammatory cytokine interferon (IFN)-γ upon activation with αCD3 + αCD28 for 4 h (*see* Fig. 2b). Similar analyses can also be performed with Flow-FISH on human T cells [29].

Flow-FISH can also reveal how posttranscriptional events alter mRNA and protein levels. We and others have shown that germline deletion of AU-rich elements in the 3′ untranslated region (UTR) of murine IFN-γ (ARE-Del, *see* Fig. 2c) results in augmented and prolonged cytokine production [24, 34]. The protein production was determined to be due to alterations in *Ifng* mRNA stabilization, and increased translation [24, 34]. Interestingly, this superior cytokine production by ARE-Del T cells even occurs in dysfunctional tumor-infiltrating T cells that normally lose their capacity to produce cytokines in the suppressive tumor microenvironment [25]. Indeed, comparative Flow-FISH analysis on activated wild-type (WT) and ARE-Del T cells show substantially higher *Ifng* mRNA and IFN-γ protein levels in ARE-Del T cells compared to WT T cells (*see* Fig. 2d).

Combined, Flow-FISH is an effective tool to simultaneously measure mRNA and protein production in T cells. This protocol describes in a step-by-step fashion how to perform a controlled Flow-FISH experiment.

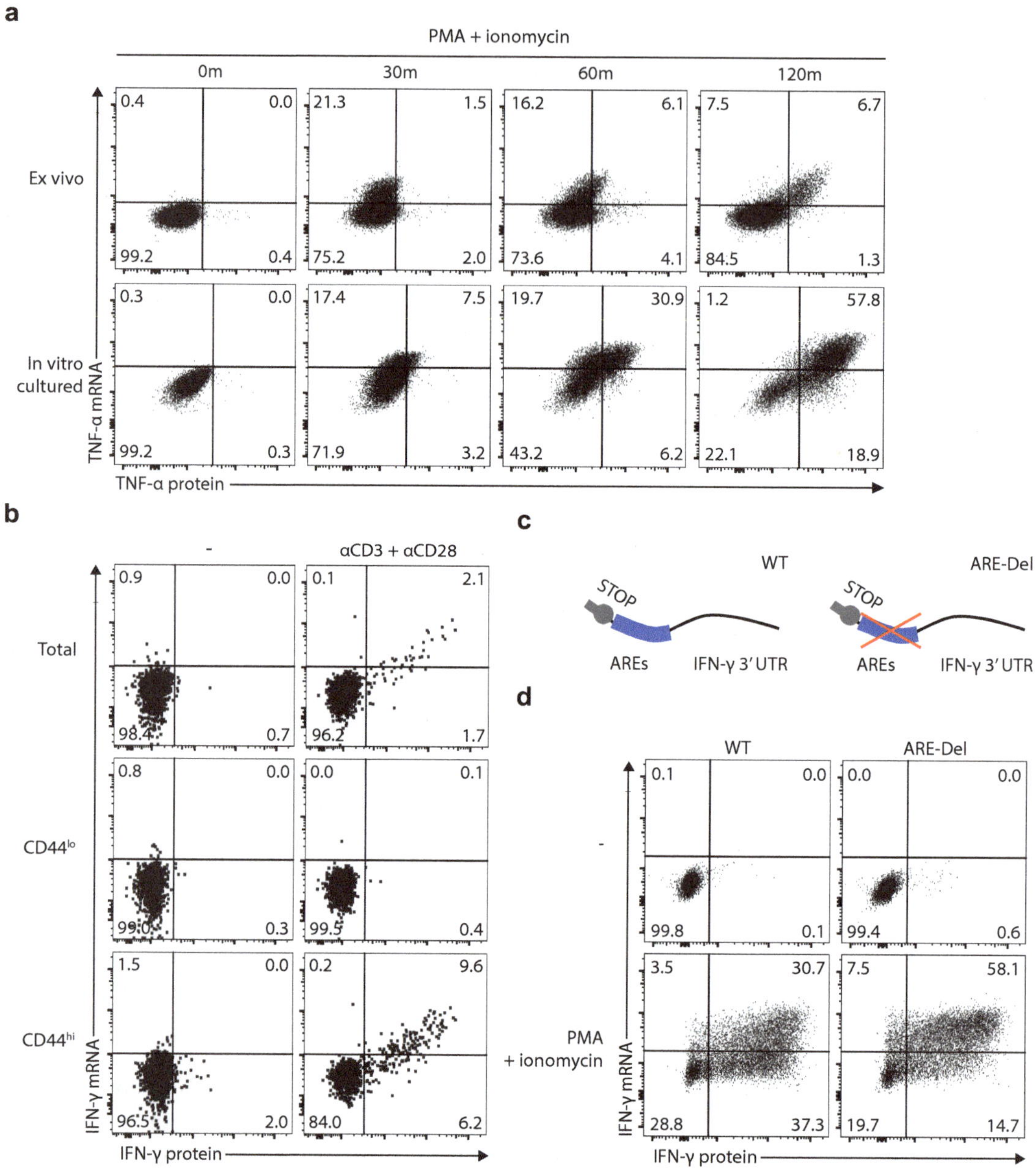

Fig. 2 Possible applications for Flow-FISH. (**a**) Human T cells from one donor were analyzed directly after thawing, or after 2d αCD3 + αCD28 activation and subsequent in vitro culture for *TNFA* mRNA and TNF-α protein levels by Flow-FISH upon PMA + ionomycin activation for indicated time points in the presence of monensin. (**b**) T cells from a murine spleen were enriched by CD8-negative MACS selection and activated for 4 h with αCD3 + αCD28, or left untreated (−), both in the presence of monensin. *Ifng* mRNA and IFN-γ protein levels were measured by Flow-FISH for all T cells, and CD44^{hi} memory-like T and CD44^{lo} naïve T cells were gated using extracellular markers. (**c**) Graphical representation of the *Ifng* locus of WT mouse strain, and of ARE-Del mice that bear a germ-line deletion of AU-rich elements in the 3′UTR of the Ifng gene [34]. (**d**) CD8^{+} OT-I T cells from WT and ARE-Del mice were activated for 4 h with PMA + ionomycin or left untreated (−), both in the presence of monensin. *Ifng* mRNA and IFN-γ protein levels were measured by Flow-FISH

2 Materials

2.1 T Cell Activation

1. (Isolated) human/murine T cells (*see* **Notes 1** and **2**).
2. Medium: Iscove's Modified Dulbecco's Medium (IMDM), supplemented with 8% heat-inactivated fetal calf serum (FCS), 2 mM L-glutamine, 20 U/mL penicillin G sodium, 20 μg/mL streptomycin sulfate, and for murine T cells 15 μM 2-mercaptoethanol.
3. Stimuli: αCD3 + αCD28, PMA + Ionomycin, target cells expressing the antigen, and soluble peptide [GP_{33}, NP_{396}, or $OVA_{257-264}$], or peptide pools (*see* **Note 3**).
4. Monensin (Thermo Fisher Scientific).
5. Plates and tubes: Polystyrene 96-well F-bottom or V-bottom plates or 1.5 mL Lo-Bind Eppendorf tubes (*see* **Note 4**).

2.2 Staining with Antibodies and FISH Probes

1. FACS buffer: 1× Phosphate-buffered saline (PBS) supplemented with 1% FCS and 2 mM EDTA. Store at 4 °C.
2. Cell surface antibodies for separating T cell populations (*see* **Notes 5–8**).
3. Fixable live/dead dye (i.e., Near-IR Dead Cell Stain Kit, Thermo Fisher Scientific).
4. Fixation/Permeabilization Solution kit (BD Biosciences).
5. RNAse A/B/C inhibitor (New England Biolabs) (*see* **Note 9**).
6. Perm/Wash solution: Dilute BD Perm/Wash™ buffer 1:10 in RNAse-free water. Store at 4 °C. The buffer can be used for subsequent experiments. Before use, take the necessary amount and add 4 IU/mL RNAse inhibitor (*see* **Note 10**).
7. Intracellular protein antibodies: αIFN-γ-eF450 (eBioscience clone 4S.B3), αTNF-α-BV785 (Biolegend clone MAb11), or αIFN-γ-PE (clone XMG1.2, eBioscience) (*see* **Notes 5**, **11**, and **12**).
8. FISH probes (custom design, *see* **Notes 13–19**).
9. 20× SSC buffer: RNAse-free water, 3 M sodium chloride, and 0.3 M sodium citrate. Store at 4 °C. The buffer can be used for subsequent experiments. If the buffer contains crystals, prepare fresh.
10. Flow-FISH wash buffer: 30 mL RNAse-free water, 5 mL de-ionized formamide (Sigma Aldrich), and 5 mL 20× SSC. Before use, add 40 IU RNAse inhibitor/mL (*see* **Note 9**). Prepare fresh for each experiment for optimal results.
11. Flow-FISH hybridization buffer: Combine 8 mL RNAse-free water, 1 mL de-ionized formamide, 1 mL 20× SSC, and 1 g dextran sodium sulfate salts (Sigma Aldrich). Of note, dextran

sodium sulfate salts will require thorough mixing or vortexing to dissolve. Can be stored at 4 °C and used in sequential experiments. Before use, take the necessary amount and add 40 IU RNAse inhibitor/mL (*see* **Note 10**).

12. 1.5 mL Lo-Bind Eppendorf tubes.
13. 96-Well V-bottom plates.
14. 5 mL Polystyrene round-bottom tubes (Corning, 352058).
15. RNAse-free pipette tips (*see* **Note 10**).
16. Swing-out centrifuge (*see* **Note 20**).
17. Plate centrifuge.
18. Thermocycler.

3 Methods

3.1 Stimulation and Extracellular Staining of Human and Murine CD8⁺ T Cells

1. Activate 3×10^5 [human] or 1×10^6 cells [murine] in 200 μL medium containing the stimulus of choice and 2 μM monensin in a sterile 96-well plate according to standard operating procedure or as described in [29, 31]. Include a sample without the stimulus as control. Cover the plate with a lid and culture cells for the desired amount of time in a humidified incubator at 37 °C + 5% CO_2 (*see* **Notes 1–4**).
2. Remove plate from incubator. Depending on the preference of the experimenter, samples can be transferred into tubes now or at Subheading 3.2, **step 3** [human]/Subheading 3.3, **step 6** [murine]. Otherwise, perform surface antibody staining in the stimulation vessel. In case plate-bound antibodies were used for activation, transfer cells to tubes or to a 96-well V-bottom plate. Spin for 3 min at 650 × *g*, maximum acceleration and brake, at 4 °C. Of note, all subsequent centrifugation steps are all performed with maximum acceleration and brake. Remove supernatant.
3. Add desired surface antibodies as for regular flow cytometry in 30 μL FACS-buffer and resuspend by pipetting. Incubate for 20 min at 4 °C in the dark (*see* **Notes 5–7**).
4. Add 150 μL FACS-buffer and spin for 3 min at 650 × *g* at 4 °C. Remove supernatant.
5. Add 50 μL Perm/FIX solution. Resuspend the cell pellet either by briefly vortexing or pipetting and incubate for 20–30 min at 4 °C in the dark (*see* **Note 10**).

The protocol for human and murine T cells diverges here. The original protocol developed for human T cells [29] required slight alterations to preserve the protein staining of cytokines in murine T cells [31].

3.2 Intracellular mRNA and Protein Staining of Human CD8$^+$ T Cells

1. During fixation, prepare the hybridization mix by denaturing FISH probes in 20 μL RNAse-free water. Heat to 65 °C for 5 min in a thermocycler (*see* **Notes 13–19**).
2. After cooling down to room temperature, add the intracellular antibodies to the denatured FISH probes and add 4 IU/mL RNAse inhibitor. Incubate at RT in the dark for 5 min to allow the neutralization of RNAses (*see* **Notes 5** and **11**).
3. Prepare hybridization solution by diluting the denatured FISH probes and intracellular antibodies from Subheading 3.3, **step 2**, in RNAse inhibitor pretreated hybridization buffer. Adjust for the number of samples and the final concentration of probes to be added to the sample, as determined by a probe titration assay (*see* **Note 17**); i.e., *for 5 samples, add 80 μL hybridization buffer to the 20 μL containing 1 μL of probes from* ***step 1***.
4. After fixation, add 150 μL RNAse inhibitor pretreated Perm/Wash solution to the cells and transfer to 1.5 mL Lo-bind Eppendorf tubes. Add 1 mL RNAse inhibitor pretreated Flow-FISH wash buffer and spin cells for 5 min at 570 × *g* at room temperature in a swing-out centrifuge (*see* **Note 20**).
5. Remove supernatant while leaving a small "dead" volume of ±50 μL, as to not disturb the cell pellet and thus limit cell loss. Add 50 μL of hybridization mix containing the FISH probes and the intracellular antibodies as prepared in **step 3**. Vortex 2 s to resuspend the pellet or scratch the bottom of the tube on a rack.
6. Incubate overnight at 37 °C + 5% CO_2 in a humidified incubator.
7. Wash cells by adding 1 mL RNAse inhibitor pretreated Flow-FISH wash buffer and spin cells for 10 min at 570 × *g* at room temperature in a swing-out centrifuge.
8. Remove supernatant while leaving ±100 μL, as to not disturb the cell pellet. Resuspend the cell pellet in the residual volume and transfer to a 5 mL polystyrene round-bottom tube and measure mRNA and protein levels on a suitable flow cytometer.

3.3 Intracellular mRNA and Protein Staining of Murine CD8$^+$ T Cells

1. During fixation, pipette the required amount of intracellular antibodies into RNAse-free tubes (*see* **Notes 5** and **12**). Deactivate RNAses present in the antibodies by adding 4 IU/mL RNAse inhibitor to intracellular antibodies and incubate at 4 °C for 10 min. Denature FISH probes in 20 μL RNAse-free water by heating to 65 °C for 5 min in a thermocycler (*see* **Notes 13–19**).
2. After fixation, add 150 μL RNAse inhibitor pretreated Perm/Wash solution to the cells and spin for 3 min at 650 × *g* at 4 °C. Remove supernatant.

3. Perform intracellular staining by adding desired intracellular antibodies prepared in **step 1** in 30 μL RNAse inhibitor pretreated Perm/Wash solution and resuspend by pipetting. Incubate for 20 min at 4 °C in the dark.
4. Wash cells with 150 μL RNAse inhibitor pretreated Perm/Wash solution and spin cells for 3 min at 650 × *g* at 4 °C. Remove supernatant.
5. Wash cells twice with 200 μL RNAse inhibitor pretreated Flow-FISH wash buffer. Between washes, spin cells for 3 min at 650 × *g* at 4 °C. Remove supernatant.
6. Prepare hybridization solution by diluting the denatured FISH probes from **step 1** in RNAse inhibitor pretreated hybridization buffer. Adjust for the amount of samples and the final concentration of probes to be added to the sample, as determined by a probe titration assay (*see* **Note 17**); i.e., *for 5 samples, add 80 μL hybridization buffer to the 20 μL containing 1 μL of probes from* ***step 1***.
7. Resuspend cells in 50 μL RNAse inhibitor pretreated Flow-FISH wash buffer and transfer to 1.5 mL Lo-Bind Eppendorf tube. Add 50 μL of hybridization buffer supplemented with FISH probes as prepared in **step 6**.
8. Incubate overnight at 37 °C + 5% CO_2 in a humidified incubator.
9. Prior to acquisition, wash cells by adding 1 mL RNAse inhibitor pretreated Flow-FISH wash buffer and spin cells for 10 min at 570 × *g* at room temperature in a swing-out centrifuge (*see* **Note 20**). Remove supernatant while leaving a small "dead" volume of ±100 μL, as to not disturb the cell pellet.
10. Resuspend the cell pellet by pipetting in the residual volume and transfer to a 5 mL polystyrene round-bottom tube. Measure mRNA and protein levels on a suitable flow cytometer.

4 Notes

1. The authors have successfully studied the cytokine mRNA and protein levels in T cells isolated from fresh and cryopreserved human PBMCs, and from different mouse organs. Both unsorted bulk single-cell solutions, FACS/MACS-isolated T cells and cultured T cells were used.
2. For reproducible results, 3×10^5 [human] or 1×10^6 [murine] cells per condition are recommended to limit cell loss during this assay. Authors found that cell loss can be up to 30–50% of the input due to, e.g., fragility and stickiness of cells to tubes during the procedure. If studying lower cells numbers,

irrelevant cells can be spiked in to prevent loss of the cells of interest. When performing Flow-FISH on other cell types, the required cell numbers may have to be reassessed.

3. For both human and murine CD8$^+$ T cells, authors use 10 ng/mL PMA and 1 μM ionomycin (both Sigma Aldrich), or 1 μg/mL (human, clone Hit3a)/2 μg/mL (murine, clone 17.A2, Bioceros) αCD3 and 1 μg/mL αCD28 (human clone CD28.2, murine clone PV-1). When using peptide (pools), authors use between 1 and 5 μg/mL.
4. Authors prefer activation in 96-well V-bottom plate (human and murine) or 1.5 mL Lo-Bind Eppendorf tubes (human). If required, 96-well F- or U-bottom plates are also suitable, but might reduce cell numbers due to having to pass cells to a suitable vessel for staining procedures.
5. Not all fluorophores are compatible with the buffers used in this protocol. For instance, some tandem dyes may disintegrate. Table 1 depicts the fluorophores that the authors have tested.
6. Human CD8$^+$ T cells were stained with Near-IR viability dye (BD Biosciences, 1:800) and αCD8-BV605 (Biolegend clone RPA-T8, 1:200). When studying different T cell populations, this panel can be expanded upon by including, i.e., αCD4, αCD27, and/or αCD45RA [29].
7. Murine CD8$^+$ T cells were stained with Near-IR viability dye (1:800), αCD8a-AF488 (Biolegend clone 53-6.7, 1:200), and αCD44-PE-Cy7 (Biolegend clone IM7, 1:300).
8. Labeling T cells with APC- and/or PE-labeled MHC class I tetramers could be compatible with the Flow-FISH protocol and may be used to study antigen-specific T cells.

Table 1
Fluorophores suitable for Flow-FISH experiments

Suitable		Not suitable
AF488	BV605	PerCP-Cy5.5
AF700	BV785	PE-Cy5.5
APC	eF450	Qdots
APC-Cy7	FITC	
BV421	PE	
BV510	PE-Cy7	

AF Alexa Fluor, *APC* allophycocyanin, *BV* Brilliant Violet, *eF* eFluor, *FITC* fluorescin, *PE* phycoerythrin

9. Authors recommend using an RNAse inhibitor without requirements for DTT, as DTT can affect the FISH staining.
10. Due to the cell permeabilization, RNAs are exposed to RNAses from the outside. Therefore, supplementing buffers and reagents with RNAse inhibitors and the use of RNAse-free tips is essential from this step onward.
11. Human T cells were stained with αIFN-γ-eF450 (eBioscience clone 4S.B3) or αTNF-α-BV785 (Biolegend clone MAb11). All antibody dilutions: 1:100. When studying other intracellular proteins of interest, this panel can be expanded upon by including, i.e., αIL-2 [29].
12. Murine T cells were stained with αIFN-γ-PE or PE-Cy7 (clone XMG1.2, eBioscience, 1:200. When studying other intracellular proteins of interest, this panel can be expanded upon by including, i.e., αTNF-α and αIL-2 [31].
13. Best results were achieved when measuring activation-induced gene products. This also facilitates the probe setup and probeset validation.
14. Authors used Quasar 570 or 670-labeled probes (Biosearchtech) to simultaneously measure mRNA and protein levels of more than one gene product [29]. Probes can also be custom-labeled [35], which allows for the expansion of the fluorophore panel and hence the number of RNAs that can be simultaneously measured.
15. A minimum of 25 unique probes per target is recommended to achieve optimal signal-to-noise ratio [36]. Therefore, smFISH is limited to RNA molecules with a length of at least 550 nucleotides.
16. Online tools can be used for probe design, e.g., https://www.biosearchtech.com. Authors verified probe specificity with BlastN (NCBI), and eliminated all probes that showed >90% homology in the same species with a second target, in particular when this gene was highly expressed in the cells of interest. To determine gene expression in immune cells, authors used ImmGen (https://www.immgen.org).
17. Authors determined the optimal probe concentration in a titration assay (*see* Fig. 3a). Both human and murine mRNA probes for IFN-γ and human mRNA probes for TNF-α, were used at a final probe concentration of 15 nM, equating to ~1 μL of probes (at a concentration of 15 μM)/5 samples. Of note, the concentration will have to be adjusted to the number of samples and cells used.
18. To determine background staining by the RNA probes, a competition assay with unlabeled cold probes can be performed (*see* Fig. 3b).
19. Fluorescence intensity and background fluorescence can be assessed with a nonrelevant probeset labeled with an identical fluorophore. A nonspecific probeset targeting a gene that is not

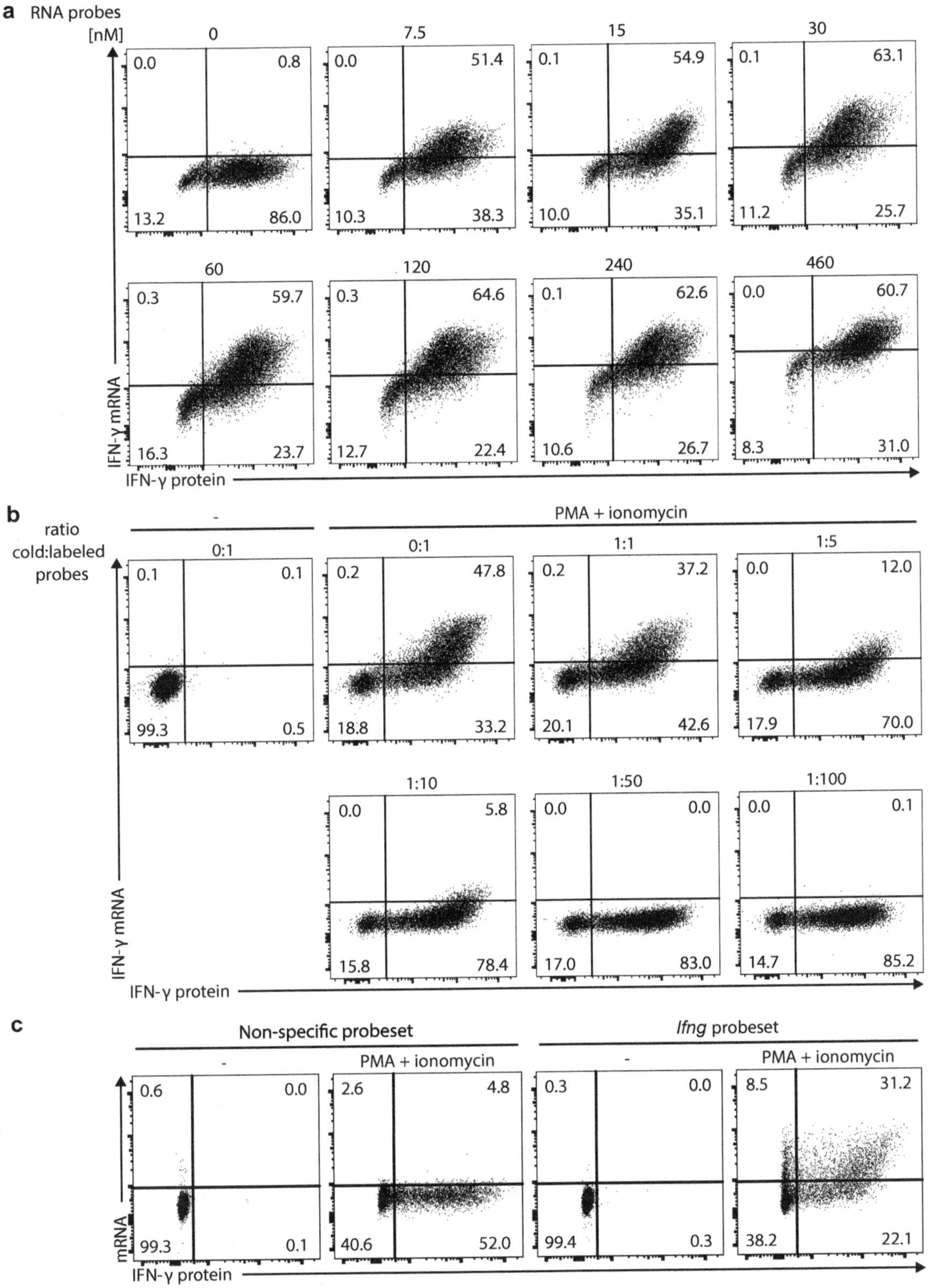

Fig. 3 Validation assays for Flow-FISH. $CD8^+$ OT-I T cells were activated for 4 h with PMA + ionomycin. Nonactivated cells stained with identical concentrations of *Ifng* probes were used to set the gate. All cells were cultured in the presence of monensin. (**a**) The optimal concentration for the *Ifng* mRNA staining was determined by adding increasing amounts of labeled probes. (**b**) The probe-signal for the *Ifng* probeset was validated by adding in increasing amounts of unlabeled sequence-identical probes. (**c**) *Ifng* probeset specificity was determined by using a non-related probeset directed against *PHOX2B* from a different species (human)

expressed in the cell type of interest, or that is from a different species, should be used (*see* Fig. 3c).

20. Using a swing-out centrifuge significantly increases the yield of cells after centrifugation.

Acknowledgments

We thank A. Guislain, M. Hansen, and B. Popovic for critical reading of this manuscript. This work was supported by the Landsteiner Foundation of Blood Transfusion Research (LSBR) [LSBR Fellowship 1373] and by the Dutch Science Foundation [VIDI Grant 917.14.214] to M.C.W. Julian J. Freen-van Heeren and Benoit P. Nicolet contributed equally to this work.

References

1. Pilarski LM, Carayanniotis G (1985) Generation of cytotoxic T cells specific for minor histocompatibility antigens by cross challenge in vitro with H-2 disparate adherent cells. J Immunol 135:3686–3690
2. Parker DC (1993) T cell-dependent B-cell activation. Annu Rev Immunol 11:331–360. https://doi.org/10.1146/annurev.iy.11.040193.001555
3. Medzhitov R, Janeway CA (2002) Decoding the patterns of self and nonself by the innate immune system. Science 296:298–300. https://doi.org/10.1126/science.1068883
4. Akira S, Uematsu S, Takeuchi O (2006) Pathogen recognition and innate immunity. Cell 124(4):783–801. https://doi.org/10.1016/j.cell.2006.02.015
5. Naito T, Tanaka H, Naoe Y, Taniuchi I (2011) Transcriptional control of T-cell development. Int Immunol 23:661–668. https://doi.org/10.1093/intimm/dxr078
6. Chen L, Flies DB (2013) Molecular mechanisms of T cell co-stimulation and co-inhibition. Nat Rev Immunol 13:227–242. https://doi.org/10.1038/nri3405
7. Rothenberg EV (2014) The chromatin landscape and transcription factors in T-cell programming. Trends Immunol 35:195–204. https://doi.org/10.1016/j.neuroimage.2013.08.045
8. Harty JT, Tvinnereim AR, White DW (2000) $CD8^+$ T cell effector mechanisms in resistance to infection. Annu Rev Immunol 18:275–308. https://doi.org/10.1146/annurev.immunol.18.1.275
9. Brehm MA, Daniels KA, Welsh RM (2005) Rapid production of TNF-alpha following TCR engagement of naive CD8 T cells. J Immunol 175:5043–5049. https://doi.org/10.4049/jimmunol.175.8.5043
10. Dinarello CA (2007) Historical review of cytokines. Eur J Immunol 37:S34–S45. https://doi.org/10.1002/eji.200737772
11. Zhu J, Paul WE (2008) CD4 T cells: fates, functions and faults. Blood 112:1557–1568. https://doi.org/10.1182/blood-2008-05-078154
12. Murali-Krishna K, Altman JD, Suresh M et al (1998) Counting antigen-specific CD8 T cells: a reevaluation of bystander activation during viral infection. Immunity 8:177–187. https://doi.org/10.1016/S1074-7613(00)80470-7
13. Huse M, Lillemeier BF, Kuhns MS et al (2006) T cells use two directionally distinct pathways for cytokine secretion. Nat Immunol 7:247–255. https://doi.org/10.1038/ni1304
14. Peixoto A, Evaristo C, Munitic I et al (2007) CD8 single-cell gene coexpression reveals three different effector types present at distinct phases of the immune response. J Exp Med 204:1193–1205. https://doi.org/10.1084/jem.20062349
15. Denton AE, Russ BE, Doherty PC et al (2011) Differentiation-dependent functional and epigenetic landscapes for cytokine genes in virus-specific CD8 + T cells. Proc Natl Acad Sci 108:15306–15311. https://doi.org/10.1073/pnas.1112520108
16. Han Q, Bagheri N, Bradshaw EM et al (2012) Polyfunctional responses by human T cells result from sequential release of cytokines.

Proc Natl Acad Sci 109:1607–1612. https://doi.org/10.1073/pnas.1117194109
17. Mahata B, Zhang X, Kolodziejczyk AA et al (2014) Single-cell RNA sequencing reveals T helper cells synthesizing steroids De Novo to contribute to immune homeostasis. Cell Rep 7:1130–1142. https://doi.org/10.1016/j.celrep.2014.04.011
18. Patel AP, Tirosh I, Trombetta JJ et al (2014) Single-cell RNA-seq highlights intratumoral heterogeneity in primary glioblastoma. Science 344:1396–1401. https://doi.org/10.1126/science.1254257
19. Tirosh I, Izar B, Prakadan SM et al (2016) Dissecting the multicellular ecosystem of metastatic melanoma by single-cell RNA-seq. Science 352:189–196. https://doi.org/10.1126/science.aad0501
20. Cuadrado E, van den Biggelaar M, de Kivit S et al (2018) Proteomic analyses of human regulatory T cells reveal adaptations in signaling pathways that protect cellular identity. Immunity 48:1046–1059, e6. https://doi.org/10.1016/j.immuni.2018.04.008
21. Salerno F, Paolini NA, Stark R et al (2017) Distinct PKC-mediated posttranscriptional events set cytokine production kinetics in CD8 + T cells. Proc Natl Acad Sci 114:9677–9682. https://doi.org/10.1073/pnas.1704227114
22. Déry RE, Lin TJ, Befus AD et al (2000) Redundancy or cell-type-specific regulation? Tumour necrosis factor in alveolar macrophages and mast cells. Immunology 99:427–434. https://doi.org/10.1046/J.1365-2567.2000.00982.X
23. Stoecklin G, Lu M, Rattenbacher B, Moroni C (2003) A constitutive decay element promotes tumor necrosis factor alpha mRNA degradation via an AU-rich element-independent pathway. Mol Cell Biol 23:3506–3515. https://doi.org/10.1128/MCB.23.10.3506-3515.2003
24. Salerno F, Engels S, van den Biggelaar M et al (2018) Translational repression of pre-formed cytokine-encoding mRNA prevents chronic activation of memory T cells. Nat Immunol 19:828–837. https://doi.org/10.1038/s41590-018-0155-6
25. Salerno F, Guislain A, Freen-van Heeren JJ et al (2018) Critical role of post-transcriptional regulation for IFN-γ in tumor-infiltrating T cells. Oncoimmunology 8:e1532762. https://doi.org/10.1080/2162402X.2018.1532762
26. Nicolet BP, Salerno F, Wolkers MC (2017) Visualizing the life of mRNA in T cells. Biochem Soc Trans 45:563–570. https://doi.org/10.1042/BST20170003
27. Freen-van Heeren JJ, Nicolet BP, Wolkers MC (2018) Measuring T cell responses by flow cytometry-based fluorescence in situ hybridization. Crit Rev Immunol 38:131–143. https://doi.org/10.1615/CritRevImmunol.2018025938
28. Porichis F, Hart MG, Griesbeck M et al (2014) High-throughput detection of miRNAs and gene-specific mRNA at the single-cell level by flow cytometry. Nat Commun 5:5641. https://doi.org/10.1038/ncomms6641
29. Nicolet BP, Guislain A, Wolkers MC (2017) Combined single-cell measurement of cytokine mRNA and protein identifies T cells with persistent effector function. J Immunol 198:962–970. https://doi.org/10.4049/jimmunol.1601531
30. Arrigucci R, Lakehal K, Vir P et al (2018) Active tuberculosis is characterized by highly differentiated effector memory Th1 cells. Front Immunol 9:1–9. https://doi.org/10.3389/fimmu.2018.02127
31. Salerno F, Freen-van Heeren JJ, Guislain A et al (2019) Costimulation through TLR2 drives polyfunctional $CD8^+$ T cell responses. J Immunol 202:714–723. https://doi.org/10.4049/jimmunol.1801026
32. Broeren CPM, Gray GS, Carreno BM, June CH (2000) Costimulation light: activation of $CD4^+$ T cells with CD80 or CD86 rather than anti-CD28 leads to a Th2 cytokine profile. J Immunol 165:6908–6914. https://doi.org/10.4049/jimmunol.165.12.6908
33. Yu SF, Zhang YN, Yang BY, Wu CY (2014) Human memory, but not naive, $CD4^+$ T cells expressing transcription factor T-bet might drive rapid cytokine. J Biol Chem 289:35561–35569. https://doi.org/10.1074/jbc.M114.608745
34. Hodge DL, Berthet C, Coppola V et al (2014) IFN-gamma AU-rich element removal promotes chronic IFN-gamma expression and autoimmunity in mice. J Autoimmun 53:33–45. https://doi.org/10.1016/j.jaut.2014.02.003
35. Gaspar I, Wippich F, Ephrussi A (2017) Enzymatic production of single-molecule FISH and RNA capture probes. RNA 23:1582–1591. https://doi.org/10.1261/rna.061184.117
36. Raj A, van den Bogaard P, Rifkin SA et al (2008) Imaging individual mRNA molecules using multiple singly labeled probes. Nat Methods 5:877–879. https://doi.org/10.1038/nmeth.1253

Chapter 23

Microscopic Methods for Analysis of Macrophage-Induced Tunneling Nanotubes

Kiersten P. Carter, Jeffrey E. Segall, and Dianne Cox

Abstract

Macrophages are known to play multiple roles in the breast cancer microenvironment including the promotion of tumor cell invasion that is dependent on soluble factors or through direct contact. Macrophages can also enhance the production of Tunneling Nanotubes (TNTs) in tumor cells which can be mimicked using macrophage-conditioned medium. TNTs are long thin F-actin structures that connect two or more cells together that have been found in many different cell types including macrophages and tumor cells and have been implicated in enhancing tumor cells functions, such as invasion. Here we describe basic procedures used to stimulate tumor cell TNT formation through macrophage-conditioned medium along with methods for quantifying TNTs.

Key words Tunneling nanotubes, Macrophages, Tumor cell, Microscopy, Conditioned medium

1 Introduction

Metastasis is the leading cause of death in breast cancer. It has been shown that tumor progression can be enhanced when macrophages interact with tumor cells, resulting in an increase in migration, co-invasion, and intravasation of the tumor cells leading to metastasis [1, 2]. Macrophages are immune cells that respond to inflammation through cytokines secreted by the resident tissue. They aid in removal of debris and can secrete cytokines that either recruit other immune cells or dampen the immune response [3]. Additionally, tumor-associated macrophages have been shown to take part in a paracrine interaction with tumor cells where tumor cell secretion of colony-stimulating factor 1 (CSF1) induces macrophages to secrete factors such as epidermal growth factor (EGF) that promote tumor invasion and progression [4, 5].

It has recently been shown that macrophages and tumor cells also employ a novel means of communication through structures known as tunneling nanotubes (TNTs) or membrane nanotubes [6]. TNTs are long thin, membranous F-actin containing

Ivana Vancurova and Yan Zhu (eds.), *Immune Mediators in Cancer: Methods and Protocols*, Methods in Molecular Biology, vol. 2108, https://doi.org/10.1007/978-1-0716-0247-8_23, © Springer Science+Business Media, LLC, part of Springer Nature 2020

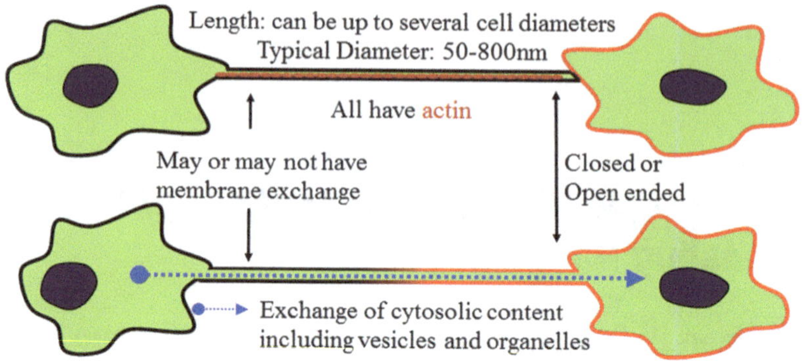

Fig. 1 Schematic illustration of TNTs showing both open and closed TNTs

structures that connect two cells and allow transfer of signals. They can be hundreds of microns long but vary in diameter from 50 to 800 nm and can either be closed (no cytoplasmic connection between cells) or open (cytoplasmic connection between cells) (diagramed in Fig. 1). When TNTs are open they can transport cytoplasmic signals, mRNA, miRNA, vesicles, and other organelles between cells. In addition, TNTs can be homotypic (connecting to cells of the same type) or heterotypic (connecting to cells of different types). For example, when in coculture tumor cells and macrophages can form heterotypic TNTs that are important for co-invasion [7]. It has also been shown that macrophage-conditioned medium can stimulate homotypic TNTs in breast tumor cells in vitro [8, 9]. However, quantitation of TNTs can be challenging. Some studies quantify the number of TNT-like protrusions per cell [10], in others every TNT connection per cell is counted [8], while we and others only count the number of TNT-connected cell pairs [11]. Additionally, some studies utilize fixation and subsequent immunofluorescent microscopy to identify TNTs, which is known to reduce TNT numbers through breakage especially for the thinner TNTs. These differences make it difficult to compare results between studies. Here we describe a method to quantify TNTs by live cell imaging microscopy as an attempt for standardization of TNT scoring.

2 Materials

1. Murine monocyte/macrophage RAW264.7 subline LR5 [12] (*see* **Note 1**).
2. Macrophage medium: RPMI 1640 containing L-glutamine, 10% heat-activated newborn serum, 1% penicillin/streptomycin solution.
3. Rat adenocarcinoma MTLn3 cells (*see* **Note 2**).

4. MTLn3 medium—Minimal Essential Medium (α-MEM): containing L-glutamine, 5% fetal bovine serum (FBS), 1% penicillin/streptomycin (*see* **Note 3**).
5. Sterile 10 mM EDTA/PBS (pH 7.4).
6. 15 mL Falcon tubes.
7. 0.22 μm Syringe filter.
8. Eppendorf centrifuge 58 10 R.
9. 10 cm Tissue culture-treated dishes.
10. 35 mm Glass Bottom No. 1.5, uncoated, gamma-irradiated Mat-Tek dishes.
11. Hemocytometer.
12. 0.05% Trypsin, 0.53 mM EDTA without sodium bicarbonate.
13. Buffer with Divalent (BWD): 20 mM HEPES, 125 mM NaCl, 5 mM KCl, 5 mM dextrose, 10 mM $NaHCO_3$, 1 mM KH_2PO_4, 1 mM $CaCl_2$, and 1 mM $MgCl_2$, pH 7.4.
14. Inverted fluorescent microscope: We use an Olympus IX71 inverted microscope with planapo phase contrast 60× NA objective with a Cooke Sensicam and Photometrics Coolsnap, HQ.

3 Methods

3.1 Preparation of Macrophage-Conditioned Medium

1. Thaw frozen vial of RAW/LR5 macrophages by placing in a 37 °C water bath for 2–3 min.
2. Dilute DMSO by adding mostly thawed cell suspension to 15 mL Falcon tube with 9 mL of appropriate medium.
3. Centrifuge at 400 × *g*, 25 °C, for 3 min.
4. Aspirate supernatant and resuspend pellet in 10 mL of macrophage medium, place cell solution into a 10 cm tissue culture-treated dish in incubator at 37 °C with 5% CO_2.
5. Wait until cells reach 70–80% confluence (*see* **Note 4**).
6. Harvest cells by quickly rinsing cells once with PBS to remove floating cells and medium components followed by incubation in 2 mL of sterile 10 mM EDTA/PBS at 37 °C/5% CO_2 for approximately 5–10 min until cells are detached.
7. Add 2 mL of macrophage medium to plate and transfer the 4 mL of cell suspension to a 15 mL Falcon tube and centrifuge at 400 × *g*, 25 °C, for 3 min.
8. Aspirate supernatant and resuspend pellet in 1 mL of macrophage medium.
9. Determine the cell concentration using the hemocytometer.

10. Plate RAW/LR5 cells in MTLn3 medium so that the cells are at approximately 90% confluency. For RAW/LR5 cells, we normally plate 9×10^5 cells per 10 cm dish but this number would vary depending on the type of macrophages used and the size of dish (*see* **Note 5**).
11. Incubate at 37 °C in a 5% CO_2 incubator overnight.
12. Next day, collect medium without lifting cells using a 10 mL syringe and filter with a 0.22 μm syringe filter. After filtering, the macrophage-conditioned medium can be used immediately, placed in −20 °C freezer for use later in the week, or kept at −80 °C for long-term storage.

3.2 Tumor Cell TNT Induction with Macrophage-Conditioned Medium

1. Thaw rat adenocarcinoma MTLn3 cells as described in Subheading 3.1, **steps 1–3**, but using MTLn3 medium.
2. Grow cells in a 10 cm plate in 10 mL of MTLn3 medium in a 37 °C incubator with 5% CO_2 until cells reach 70–80% confluence. Be careful not to allow cells to become too confluent (*see* **Note 4**).
3. Aspirate medium and wash with 2 mL of 1× PBS. Lift cells using 2 mL of 0.05% Trypsin, 0.53 mM EDTA. Wait 10–15 min or until cells are in suspension.
4. Add 2 mL of MTLn3 medium to plate to inactivate the trypsin and transfer the 4 mL of cell suspension to a 15 mL Falcon tube.
5. Centrifuge at 400 × *g* at 25 °C for 3 min and aspirate supernatant. Resuspend pellet in 1 mL of MTLn3 medium.
6. Plate 1×10^5 tumor cells in a 35 mm Glass Bottom No. 1.5, uncoated, gamma-irradiated Mat-Tek dish per condition.
7. To determine the basal number of tumor cell TNTs, MTLn3 cells are plated in 2 mL of MTLn3 medium and placed in a 37 °C incubator with 5% CO_2 overnight.
8. To determine the effect of macrophage-conditioned medium on tumor cell, TNTs-MTLn3 cells are plated in a 50:50 ratio of MTLn3 medium:macrophage-conditioned medium. Place dish in a 37 °C incubator with 5% CO_2 overnight.

3.3 Live Cell Imaging of Tumor Cell TNTs

As noted by us and others, TNTs can be very fragile, and many are broken during fixation. Therefore, we prefer to utilize the live cell imaging method described below. An example of a live cell image of a TNT is shown in Fig. 2. It is possible to use fixation followed by fluorescent staining (*see* **Note 6**).

1. Replace medium with BWD to avoid autofluorescence due to components in the medium.

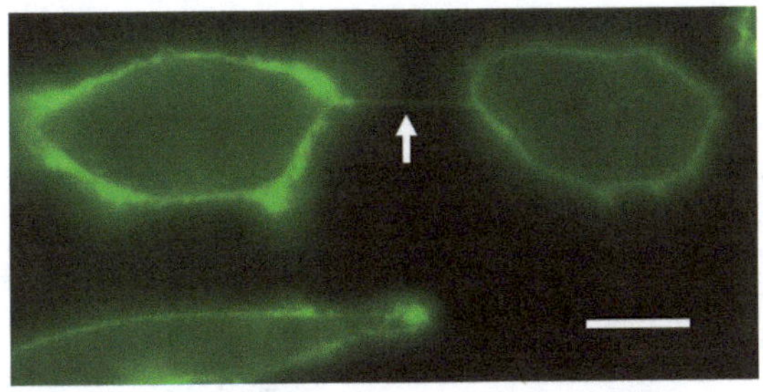

Fig. 2 Live cell confocal imaging of MTLn3 cells treated with macrophage-conditioned medium and stained with Alexa488 WGA. Cells appear to be out of focus since the image is focused in the plane of the TNT which is suspended above the substrate. Arrow indicates a TNT. Scale bar = 10 μm

2. TNTs can be identified by phase contrast microscopy, but it is preferable to include a fluorescent dye that labels the plasma membrane by adding 1 μg/mL Alexa Fluor™ conjugated Wheat Germ Agglutinin or 1:1000 dilution of FM1-43FX directly into the BWD in the Mat-Tek dish immediately before imaging. It is also possible to use tumor cells expressing a genetically encoded fluorescent protein targeted to the membrane, such as mCherry, with a fused CAAX motif [7].
3. Place the dish on the stage of an Olympus IX71 fluorescent microscope using a 60× oil NA 1.43 objective.
4. Focus lens using the coarse focus until cells are in view, and then use the fine focus adjustment until cells can be clearly seen attached to the substrate. Search the field for thin, tubular structures. To verify that a structure is a TNT at least part of the structure must be off of the substrate, move the fine focus adjustment above and below the plane of focus. When going in and out of the plane of focus, you will see part of the structure fade away while the other part of the structure becomes visible indicating that part of the structure is above the substrate (*see* **Note** 7).

3.4 Quantification of Tunneling Nanotubes

TNTs are identified and quantified as long thin connections between two cells that are at least 8 μm in length where at least part of the TNT is not in contact with the substrate (as described in [7, 13]). In some cases, the kinetics of TNT precursors or protrusions can be analyzed (*see* **Note 8**).

1. Cells counted as negative for TNTs must be within one cell body length of another cell without touching any other cell.
2. Each cell containing a TNT that is connected to another cell is counted as positive. A minimum of 128 cells are normally counted per sample and at least three independent experiments are needed for statistical analysis. The data reported are the

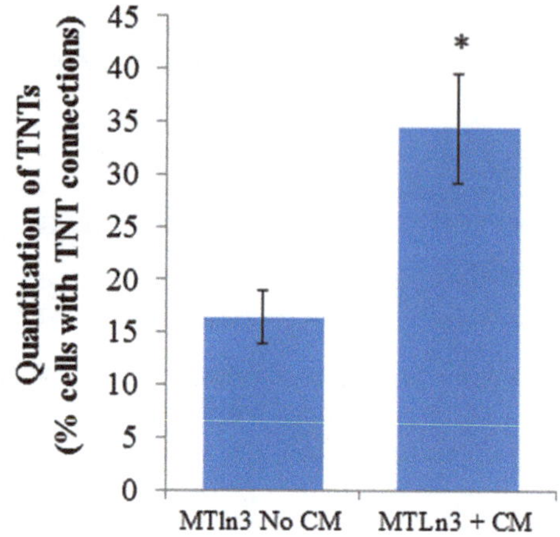

Fig. 3 MTLn3 cells untreated or treated with macrophage-conditioned medium overnight stained with Alexa488 WGA for live cell imaging. Cells connected via a TNT to other cells were quantified as described in Subheading 3.4 and plotted as the percentage of cells with TNTs. $n = 3$, $^{*}p < 0.05$

average number of cells that are connected or % of cells with TNTs. An example of this quantitation is shown in Fig. 3.

3. Alternatively, the number of TNTs present can be identified as described above and quantified but reported as the number of TNTs per 100 cells.

4 Notes

1. Primary murine bone marrow or human monocyte-derived macrophages have also been successfully used.
2. We have successfully employed other cancer cell lines in this method.
3. If there is no CO_2 control for microscope, 10 mM HEPES can be added to the medium, or Leibovitz's L-15 medium can be used to maintain appropriate pH control.
4. To improve consistency between experiments we have found that it is best to start with healthy cells, so it is essential not to overgrow the cells.
5. The number of macrophages to be plated is variable, and depends on the macrophage type and should be adjusted for 90% confluency. Additionally, when using other tumor cell lines in this assay it is essential to generate the macrophage-conditioned medium in the appropriate medium for each line to be used in the assay.
6. We have found that fixation using 3.7% formaldehyde in BWD preserves approximately 50% of the TNTs. However, fixation

permits the use of other microscopy techniques such as confocal and super resolution imaging by structured illumination microscopy [7, 13]. We routinely use fluorescently labeled phalloidin and Wheat Germ Agglutinin to identify F-actin containing membrane covered connections but other methods can be used including labeling vesicles with a Cell tracker dye [7].

7. Several characteristics are used to distinguish TNTs from similar structures such as filopodia such as length and attachment to the substrate. Another indicator of a TNT is the presence of cargo that can be seen as bulges in the structure or labeled with a vesicle marker.

8. Other possible definitions of TNTs have been used. TNT precursors have been identified as long protrusions that are off the substratum, and reach a minimum of 8 μm in length during the imaging period and eventually touch another cell.

References

1. Sharma VP, Beaty BT, Cox D et al (2014) An in vitro one-dimensional assay to study growth factor-regulated tumor cell-macrophage interaction. Methods Mol Biol 1172:115–123
2. Yang M, McKay D, Pollard JW et al (2018) Diverse functions of macrophages in different tumor microenvironments. Cancer Res 78:5492–5503
3. Davies LC, Taylor PR (2015) Tissue-resident macrophages: then and now. Immunology 144:541–548
4. Wyckoff J, Wang W, Lin EY et al (2004) A paracrine loop between tumor cells and macrophages is required for tumor cell migration in mammary tumors. Cancer Res 64:7022–7029
5. Dang W, Qin Z, Fan S et al (2016) miR-1207-5p suppresses lung cancer growth and metastasis by targeting CSF1. Oncotarget 7:32421–32432
6. Lou E, Gholami S, Romin Y et al (2017) Imaging tunneling membrane tubes elucidates cell communication in tumors. Trends Cancer 3:678–685
7. Hanna SJ, McCoy-Simandle K, Leung E et al (2019) Tunneling nanotubes, a novel mode of tumor cell-macrophage communication in tumor cell invasion. J Cell Sci 132(3). pii: jcs223321. https://doi.org/10.1242/jcs.223321
8. Patheja P, Sahu K (2017) Macrophage conditioned medium induced cellular network formation in MCF-7 cells through enhanced tunneling nanotube formation and tunneling nanotube mediumted release of viable cytoplasmic fragments. Exp Cell Res 355:182–193
9. Carter KP, Hanna S, Genna A et al (2019) Macrophage induced tumor cell tunneling nanotubes enhance tumor cell 3D invasion. Cancer Rep, 28 August 2019. https://doi.org/10.1002/cnr2.1213
10. Eugenin EA, Gaskill PJ, Berman JW (2009) Tunneling nanotubes (TNT): a potential mechanism for intercellular HIV trafficking. Commun Integr Biol 2:243–244
11. Saenz-de-Santa-Maria I, Bernardo-Castineira-C, Enciso E, Garcia-Moreno I et al (2017) Control of long-distance cell-to-cell communication and autophagosome transfer in squamous cell carcinoma via tunneling nanotubes. Oncotarget 8:20939–20960
12. Cox D, Chang P, Zhang Q et al (1997) Requirements for both Rac1 and Cdc42 in membrane ruffling and phagocytosis in leukocytes. J Exp Med 186:1487–1494
13. Hanna SJ, McCoy-Simandle K, Miskolci V et al (2017) The role of Rho-GTPases and actin polymerization during macrophage tunneling nanotube biogenesis. Sci Rep 7:8547

Chapter 24

Optogenetics: Rho GTPases Activated by Light in Living Macrophages

Maren Hülsemann, Polina V. Verkhusha, Peng Guo, Veronika Miskolci, Dianne Cox, and Louis Hodgson

Abstract

Genetically encoded optogenetic tools are increasingly popular and useful for perturbing signaling pathways with high spatial and temporal resolution in living cells. Here, we show basic procedures employed to implement optogenetics of Rho GTPases in a macrophage cell line. Methods described here are generally applicable to other genetically encoded optogenetic tools utilizing the blue-green spectrum of light for activation, designed for specific proteins and enzymatic targets important for immune cell functions.

Key words Rho GTPases, Optogenetics, Photoactivatable proteins, LOV2

1 Introduction

Optogenetic manipulation of living cells during imaging experiments enables perturbation of a pathway while in direct observation of the resulting cellular behavior. This is a powerful approach because the specific perturbation and the resulting modulation of the cellular phenotype can be quantified immediately and continuously in single cells during live imaging. In addition to optogenetic perturbations, recent advances in fluorescent biosensors for detecting protein activations and posttranslational modification statuses could be used either in combination within a set of imaging studies or directly and concurrently with optogenetic perturbations to provide researchers with the ability to "probe" and "perturb" in living cells for the first time. The most common tools available in the field thus far have been based on the light-oxygen-voltage (LOV) 2-Jα system [1–8], cryptochrome-2 (CRY2), and channelrhodopsins [2, 9]. These tools require blue-green light for photoactivation, and exhibit different quantum efficiencies and half-lives of light-based conformational switching as the key mechanism of these optogenetic applications.

Ivana Vancurova and Yan Zhu (eds.), *Immune Mediators in Cancer: Methods and Protocols*, Methods in Molecular Biology, vol. 2108, https://doi.org/10.1007/978-1-0716-0247-8_24, © Springer Science+Business Media, LLC, part of Springer Nature 2020

In our works, we have focused on studying the Rho family GTPase functions in living cells, including breast tumor cells [10–13] and macrophages [14–16], and applied optogenetic tools to directly perturb pathways important in cell invasion and motility [12]. Here, we outline a procedure for performing optogenetic imaging experiments in macrophage cell line, using photoactivatable (PA)-GTPase system [4]. We also note that approaches outlined here can be generalized to most optogenetic systems which can be activated by the blue-green spectrum of light, targeting Rho GTPase pathways. These approaches could include multicomponent dimerizer systems such as the LOVTRAP [1, 17], and the extrinsic order/disorder-based optogenetic systems wherein LOV-domain is directly inserted into the catalytic interface of a molecule to modulate enzymatic function [18]. In this report, we will present a primary application example of the PA-Cdc42 system in a macrophage cell line.

2 Materials

2.1 Cell Culture and Transfection

1. Cell lines: RAW/LR5 monocyte/macrophage cell line [19] (*see* **Note 1**).
2. RPMI medium with L-Glutamine 300 mg/L, supplemented with 10% newborn calf serum (NCS), penicillin (100 IU)/streptomycin (100 μg/mL).
3. Opti-MEM medium.
4. Plasmids: The photoactivatable GTPases (PA-Cdc42, PA-Rac1) [4] and GEFs [17, 18] in pTriEX-backbone or in other mammalian expression plasmids. Empty pCDNA or other appropriate empty mammalian expression plasmid which will be used as a transfection control. Appropriate control mutant versions of PA-GTPase, including C450A mutant (dark mutant). PA-GTPases [4] and PA-GEF based on LOV-TRAP [17] or direct insertion of LOV2 in the GEF-domain [18], are available from Addgene.
5. FuGENE HD transfection reagent.
6. DPBS, calcium and magnesium free: 0.2 g/L KCl, 0.2 g/L KH_2PO_4, 8 g/L NaCl, 1.15 g/L Na_2HPO_4 (anhydrous).
7. 10 mM EDTA in DPBS, made from diluting 0.5 M EDTA (pH 8) in DPBS.
8. 6-Well tissue culture plates.
9. 12-Well tissue culture plates.
10. 15 and 50 mL polypropylene tubes.
11. 6 and 10 cm cell culture dishes.

2.2 Imaging Experiments

1. 25 mm Round coverslips #1.5 thickness.
2. BWD buffer [15, 19]: 20 mM HEPES, pH 7.4, 125 mM NaCl, 5 mM KCl, 5 mM glucose, 10 mM $NaHCO_3$, 1 mM KH_2PO_4, 1 mM $CaCl_2$, 1 mM $MgCl_2$, pH 7.4.
3. BWD buffer containing 5% fetal bovine serum (FBS).
4. Live cell imaging chamber [11, 20, 21], Attofluor chamber system (Invitrogen) or other compatible live-cell chamber system that can accommodate 25 mm coverslips, or CellView glass bottom culture dishes (Greiner-Bio-one), or Mattek dishes (Mattek.com).
5. Mineral oil.
6. 200-proof ethanol.
7. Fluorescence inverted microscope capable of timelapse fluorescence imaging, fitted with photoactivation illuminator (IX2-RFAW: Olympus) (*see* **Note 2**) (Fig. 1).

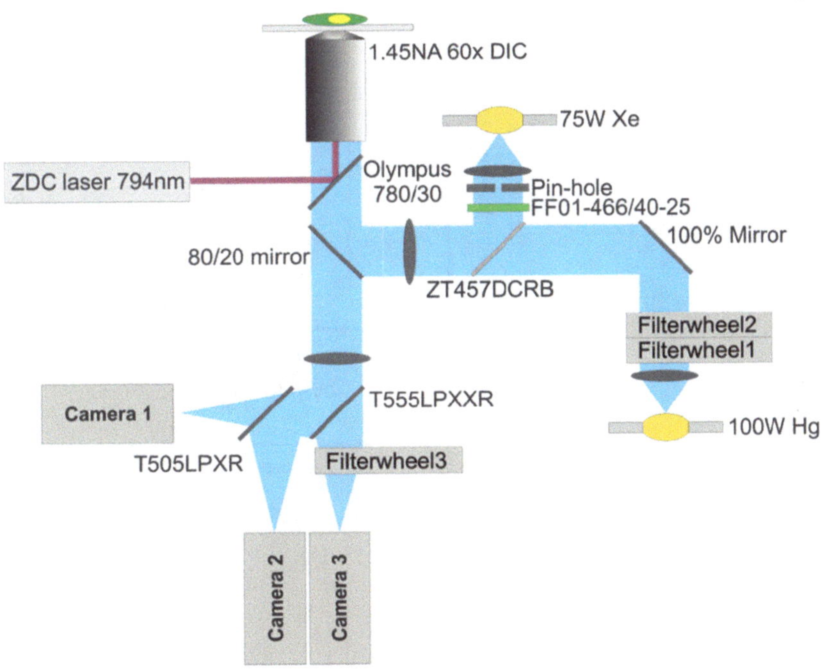

Fig. 1 Schematic drawing of the inverted microscope used for live cell imaging and optogenetic activation of Rho GTPases. The microscope as depicted is configured for simultaneous CFP-YFP FRET biosensor imaging and DIC/red/far-red/near-infrared imaging setup. Filterwheel 1: switches the neutral density filters; Filterwheel 2: switches the excitation band-pass filters; Filterwheel 3: switches the emission band-pass filters. Microscope is equipped with ZeroDrift Compensation (ZDC) mechanism (Olympus) utilizing a 794 nm laser source, illuminating the specimen plane via an Olympus 780/30 nm notch filter. Photoactivation of PA-GTPase is performed via a pin-hole and through a 466/40 nm band-pass filter. This is combined with the main fluorescence excitation light train via a notch filter centered at 457 nm. The main fluorescence turret of the microscope contains a custom 80/20 (transmittance/reflection) mirror (Chroma). Details of the construction and specification of this microscope can be found elsewhere [21]

8. Optionally, a fluorescence inverted microscope capable of time-lapse imaging of Förster resonance energy transfer (FRET) biosensors [21], fitted with photoactivation illuminator (IX2-RFAW: Olympus).
9. Bandpass filter for photoactivation of LOV2 domain: FF01-466/40–25 (Semrock) (Fig. 2a).
10. Custom dichromatic notch filter for the photoactivation illuminator system: ZT457DCRB, 3 mm thickness (Chroma Technology) (Fig. 2b).
11. 16 mm Round, mounted pin-hole inserts of various sizes for the fluorescence microscope (Melles Griot).
12. Optionally, an Olympus Fluoview1000 multi-photon microscope system.

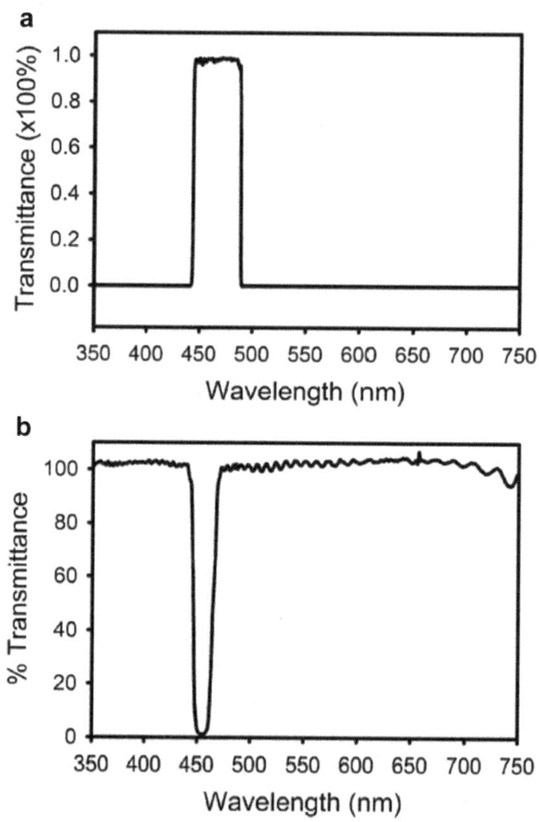

Fig. 2 (**a**) Transmittance specification of the FF01-466/40–25 mm filter (Semrock) used for photoactivation of LOV2-Jα-based optogenetic systems. (**b**) Transmittance specification of the notch filter centered at 457 nm (Chroma) used to mix the photoactivation light into the main excitation light train

3 Methods

3.1 Transient Transfection of Optogenetic Components in RAW/LR5 Cells

For transfection of optogenetic components, individual optimizations of transfection conditions are required to achieve best results. As an example, we will use our protocol for the PA-Cdc42 (*see* **Note 3**) [4].

1. (Day 1) Plate RAW/LR5 cells in a 12-well plate the day before transfection so that they will be approximately 60–80% confluent for transfection the next day.
2. (Day 2) Let FuGENE HD (*see* **Note 4**) and OptiMEM come to room temperature (RT), ~10 min.
3. Prepare FuGENE HD transfection mix (DNA:FuGENE HD ratio 1:3). In 100 μL of OptiMEM, add 1 μg PA-Cdc42 (*see* **Notes 5** and **6**), vortex for 10 s; add 3 μL of FuGENE HD, and pipet to mix (do not vortex). Incubate at RT for 15 min. The transfection mix should be scaled up or down based on surface area of the tissue culture vessel, if different cell numbers are required.
4. While the transfection mix incubates, rinse cells once with DPBS and add 500 μL of complete medium for transfection.
5. Add transfection mix dropwise to the plate. Swirl gently to mix.
6. Incubate the plate for 2–3 h (*see* **Note 7**) at 37 °C and 5% CO_2.
7. After incubation, transfer the medium from cells to a 15 mL tube to collect cells that may have detached during the incubation. Then lift adherent cells by adding 10 mM EDTA/DPBS to the well and incubate for 5 min at 37 °C and 5% CO_2. Tap gently to lift cells and transfer to the same 15 mL tube. Rinse the dish once with complete medium to collect all cells and add again to the 15 mL tube. Spin cells at 300 × *g* for 3 min.
8. Aspirate the supernatant and resuspend the cell pellet in 2 mL of complete medium.
9. Set up sterile 25 mm round coverslips in 6-well plate (*see* **Note 8**). Plate at 4×10^4 cells/coverslip (*see* **Note 9**). Alternatively, Mattek or CellView chambers can be used.
10. Let cells recover on the coverslips overnight at 37 °C and 5% CO_2.
11. (Day 3) Next day, set up for optogenetic experiments.

3.2 Imaging and Optogenetic Activation of PA-GTPase

For live cell imaging and optogenetic activation, optimization of illumination condition is required to achieve the best response.

1. Mount the coverslips containing cells onto live-cell imaging chamber (Attofluor chamber or the sealed chamber system) [21]. Alternatively, CellView or Mattek dishes can be used as well, and add BWD buffer with 5% FBS to sufficiently fill the chambers (*see* **Note 10**).

2. Using a 60× magnification objective lens (60× DIC N/A 1.45), set up for Köhler illumination and differential interference contrast (DIC) imaging.
3. In a cell-free field of view, open the photoactivation shutter momentarily and determine the location of the illumination spot. If the location of the spot is suboptimal (i.e., not well centered in the field of view), move the pin-hole by adjusting the positional adjustment screws at the photoactivation illuminator. Once the spot is centered in the field of view, mark this spot using the region tool and save such a region so that it can be loaded onto the image during image acquisition (*see* **Note 11**).
4. Observe and quickly identify in mVenus (515 nm excitation, 528 nm emission) fluorescence, cells positive for PA-Cdc42 expression after transfection (*see* **Notes 12** and **13**).
5. Set up for timelapse imaging in DIC (*see* **Note 14**). It is not necessary to image mVenus in the timelapse sequence as this is only a marker of expression of PA-Cdc42.
6. Locate an appropriate cell in the field of view, load the region that indicates the location of the photoactivation spot, and then move the stage so that the cell is appropriately moved into the photoactivation spot (*see* **Note 15**).
7. Start the timelapse experiment, usual frame rate for RAW/LR5 cells is 10 s intervals or shorter. Establish a stable basal condition by imaging for some time without photoactivation (*see* **Note 16**).
8. Photoactivation is initiated by pulsing the photoactivation light at 457 nm on/off at specific intervals (*see* **Notes 17–20**) (Fig. 3).

4 Notes

1. RAW/LR5 cell line can be readily made to express FRET biosensors for Rho GTPases [15, 22], including those that fluoresce in near infrared (NIR) [23]. This is advantageous because NIR FRET biosensor can be used together with other optogenetic tools that require blue/green light for photo-uncaging [23]. The description of biosensors based on CFP-YFP FRET and NIR FRET systems is beyond the scope of this work, but RAW/LR5 cells stably expressing the tet-OFF tTA are available [15]; thus, inducible NIR-FRET biosensor cell line can be readily produced following previously published [22] protocols.
2. If interested in imaging FRET biosensor measurements at the same time as performing optogenetic manipulation, the microscope should be fitted with optimized imaging components for

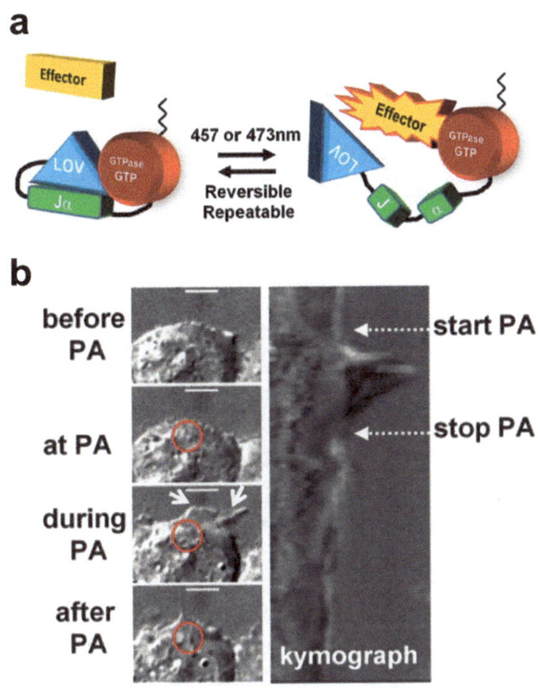

Fig. 3 (**a**) Schematic cartoon of a PA-GTPase. A constitutively active mutant of Rho GTPase is caged by LOV2-Jα in the dark state. Upon irradiation by 457 or 473 nm light, conformational shift within the LOV2-Jα reversibly uncages the activated GTPase, targeting downstream effectors. (**b**) DIC images of a macrophage transiently transfected with PA-Cdc42 and photoactivated within a 3.3 μm area indicated by a red circle. *PA* photoactivation. White arrows indicate protrusions. Kymograph was measured along a line drawn perpendicular to the leading edge (not shown). Scale bar = 5 μm

biosensor measurements, in addition to the photoactivation module for the optogenetic tools [21].

3. PA-Cdc42 as published in [4] contains an F56W mutation. This mutation is found in the β3 sheet in front of Switch II domain important for effector binding. The analysis in [4] revealed that tryptophan at this location was required to form a stable salt-bridge with the LOV2-Jα in the dark-state. This enhanced the stability of the caged state of PA-Cdc42. Rac1 natively contains a tryptophan at this location. A caveat, as noted in [4], is that because of this Rac1-like mutation in PA-Cdc42, the downstream effector signaling may be biased toward the Rac1-like pathway as opposed to Cdc42. Indeed, we find that repeated photoactivation of PA-Cdc42 in macrophages leads to cell protrusions that are more lamellipodia-like. Thus, users are cautioned to note the potential consequences of these mutations that may be present in these constructs which could produce spurious effects.
4. FuGENE HD and Opti-MEM must be at room temperature, or transfection efficiency will be significantly impacted.

5. Macrophage cell lines are challenging to transfect in general. We have had the most success with FuGENE HD, giving a transfection efficiency of approximately 10%. However, the transfection efficiency also varies greatly depending on the cDNA. The amount of DNA and the DNA:FuGENE HD ratio have been optimized for RAW/LR5 cells. For other cell types, DNA and FuGENE HD amounts should be optimized.
6. PA-Rac1 and PA-Cdc42 require optimization of expression levels. Too much expression leads to constitutive activation and loss of optogenetic control. Therefore, we advise that the amount of DNA should be titrated down, using an empty pCDNA to maintain the same amount of DNA transfected at all times. LOVTRAP-GEF system also requires optimization of transfection ratios. We have found that 10:1 ratio of pTriEX-N-TOM20-LOV2 and pTriEx-mVenus-Zdk1-VAV2 DHPHC1 [1, 17] produces good optogenetic activation in living cells.
7. Overnight incubation of the cells increases transfection efficiency, while cell health is adversely affected and pre-activation can also be a problem. For a simple protein expression analysis an overnight incubation is tolerable. However, for downstream cellular assays we routinely opt for shorter transfection times, in the order of 2–3 h.
8. Keep stock of 25 mm round coverslips in 200-proof ethanol and flame them to sterilize.
9. 4×10^4 cells/coverslip is a starting cell density for imaging. Optimal plating density for imaging should be determined individually.
10. In the case of open chamber systems, mineral oil can be layered onto the BWD medium to protect it from evaporation and gas exchange. The sealed chamber system does not require the oil because it uses a clean coverslip to seal the upper side of the chamber [21].
11. The pin-hole size at the specimen plane can be calculated by the following equation:

$$\text{Exposed area on the specimen} = (\text{Pin-hole diameter})/(\text{objective magnification})$$

We are using a 200 μm diameter pin-hole insert. This translates to 3.33 μm diameter activation spot at the specimen plane under 60× magnification. We found this size to be ideal for targeting relatively small cells such as macrophages, or small structures within larger cells such as the invadopodium in breast tumor cells [12]. Users should determine the best geometries of optogenetic activation conditions based on the size and shape of the targeted structures or the size of the targeted cells.

12. PA-Cdc42 was originally produced with mVenus as the expression tag, and PA-Rac1 with mVenus or mCherry [3]. We have changed the expression marker to mtagBFP2 for PA-Rac1 to make it compatible with fluorescence imaging conditions that require red fluorescence for other cellular markers [12].
13. Fluorescence excitation of mVenus (515 nm) will cause photoactivation of PA-GTPases that are tagged with mVenus. Thus, observations in the mVenus channel (or EGFP channel can be used as well) should be kept to an absolute minimum, just enough to quickly find cells positive for transfection. Once a cell is found, immediately switch to DIC and perform adjustments for cell placement within the field of view to target the uncaging spot in the field of view. This problem can be circumvented by switching the tag to mtagBFP2 and exciting it at 395 nm, or mCherry (585 nm) if longer wavelengths can be used. Trans-illumination light train for DIC may include a green filter by default. This should be removed and ideally replaced with a bandpass filter in red. We use a 632/32 nm bandpass glass filter for DIC imaging.
14. The choice of fluorescence wavelengths available for timelapse imaging will be limited by the requirement for PA-GTPase uncaging.
15. The location of photoactivation depends on the function of the GTPase that you want to study. In the example given in this section, we placed the spot at the edge of a cell to induce edge protrusions. In other examples in different cell type, we have placed the spot at intracellular structure that is away from the edge [12]. Therefore, adjusting the size of the pin-hole and its location becomes very important to target signaling events at specific locations.
16. We routinely observe cells for approximately 5–15 min prior to start of the photoactivation to establish a stable pre-activation baseline response.
17. Because the wild-type PA-GTPase has a ½-life of relaxation of approximately 43 s [3], we cycled the illumination of 1 s at 457 nm light followed by 30 s of dark state. By repeating this cycle, we achieve continuous activation of PA-GTPase [12]. It is advisable, however, to optimize this condition appropriately depending on the experimental requirements. In the case of the LOVTRAP-GEF experiments [23], we have instead irradiated the whole field of view using continuous irradiation as the ½-life of the LOVTRAP system based on the wild-type LOV2 was shorter (18.5 s for return to mitochondria) [1, 17]. To control the cycling of the activation light, a script can be written in Metamorph software which controls the microscope system, to automate this process during a timelapse experiment.

18. Control experiments with a dark mutant of PA-GTPase (C450A), unable to be photoactivated, should be performed under similar conditions to ascertain that the phenotype being observed is specific to optogenetic uncaging of PA-GTPase [4]. Additional control experiments could include: (a) photoactivation within regions away from the targeted zones of interest (e.g., the leading edge, cell body, vs. nucleus); and (b) photoactivation of cells without expression of the optogenetic components to determine the effects of the light illumination.
19. PA-GTPase can be activated using multi-photon microscopy modality irradiating at 915 nm light (Fig. 4). This could be a

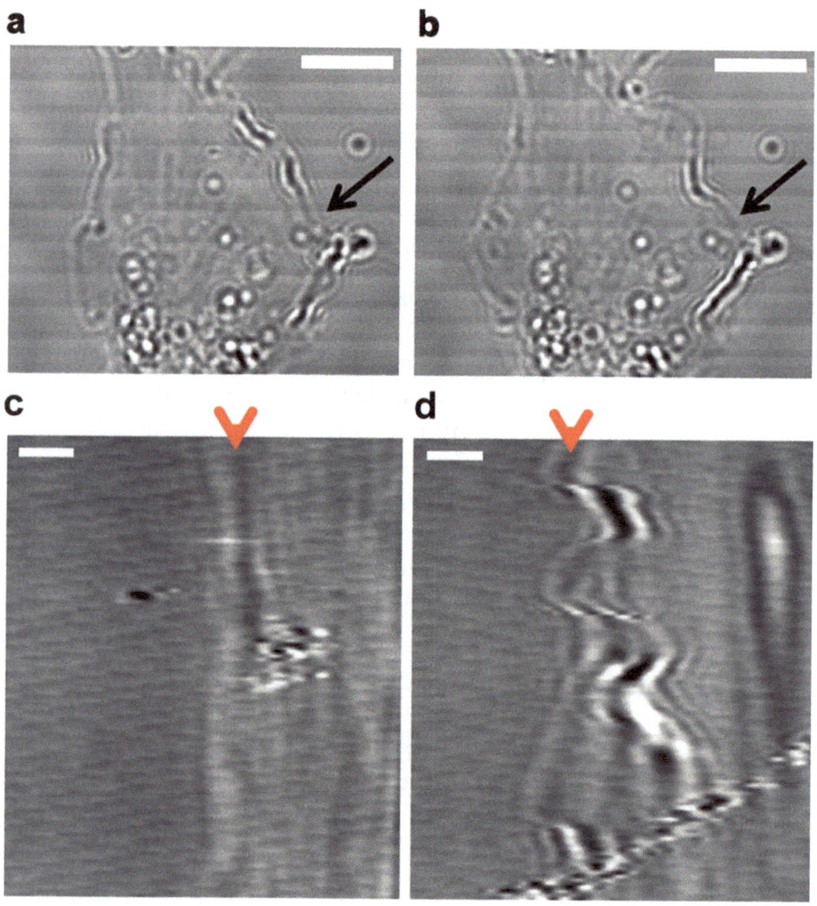

Fig. 4 Photo-uncaging of PA-Rac1 in mouse embryonic fibroblasts (MEF) using a two-photon excitation at 915 nm, shown as an example. (**a**, **c**) Without photoactivation; (**b**, **d**) with photoactivation. Global uncaging excitation was used to image the bright-field. MEFs stably expressing the PA-Rac1 were imaged on an Olympus Fluoview1000 multi-photon system. Black arrows indicate locations of lamellipodial protrusion as a function of photouncaging at 915 nm. Kymographs show the changes in edge motion (red arrow head, location of the edge) with and without two-photon-uncaging. White bar in (**a**, **b**) 20 μm and in (**c**, **d**) 5 μm

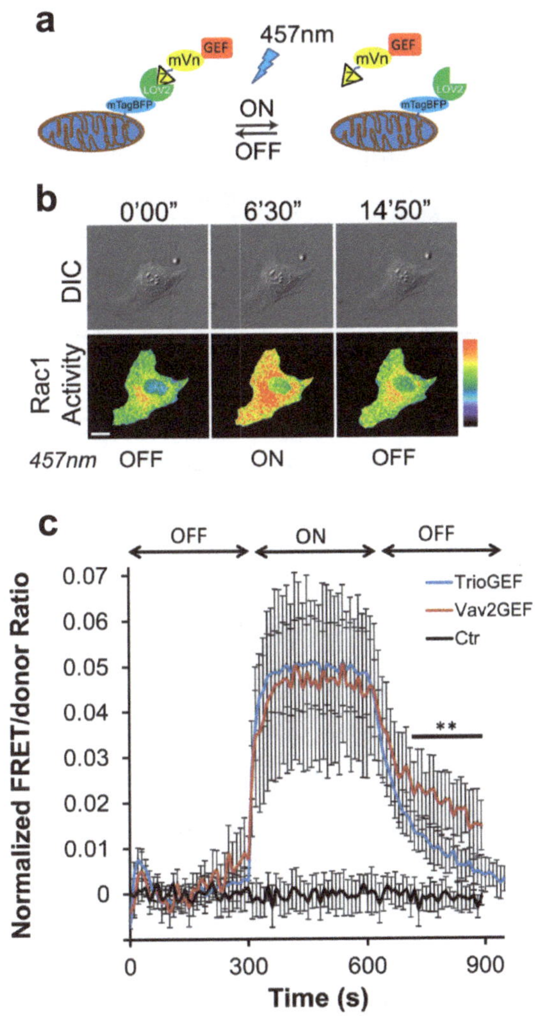

Fig. 5 Concurrent measurement of Rac1 activity during LOVTRAP optogenetics, reproduced from Shcherbakova et al. 2018 Nature Chemical Biology [23]. (**a**) Schematic drawing of the LOVTRAP system. Mitochondrially targeted mtagBFP-LOV2wt sequesters the GEF-domain of interest attached to Zdk1 molecule. Upon photoactivation with 457 nm light, Zdk1-GEF is released and acts on the target GTPase, followed by dark relaxation upon cessation of illumination. (**b**) An example panel of a MEF undergoing photoactivation of LOVTRAP and concurrent measurements of Rac1 activity using the NIR-Rac1 biosensor. NIR-Rac1 biosensor image sets were acquired every 10 s. 457 nm illumination (cycles of 4 s-on, 6 s-off) was started at 300 s and ended at 600 s time points. White bar = 20 μm. Pseudocolor limits are 1.0 to 1.74 (black to red). (**c**) Quantification of Rac1 activity measured concurrently with the LOVTRAP-TrioGEF and -VavGEF photoactivation. During the "on" phase of the 457 nm illumination, Rac1 activity levels are significantly elevated compared to the control which received no 457 nm illumination. $n = 17$ independent photoactivation experiments for LOVTRAP-TrioGEF, $n = 10$ independent photoactivation experiments for LOVTRAP-VavGEF, $n = 10$ independent mock-photoactivation experiments for the control condition, all shown with mean ± SEM. The original Vav2 GEF LOVTRAP results in slower decay of Rac1 activity during the dark relaxation compared to the TrioGEF LOVTRAP, pointing to differential ability of GEFs to modulate Rho GTPase activities, $^{**}p < 0.01$

useful approach to optogenetically target macrophages in in vivo imaging experiments.

20. Optogenetic activation of Rho-targeting GEF via LOVTRAP [1] can be used together with a compatible FRET biosensor that utilizes near-infrared fluorescent proteins [23]. This method allows direct observation of the perturbation of Rho GTPase activity during blue-green optogenetic perturbation of an upstream signal regulator (Fig. 5).

Acknowledgements

This work was supported by National Institutes of Health grant T32GM007491 to V.M., R01GM129098 and R01GM132098 to L.H. National Cancer Institute P30CA013330 for Analytical Imaging Facility support. Irma T. Hirschl Career Scientist Award to L.H. pTriEX-mVenus-PA-Cdc42 (Addgene #75263), pTriEX-mVenus-PA-Rac1 (Addgene #22007), pTriEX-PA-Rac1 C450R (Addgene #22025), pTriEX-NTOM20-LOV2 WT (Addgene #81009) and pTriEx-mVenus-Zdk1-VAV2 DH/PH/C1 (Addgene #81133) were gifts from Dr. Klaus Hahn (UNC-Chapel Hill).

References

1. Wang H, Hahn KM (2016) LOVTRAP: a versatile method to control protein function with light. Curr Protoc Cell Biol 73:21.10.1–21.10.14. https://doi.org/10.1002/cpcb.12
2. Shcherbakova DM, Shemetov AA, Kaberniuk AA, Verkhusha VV (2015) Natural photoreceptors as a source of fluorescent proteins, biosensors, and optogenetic tools. Annu Rev Biochem 84:519–550. https://doi.org/10.1146/annurev-biochem-060614-034411
3. Wu YI, Wang X, He L, Montell D, Hahn KM (2011) Spatiotemporal control of small GTPases with light using the LOV domain. Methods Enzymol 497:393–407. https://doi.org/10.1016/B978-0-12-385075-1.00016-0
4. Wu YI, Frey D, Lungu OI, Jaehrig A, Schlichting I, Kuhlman B, Hahn KM (2009) A genetically encoded photoactivatable Rac controls the motility of living cells. Nature 461(7260):104–108
5. Christie JM, Gawthorne J, Young G, Fraser NJ, Roe AJ (2012) LOV to BLUF: flavoprotein contributions to the optogenetic toolkit. Mol Plant 5(3):533–544. https://doi.org/10.1093/mp/sss020
6. Losi A, Gartner W (2012) The evolution of flavin-binding photoreceptors: an ancient chromophore serving trendy blue-light sensors. Annu Rev Plant Biol 63:49–72. https://doi.org/10.1146/annurev-arplant-042811-105538
7. Pudasaini A, El-Arab KK, Zoltowski BD (2015) LOV-based optogenetic devices: light-driven modules to impart photoregulated control of cellular signaling. Front Mol Biosci 2:18. https://doi.org/10.3389/fmolb.2015.00018
8. Zhang K, Cui B (2015) Optogenetic control of intracellular signaling pathways. Trends Biotechnol 33(2):92–100. https://doi.org/10.1016/j.tibtech.2014.11.007
9. Chernov KG, Redchuk TA, Omelina ES, Verkhusha VV (2017) Near-infrared fluorescent proteins, biosensors, and optogenetic tools engineered from phytochromes. Chem Rev 117(9):6423–6446. https://doi.org/10.1021/acs.chemrev.6b00700
10. Bravo-Cordero JJ, Oser M, Chen X, Eddy R, Hodgson L, Condeelis J (2011) A novel spatiotemporal RhoC activation pathway locally regulates cofilin activity at invadopodia. Curr Biol 21(8):635–644. pii: S0960-9822(11)00311-3

11. Bravo-Cordero JJ, Moshfegh Y, Condeelis J, Hodgson L (2013) Live cell imaging of RhoGTPase biosensors in tumor cells. Methods Mol Biol 1046:359–370. https://doi.org/10.1007/978-1-62703-538-5_22
12. Moshfegh Y, Bravo-Cordero JJ, Miskolci V, Condeelis J, Hodgson L (2014) A Trio-Rac1-Pak1 signalling axis drives invadopodia disassembly. Nat Cell Biol 16(6):574–586. https://doi.org/10.1038/ncb2972
13. Donnelly SK, Cabrera R, Mao SPH, Christin JR, Wu B, Guo W, Bravo-Cordero JJ, Condeelis JS, Segall JE, Hodgson L (2017) Rac3 regulates breast cancer invasion and metastasis by controlling adhesion and matrix degradation. J Cell Biol 216(12):4331–4349. https://doi.org/10.1083/jcb.201704048
14. Hanna S, Miskolci V, Cox D, Hodgson L (2014) A new genetically encoded single-chain biosensor for Cdc42 based on FRET, useful for live-cell imaging. PLoS One 9(5): e96469. https://doi.org/10.1371/journal.pone.0096469
15. Miskolci V, Wu B, Moshfegh Y, Cox D, Hodgson L (2016) Optical tools to study the isoform-specific roles of small GTPases in immune cells. J Immunol 196(8):3479–3493. https://doi.org/10.4049/jimmunol.1501655
16. Hanna SJ, McCoy-Simandle K, Miskolci V, Guo P, Cammer M, Hodgson L, Cox D (2017) The role of rho-GTPases and actin polymerization during macrophage tunneling nanotube biogenesis. Sci Rep 7(1):8547. https://doi.org/10.1038/s41598-017-08950-7
17. Wang H, Vilela M, Winkler A, Tarnawski M, Schlichting I, Yumerefendi H, Kuhlman B, Liu R, Danuser G, Hahn KM (2016) LOVTRAP: an optogenetic system for photo-induced protein dissociation. Nat Methods 13 (9):755–758. https://doi.org/10.1038/nmeth.3926
18. Dagliyan O, Tarnawski M, Chu PH, Shirvanyants D, Schlichting I, Dokholyan NV, Hahn KM (2016) Engineering extrinsic disorder to control protein activity in living cells. Science 354(6318):1441–1444. https://doi.org/10.1126/science.aah3404
19. Cox D, Chang P, Zhang Q, Reddy PG, Bokoch GM, Greenberg S (1997) Requirements for both Rac1 and Cdc42 in membrane ruffling and phagocytosis in leukocytes. J Exp Med 186(9):1487–1494
20. Spiering D, Bravo-Cordero JJ, Moshfegh Y, Miskolci V, Hodgson L (2013) Quantitative ratiometric imaging of FRET-biosensors in living cells. Methods Cell Biol 114:593–609. https://doi.org/10.1016/B978-0-12-407761-4.00025-7
21. Spiering D, Hodgson L (2012) Multiplex imaging of Rho family GTPase activities in living cells. Methods Mol Biol 827:215–234. https://doi.org/10.1007/978-1-61779-442-1_15
22. Miskolci V, Hodgson L, Cox D (2017) Using fluorescence resonance energy transfer-based biosensors to probe Rho GTPase activation during phagocytosis. Methods Mol Biol 1519:125–143. https://doi.org/10.1007/978-1-4939-6581-6_9
23. Shcherbakova DM, Cox Cammer N, Huisman TM, Verkhusha VV, Hodgson L (2018) Direct multiplex imaging and optogenetics of Rho GTPases enabled by near-infrared FRET. Nat Chem Biol 14:591. https://doi.org/10.1038/s41589-018-0044-1

Part IV

Bioinformatics and Genome Editing Approaches

Chapter 25

High-Throughput RNA Interference Screen Targeting Synthetic-Lethal Gain-of-Function of Oncogenic Mutant TP53 in Triple-Negative Breast Cancer

Susumu Rokudai

Abstract

TNBC is an aggressive and metastatic subtype of breast cancer in which TP53 mutation occurs frequently and is associated with particularly poor outcome. Mutations in TP53 can disrupt the intrinsic function of the tumor suppressor as well as acquire oncogenic gain-of-function (GOF) activities. However, little is known about its oncogenic GOF mediators and functions. Targeted therapy for TNBC patients is thus one of the most urgent needs in breast cancer therapeutics, and identifying genes that have synthetic lethal interactions with mutant TP53 may be a promising approach. In this chapter, we present procedures on sequential analysis of RNA-seq followed by high-throughput RNA interference screening (HTS-RNAi screening). This approach has been utilized to identify genes with synthetic lethality of mutant TP53, providing a promising strategy for the treatment of mutant TP53 in TNBC and determining its impact on tumorigenesis.

Key words High-throughput RNA interference screens (HTS-RNAi screens), Mutant TP53, Molecular-targeting cancer therapy, Triple-negative breast cancer, Adenosine receptor

1 Introduction

Triple-negative breast cancer (TNBC), which is characterized by the absence of ER, PgR, and HER2, exhibits a relatively aggressive phenotype, therapeutic resistance, and is correlated with a poor prognosis [1, 2]. TNBC is associated with the phenotypes of cancer stem cells (CSCs) [3, 4] and epithelial-mesenchymal transition (EMT), which is characterized by the downregulation of epithelial markers and mesenchymal phenotypes with high migration ability [5]. Validation of a targeted therapy approach for patients with TNBC is thus urgently needed [6].

TNBC with mutant TP53 cells were analyzed by RNA-seq, and synthetic-lethal shRNA knockdown screening to identify genes related to the expression of mutant TP53, since TP53 mutations

Ivana Vancurova and Yan Zhu (eds.), *Immune Mediators in Cancer: Methods and Protocols*, Methods in Molecular Biology, vol. 2108, https://doi.org/10.1007/978-1-0716-0247-8_25, © Springer Science+Business Media, LLC, part of Springer Nature 2020

occur in approximately 40% of all breast cancers, with the highest frequency found in the basal-like (80%) subtypes of TNBC [7, 8].

RNA interference (RNAi) is an effective mechanism for gene silencing, whereby complementary mRNA triggers the cleavage and degradation of homologous transcript sequences. HTS-RNAi screening is an intrinsic cellular mechanism for identifying the synthetic-lethal genes of mutant TP53 and is a promising therapeutic strategy and method to determine their impact on tumorigenesis. However, one barrier often encountered with high-throughput screens is the cost and difficulty in deconvolution. Here, we present the RNA interference methods of a LentiPlex shRNA library to rapidly conduct a positive selection screen for the identification of genes with synthetic lethality of mutant TP53 in TNBC and their impact on tumorigenesis [9].

2 Materials

2.1 Cell Culture

1. The human breast cancer cell lines. TNBC cell lines (HCC70, and HCC1143) and non-TNBC cell lines (MCF-7).
2. Medium: RPMI 1640 medium supplemented with 100 U/mL penicillin-streptomycin and 10% fetal bovine serum.
3. Tissue culture plates and related tissue culture supplies.
4. CO_2 incubator: 37 °C with 5% CO_2.

2.2 Transcriptome Analysis

1. RNeasy Mini kit (Qiagen, Hilden, Germany).
2. RNA6000 Pico Kit (Agilent Technologies, Santa Clara, CA).
3. TruSeq RNA Sample Prep Kit v2 (Illumina, Inc., San Diego, CA).
4. NextSeq 500 High Output v1 Kit (Illumina, Inc.).
5. Agilent 2100 Bioanalyzer (Agilent Technologies).
6. NextSeq 500 system (Illumina, Inc.).
7. TopHat 2 alignment apps (Illumina, Inc.).
8. Cufflinks assembly apps (Illumina, Inc.).
9. Differential expression apps (Illumina, Inc.).

2.3 RNA Interference Screening (RNAi Screening)

1. MISSION LentiPlex pooled shRNA library (SHPH01-1SET; Sigma-Aldrich, St. Louis, MO) (*see* **Note 1**) [10].
2. Tissue culture plates and related tissue culture supplies.
3. Polybrene (Santa Cruz Biotechnology, Dallas, TX).
4. Puromycin dihydrochloride (Sigma-Aldrich).
5. DNA Mini Kit (Qiagen).
6. KAPA HiFi HotStart ReadyMix (Roche Diagnostics).

7. 1% TAE Agarose gel.
8. DirectLoad PCR 100 bp Low Ladder (Sigma-Aldrich).
9. Thermal cycler (Thermo Fisher Scientific).
10. Primers for the PCR of the shRNA vector:
    (sense) 5′-ATTTCTTGGCTTTATATATCTTGTGGAAAG-3′
    (anti-sense) 5′-TGTGGATGAATACTGCCATTTGTCTC-3′
11. Sequencing adapters (BIOO Scientific; Perkin Elmer).
12. PhiX control DNA (Illumina, Inc.).

3 Methods

3.1 Transcriptome Analysis

1. Prepare total RNA from TNBC cell lines (HCC70, and HCC1143) and non-TNBC cells (MCF-7) using the RNeasy Mini kit.
2. Assess the RNA quality using the Agilent RNA6000 Pico Kit and the Agilent 2100 Bioanalyzer as per the manufacturer's instructions to obtain the RNA integrity number (RIN) (*see* **Note 2**).
3. Prepare the library using the TruSeq RNA Sample Prep Kit v2 from 1 μg of total RNA according to the manufacturer's protocol.
4. Subject the resulting libraries from **step 3** to single-end sequencing of 76-bp reads using the NextSeq 500 High Output v1 Kit on the Illumina NextSeq 500 system.
5. Perform data processing and analyses using TopHat 2 alignment, Cufflinks assembly, and differential expression apps (*see* **Note 3**).

3.2 Transduction and Selection of Target Cells

1. Seed the appropriate number of cells to obtain ~50% confluence on the following day (*see* **Note 4**).
2. Allow cells to adhere by incubating overnight at 37 °C in a humidified incubator with an atmosphere of 5% CO_2.
3. Transduce the cells with shRNA lentiviral particles at multiplicity of infections that yield 30–50% infected cells. Gently swirl the plates to evenly distribute the virus across the cells.
4. Incubate for 18–20 h at 37 °C in a humidified incubator with an atmosphere of 5% CO_2.
5. The infected cells are subsequently selected using puromycin for 7 days (*see* **Note 5**).

3.3 Deconvolution from a Polyclonal Cell Population

1. Isolate genomic DNA with integrated shRNA from the cell lines generated from Subheading 3.2.

2. Set up polymerase chain reaction (PCR) using KAPA HiFi HotStart ReadyMix (2×) with primers for the shRNA vector and 3 μg of genomic DNA samples from **step 1**.
3. Run samples in a thermal cycler using the following parameters: 95 °C for 3 min, 30 cycles of (98 °C for 20 s, 60 °C for 15 s, 72 °C for 30 s).
4. Ligate sequencing adapters to the PCR amplicons with 8 cycles of PCR.
5. Perform Illumina sequencing for 150 cycles on an Illumina NextSeq500 sequencer with 10% PhiX control DNA.

3.4 Target Identification and Validation

1. Perform base calling in accordance with the manufacturer's protocol (Illumina, Inc.) to generate FASTQ files.
2. Trim and align the adapter sequences in FASTQ files to the reference shRNA sequences using Bowtie2 (*see* **Note 6**).
3. Perform normalization and statistical analysis using TCC-edgeR [11] (*see* **Note 7**). List of the candidate genes that are related to the expression of mutant TP53 (R248Q) in TNBC using synthetic-lethal shRNA knockdown screening is shown in Fig. 1 (*see* **Notes 8** and **9**). The expression levels of specific interest genes, adenosine receptors (ADORA2B, ADORA1, ADORA2A, and ADORA3) in this case, are analyzed using a Reference Expression Dataset from several noncancerous tissues (Fig. 2; *see* **Note 10**).

Fig. 1 Identified genes by shRNA-LentiPlex screening for synthetic-lethal interaction between TNBC with mutant TP53 and non-TNBC cells. Twelve synthetic lethal candidate genes (Numbers of Hits ≧ 3) were identified that had multiple hits by shRNA-LentiPlex screening. The genes are listed in descending order of 15 identified genes in regard to the number of hits between TNBC with mutant TP53 (R248Q) and non-TNBC cell lines

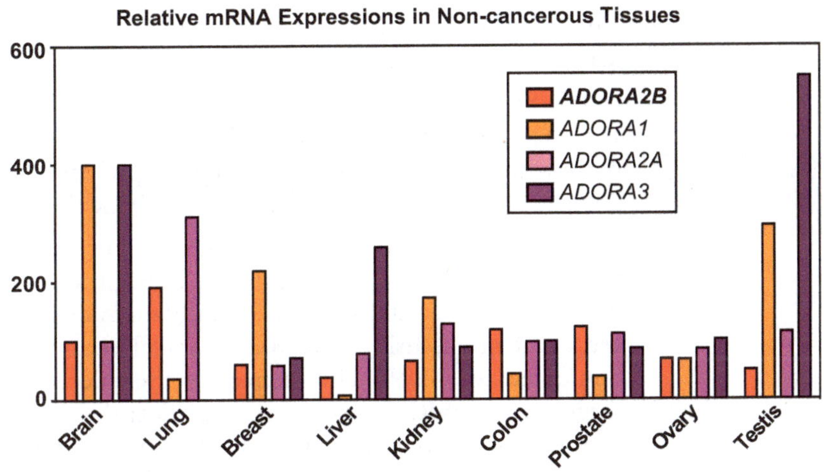

Fig. 2 The expression levels of Adenosine Receptors in Several Noncancerous Tissues. The Reference Expression dataset was used to examine the expression levels of adenosine receptors (ADORA2B, ADORA1, ADORA2A, and ADORA3) in several noncancerous tissues using RNA sequencing methods (http:/refex.dbcls.jp). Specific low-expression genes in normal organs were picked up as maximum fragments per kilobase of transcript per million (FPKM)

4 Notes

1. The MISSION LentiPlex human pooled shRNA library is a genome-wide shRNA library that covers ~15,000 genes, with 80,000 shRNA clones. On average, there are five shRNA designs for each gene target. The shRNA plasmids are processed into lentiviral particles to facilitate stable gene silencing in both dividing and quiescent cells.
2. Samples used for transcriptome analysis are recommended to have a minimum RIN value of 8.0. In the representative experiment, the average RIN value is 9.0.
3. The reads are filtered, trimmed, and aligned in the UCSC human reference genome using the Tophat2 (v2.0.7) and Bowtie1 (0.12.9) pipeline. The transcripts are assembled using Cufflinks 2.1.1, and differentially expressed transcripts are detected using Cuffdiff 2.1.1. Genes with a false-discovery rate (FDR)-adjusted *q*-value (<0.05) and $\log_2$-fold change (>5) are defined as significantly upregulated genes. In the representative experiment, UCSC human reference genome 19 (hg19) is used for alignment.
4. For our study, 4×10^5 cells/well are seeded in 6-well plates to achieve a confluence of 70% prior to transduction. This ensures that the cells are still in the exponential growth phase.
5. For our study, the average of final puromycin concentration in the media ranged from 0.5 to 1.0 μg/mL.

6. The shRNA sequence initiates with 5′-GAAACACCGG-3′. At least the next 10–20 nucleotides are available as query sequence.
7. If Bowtie output files are needed for conversion to count files, python scripts (e.g., "countBowtieHits.py" and "RTable.py") are available from the manufacturer's protocol.
8. To undertake negative-selection RNAi screening for genes of interest in TNBC cells with mutant TP53, the cells are treated with pooled lentiviral shRNAs. Abundances of shRNAs in cells are determined using massively parallel sequencing and are compared to shRNA abundances in the injected cells. Genes targeted by shRNAs that are significantly depleted during tumor growth are considered as hits and prioritized by analyzing the gene copy number data from TNBC cells.
9. TNBC cell lines carrying R248Q mutated TP53 (HCC70 and HCC1143) and non-TNBC cell line carrying wild-type TP53 (MCF-7) are analyzed by transcriptome analysis (RNA-seq). After alignment of a total of 15,346 genes to the reference sequences, a total of 12 genes (Number of Hits ≧ 2) are identified that show synthetic-lethal interaction between TNBC with mutant TP53 and non-TNBC cell lines (Fig. 1). The Cancer Genome Atlas database (cBioPortal: http://www.cbioportal.org) may also be used for the validation of prognostic significance in cancer patients.
10. The Reference Expression dataset (http://refex.dbcls.jp) is available for the identification of the expression levels of the specific interest genes in several noncancerous tissues using RNA sequencing methods. Among the candidate genes that are related to the expression of mutant TP53 (R248Q) in TNBC, ADORA2B is a G protein-coupled adenosine receptor protein known to be involved in inflammation and immune responses [12]. In line with this, ADORA2B-transduced TNBC cells shows increased tumorigenesis, and ADORA2B knockdown, along with mutant p53 knockdown, decreased metastasis both in vitro and in vivo. Together, we conclude that ADORA2B increases the oncogenic potential of basal-like TNBC with mutated TP53 and is an independent predictor of outcome. Therefore, ADORA2B may serve as both a prognostic biomarker and a therapeutic target in basal-like TNBC.

References

1. Papa A, Caruso D, Tomao S, Rossi L, Zaccarelli E, Tomao F (2015) Triple-negative breast cancer: investigating potential molecular therapeutic target. Expert Opin Ther Targets 19:55–75
2. Dent R, Trudeau M, Pritchard KI, Hanna WM, Kahn HK, Sawka CA, Lickley LA, Rawlinson E, Sun P, Narod SA (2007) Triple-negative breast cancer: clinical features and patterns of recurrence. Clin Cancer Res 13:4429–4434

3. Giatromanolaki A, Sivridis E, Fiska A, Koukourakis MI (2011) The CD44+/CD24− phenotype relates to 'triple-negative' state and unfavorable prognosis in breast cancer patients. Med Oncol 28:745–752
4. Idowu MO, Kmieciak M, Dumur C, Burton RS, Grimes MM, Powers CN, Manjili MH (2012) CD44(+)/CD24(−/low) cancer stem/progenitor cells are more abundant in triple-negative invasive breast carcinoma phenotype and are associated with poor outcome. Hum Pathol 43:364–373
5. Mani SA, Guo W, Liao MJ, Eaton EN, Ayyanan A, Zhou AY et al (2008) The epithelial-mesenchymal transition generates cells with properties of stem cells. Cell 133:704–715
6. Synnott NC, Murray A, McGowan PM, Kiely M, Kiely PA, O'Donovan N et al (2017) Mutant p53: a novel target for the treatment of patients with triple-negative breast cancer? Int J Cancer 140:234–246
7. Cancer Genome Atlas Network (2012) Comprehensive molecular portraits of human breast tumours. Nature 490:61–70
8. Walerych D, Napoli M, Collavin L, Del Sal G (2012) The rebel angel: mutant p53 as the driving oncogene in breast cancer. Carcinogenesis 33:2007–2017
9. Horigome E, Fujieda M, Handa T, Katayama A, Ito M, Ichihara A et al (2018) Mutant TP53 modulates metastasis of triple negative breast cancer through adenosine A2b receptor signaling. Oncotarget 9:34554–34566
10. Coussens MJ, Corman C, Fischer AL, Sago J, Swarthout J (2011) MISSION LentiPlex pooled shRNA library screening in mammalian cells. J Vis Exp 58. https://doi.org/10.3791/3305
11. Sun J, Nishiyama T, Shimizu K, Kadota K (2013) TCC: an R package for comparing tag count data with robust normalization strategies. BMC Bioinformatics 14:219
12. Merighi S, Mirandola P, Varani K, Gessi S, Leung E, Baraldi PG et al (2003) A glance at adenosine receptors: novel target for antitumor therapy. Pharmacol Ther 100:31–48

Chapter 26

Discovering Transcription Factor Noncoding RNA Targets Using ChIP-Seq Analysis

Vitalay Fomin and Carol Prives

Abstract

Next generation sequencing enables large-scale analysis of mRNA expression (RNA-seq), genome variance (whole genome or exome), and transcription factor binding (ChIP-seq). Here we describe a method that allows the identification of transcription factor-binding sites in the vicinity of nonprotein-coding genes.

Key words ChIP-seq, p53, Noncoding, Transcription factor, Next generation sequencing

1 Introduction

Advancements in DNA sequencing technology over the last couple of decades such as next generation sequencing has led to the realization that ~90% of the genome is transcribed even though protein-coding genes comprise only ~1–3% of the genome [1, 2]. The other ~87% of transcripts were initially considered to be "junk", but more recent studies revealed that at least some of these transcripts have important biological function(s) [3–5]. These previously un-annotated transcripts belong to an expanding family of noncoding transcripts that include: microRNAs, enhancer RNAs (eRNAs), long noncoding RNAs (lncRNAs), Piwi-interacting RNA (piRNAs), small nucleolar RNAs (snoRNAs), ribosomal ribonucleic acid (rRNA), and transfer ribonucleic acid (tRNA). It is now known as well that that the transcription of some of these noncoding transcripts—especially lncRNAs—is tissue and cell type dependent [6], suggesting that their transcription is tightly regulated. As more noncoding transcripts are being discovered it is becoming important to understand how their transcription is regulated as it can provide functional insights. A key mode by which coding and noncoding genes are regulated is by transcription factors (TFs) that bind to specific DNA sequences and such interactions are sufficiently stable that they can be documented experimentally. Such

Ivana Vancurova and Yan Zhu (eds.), *Immune Mediators in Cancer: Methods and Protocols*, Methods in Molecular Biology, vol. 2108, https://doi.org/10.1007/978-1-0716-0247-8_26, © Springer Science+Business Media, LLC, part of Springer Nature 2020

TFs are proteins that either themselves contain a sequence-specific DNA-binding domain or interact with other factors with such domains, and as a result of such interactions such TFs can activate or repress the transcription of their target genes. DNA-binding complexes containing a given TF can often be detected via antibodies bound to the TF. Such complexes can be identified in cells via the process of Chromatin Immunoprecipitation (ChIP) by combining formaldehyde cross-linking, DNA shearing, antibody binding, and recovery of bound genomic DNA fragments associated with the TF that are identified by sequencing the bound DNA. This approach has also been modified to acquire globally the genomic DNA sites bound by a given TF using massively parallel sequencing, a procedure named ChIP-Seq.

Here we provide a method to analyze ChIP-seq data geared toward the discovery of noncoding genes regulated by a TF(s) of interest. This method can be applied to any publicly or proprietary ChIP-seq data in any organism that has their genome sequenced. In this protocol we will use p53 as the TF and demonstrate the analysis of p53 ChIP-seq data from Menendez et al., paper [7].

2 Materials

The analysis shown here is done in an Ubuntu environment in a command shell but will work with other UNIX-based operating systems. Please see important remarks listed in Subheading 4 (*see* **Note 1**).

2.1 Operating System, ChIP-seq Data, and Software

1. Operating system:

   Ubuntu available https://www.ubuntu.com/download with installation instructions available here: https://tutorials.ubuntu.com/tutorial/tutorial-install-ubuntu-desktop#0.

2. ChIP-seq generated reads: Download the raw reads that we will be working with by accessing http://www.ebi.ac.uk/ena and downloading the following two files, SRR847014 and SRR847015 by clicking on them and then pressing the File 1 under the FASTQ files (FTP) category. This will result in the download of the two files (SRR847014.fastq.gz and SRR847015.fastq.gz). SRR847014.fastq.gz is the input file for the ChIP-seq and acts as the control. File 2, SRR847015.fastq.gz is a sample treated with nutlin, which induces the accumulation of p53 and increased p53 binding to its target genes.

   Unzip files by using the command `#gunzip SRR847014.fastq.gz` and `#gunzip SRR847015.fastq.gz`.

3. Bowtie2 aligner [8]: available from https://sourceforge.net/projects/bowtie-bio/files/bowtie2/2.3.5.1/; download the latest version.
4. Samtools [9]: available from http://www.htslib.org/download/.
5. HOMER [10]: Peak calling and motif finding software; available from http://HOMER.ucsd.edu/HOMER/.
6. hg19 reference genome and bowtie index: available from https://support.illumina.com/sequencing/sequencing_software/igenome.html; click on hg19 to download.
7. Integrative Genomics Viewer (IGV) [11]: available from https://igv.org/app/.

2.2 Software Installation

1. Samtool (*see* **Note 2**).

```
# tar -jxvf samtoolVersioX.tar.bz2
# cd samtoolsVersionX/
# make
# make install
```

2. Bowtie2.

```
# gunzip bowtie2-2.3.5.1-linux-x86_64.zip
```

Add directory to the path (*see* **Notes 3** and **4**).

3. Genome index (*see* **Note 5**).

```
# tar -xvzf Homo_sapiens_UCSC_hg19.tar.gz
```

4. HOMER.

Detailed instructions on how to install HOMER are found here: http://HOMER.ucsd.edu/HOMER/introduction/install.html (*see* **Note 6**).

3 Methods

3.1 Map Reads to the Genome with Bowtie2

Align the reads stored in SRR847014.fastq SRR847015.fastq files to hg19 genome with the following commands:

```
# bowtie2 -p 16 -x ~/my_chipseq_experiment/Location/of/Bowtie/Index
-q SRR847014.fastq -S Nutlin_input.sam
# bowtie2 -p 16 -x ~/my_chipseq_experiment/Location/of/Bowtie/Index
-q SRR847015.fastq -S Nutlin_p53_ChIP.sam
```

Argument explanation:

-x: The base name of the index for the reference genome and is located in the directory unpacked from Homo_sapiens_UCSC_hg19.tar.gz file. If the above instructions are followed the index should be located here: ~/my_chipseq_experiment/Homo_sapiens/UCSC/hg19/Sequ ence/Bowtie2Index, and should contain files with the bt2 extension (like genome.1.bt2).

-S: Tells Bowtie2 to export alignments in Sequence Alignment Map format (SAM) format.

-q: specifies that the input is a FASTQ file.

-p: the amount of threads to use for the mapping. Check how many threads you can use, as it varies with the type of processor the computer has (*see* **Note 3**).

3.2 Converting SAM Files into BAM Files and Sorting

1. Since SAM files are large files they are converted into Binary Alignment Map (BAM) format, which produces files that are easier to work with. The conversion is done with the following commands:

```
# samtools view -bS Nutlin_input.sam > Nutlin_input.bam
# samtools view -bS Nutlin_input.sam > Nutlin_p53_ChIP.bam
```

2. Sort Bam files with the following commands:

```
# samtools sort Nutlin_input.bam > Nutlin_input_sorted.bam
# samtools sort Nutlin_p53_ChIP.bam > Nutlin_p53_ChIP_sorted.
bam
```

3.3 TF Peak Finding

In order to reveal which genes and the chromosomal locations bound by a TF we must find the locations in the genome that have more reads aligned to than expected by pure chance.

1. Generate a tag directory which is needed by HOMER to find peaks. This step also provides some quality assessment (*see* **Note 7**). The following commands are used:

```
# makeTagDirectory Nutlin_input_HOMER_tags Nutlin_input_
sorted.bam -format bed
# makeTagDirectory Nutlin_p53_ChIP_HOMER_tags Nutlin_p53_
ChIP_sorted.bam -format bed
```

Two directories are created:

(a) Nutlin_input_HOMER_tag.

(b) Nutlin_p53_ChIP_HOMER_tags.

2. Find enriched peaks compared to control with actual peak finding/calling. The following command is used (*see* **Note 8**):

```
# findPeaks Nutlin_p53_ChIP_HOMER_tags/ -style factor -o
nutlin.peaks -i Nutlin_input_HOMER_tags/
```

Argument explanation:

The first argument (after findPeaks command) is the tag directory for the experiment, in our case it is "Nutlin_p53_-ChIP_HOMER_tags/".

-o: Specify the output file name that will contain the peaks.

-i: Specifies the location of the input/control directory, usually is the input of igG control.

-style: the type of experiment, in our case for ChIP-seq we use factor.

3.4 Peak Annotation

Peak annotation associates the peaks with gene names. Additionally it provides other useful information (*see* **Note 9**). The following command is used to annotate peaks:

```
# annotatePeaks.pl nutlin.peaks hg19 > nutlin.annotated.peaks
```

Argument explanation:

First argument (after annotatePeaks.pl command) is the peak file from the previous step, in our case it is "nutlin.peaks."

Second argument is the genome that was used to map the ChIP-seq reads, in our case it is "hg19."

Third argument indicates the output file name that contains the annotated peaks, in our case it is "nutlin.annotated.peaks" (*see* **Note 10**).

3.5 Analysis Examination and Extraction of Noncoding Transcripts

1. Export the content of nutlin.annotated.peaks to excel for sorting and analysis.
   (a) Use the following command to open a text editor.

```
# gedit nutlin.annotated.peaks
```

   (b) Press Ctrl-A to select all and then Ctrl-C to copy the information.
   (c) Press Ctrl-P in excel spreadsheet to paste the information.
2. Find all the noncoding transcripts with p53 binding.
   (a) Sort the file by gene type (the last column) in the excel sheet.
   (b) Choose all the genes with marked as ncRNA, which stands for noncoding RNA.

3.6 Visualize the Results in IGV

The following steps allow to visualize the actual peak, which consists of the mapped reads.

1. Index the BAM files from Subheading 3.2 with the following commands:

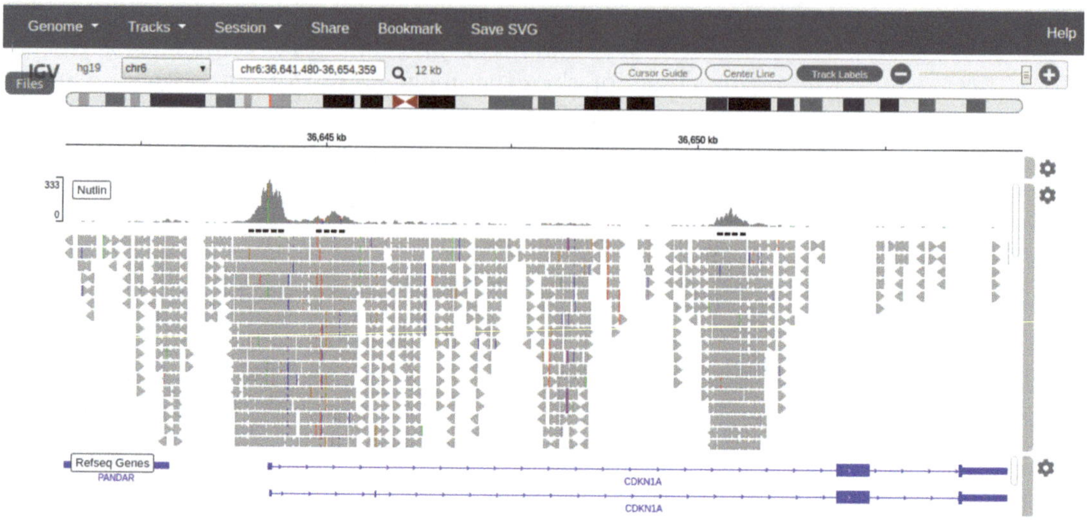

Fig. 1 Image of integrative genome viewer with p53 ChiP-seq peaks. Bam and indexed bam files were loaded into the IGV web app with the resulting Image showing CDKN1A (p21) gene with peaks representing reads that were aligned to the location of p53 binding within p21

```
# samtools index Nutlin_input.bam
# samtools index Nutlin_p53_ChIP.bam
```

Two files are generated:

(a) Nutlin_input.bam.index.

(b) Nutlin_p53_ChIP.bam.index.

2. Upload the files to the IGV browser app: https://igv.org/app/

   (a) Click on Tracks then Local File.

   (b) Choose the bam and bam.index files for upload.

3. Enter the name of gene of interest in the gene location window to visualize the peak.

In our case CDKN1A gene is a known p53 target, so enter the gene name (CDKN1A) in the gene location window and look at the peak (Fig. 1). Since peaks include both coding and noncoding genes, this protocol is applicable for coding genes as well.

4 Notes

1. Important remarks:

   (a) Before attempting the protocol it is recommended to become familiarized with ChIP and ChIP-seq methodology, which is provided in these reviews [12, 13].

(b) _Commands that are meant to be executed from the UNIX shell are prefixed with a "#," which represents the terminal/shell.

(c) In this protocol a home directory is used to store all the tools for the analysis. For convenience it is recommended to create the same directory.
   - Go to the home directory with command: # cd ~/.
   - Create a directory with command: `# mkdir my_chipseq_experiment`.
   - Download all the software mentioned in Subheading 2 into the my_chipseq_experiment/ directory (ignore if you already have everything installed).

(d) Some of the software requires additional UNIX utilities. Please follow the installation guidelines for each of the tools below and install these utilities prior to tool installation.

(e) Google is your best friend when it comes to troubleshooting software installation issues. For any error not discussed here, please google it and try to find a solution.

2. Check the System Requirements (UNIX utilities for the installation of samtool; available from https://samtools.github.io/bcftools/howtos/install.html). This website also provides extensive instruction on how to use samtools.
3. For further details and more extensive instructions please read the Bowtie2 manual available here: http://bowtie-bio.sourceforge.net/bowtie2/manual.shtml which also provides installation instructions.
4. All tools must be added to executable path, which requires to edit ~/.bashrc file and add the line PATH=$PATH:~/name/of/directory/for/the/tool. Additional tutorial and examples can be found here: https://opensource.com/article/17/6/set-path-linux.
5. You do not need to add this one to the path, but you will have to know the directory location.
6. Reading the manual in the HOMER website is strongly recommended as it provides extensive instructions and other applications of HOMER not discusses in this protocol. Website available here: http://homer.ucsd.edu/homer/index.html.
7. More information is available here: http://homer.ucsd.edu/homer/ngs/tagDir.html8.
8. For more information about findPeaks command in HOMER please read the following manual http://homer.ucsd.edu/homer/ngs/peaks.html.

9. Please read http://HOMER.ucsd.edu/HOMER/ngs/annotation.html which explains in detail all the additional information added by running annotatePeaks.pl.

10. Detailed tutorial that showshow to use HOMERwith several other options not discussed here is recommended and availablehere: http://HOMER.ucsd.edu/HOMER/ngs/index.html.

References

1. Djebali S, Davis CA, Merkel A et al (2012) Landscape of transcription in human cells. Nature 489:101–108. https://doi.org/10.1038/nature11233
2. Pertea M (2012) The human transcriptome: an unfinished story. Genes 3:344–360. https://doi.org/10.3390/genes3030344
3. Hu WL, Jin L, Xu A et al (2018) GUARDIN is a p53-responsive long non-coding RNA that is essential for genomic stability. Nat Cell Biol 20:492–502. https://doi.org/10.1038/s41556-018-0066-7
4. Engreitz JM, Pandya-Jones A, McDonel P et al (2013) The Xist lncRNA exploits three-dimensional genome architecture to spread across the X chromosome. Science 341:1237973. https://doi.org/10.1126/science.1237973
5. Fang Y, Fullwood MJ (2016) Roles, functions, and mechanisms of long non-coding RNAs in cancer. Genomics Proteomics Bioinformatics 14:42–54. https://doi.org/10.1016/j.gpb.2015.09.006
6. Gloss BS, Dinger ME (2016) The specificity of long noncoding RNA expression. Biochim Biophys Acta 1859:16–22. https://doi.org/10.1016/j.bbagrm.2015.08.005
7. Menendez D, Nguyen T-A, Freudenberg JM et al (2013) Diverse stresses dramatically alter genome-wide p53 binding and transactivation landscape in human cancer cells. Nucleic Acids Res 41:7286–7301. https://doi.org/10.1093/nar/gkt504
8. Langmead B, Salzberg SL (2012) Fast gapped-read alignment with Bowtie 2. Nat Methods 9:357–359. https://doi.org/10.1038/nmeth.1923
9. Li H, Handsaker B, Wysoker A et al (2009) The sequence alignment/map format and SAMtools. Bioinformatics 25:2078–2079. https://doi.org/10.1093/bioinformatics/btp352
10. Heinz S, Benner C, Spann N et al (2010) Simple combinations of lineage-determining transcription factors prime cis-regulatory elements required for macrophage and B cell identities. Mol Cell 38:576–589
11. Robinson JT, Thorvaldsdóttir H, Winckler W et al (2011) Integrative genomics viewer. Nat Biotechnol 29:24–26. https://doi.org/10.1038/nbt.1754
12. Furey TS (2012) ChIP-seq and beyond: new and improved methodologies to detect and characterize protein–DNA interactions. Nat Rev Genet 13(12):840–852. https://doi.org/10.1038/nrg3306
13. Landt SG, Marinov GK, Kundaje A et al (2012) ChIP-seq guidelines and practices of the ENCODE and modENCODE consortia. Genome Res 22:1813–1831. https://doi.org/10.1101/gr.136184.111

Chapter 27

Phylogenetic Analyses of Chemokine Receptors from Sequence Retrieval to Phylogenetic Trees

Juan C. Santos

Abstract

Phylogenetic trees are an essential requisite for comparative biology studies where hypotheses regarding the evolution of genes can be investigated. Trees provide visual and statistical guides to characterize the degree of relatedness among biological entities from genes to species. In a tree, ancestor-descendant relationships are represented by connections, and closely related entities share most of these links. In this chapter, I outlined a method to retrieve and label amino acid and nucleotide sequences of chemokine receptors, align them in sequence matrices, determine their best-model of molecular evolution, and estimate the corresponding phylogenetic trees with distance and maximum likelihood approaches. Most of these analyses are performed within the *R* environment, and all of these methods use open-source software.

Key words Amino acids, Nucleotides, Automatic sequence retrieval, Alignment, Homology, Substitution models, Maximum likelihood, Neighbor joining, Phylogenetic trees

1 Introduction

Most comparisons at the level of nucleotide and amino acid sequences should address the evolutionary relationships among the source populations and species before any inferences can be formulated [1]. By accounting for phylogenetic relationships, the characterization of paralogous or orthologous sequences can reveal interesting patterns that can be associated with biological adaptations and key protein functions [2]. However, direct comparisons among sequences can be biased due to phylogenetic signal, which is defined as the similarities between biological entities as a result of inherited resemblances from their ancestors [3]. To avoid such bias, phylogenetic trees are inferred as evolutionary hypotheses of ancestor-descendant relationships derived from sequence alignments, a model of nucleotide or amino acid substitutions and an optimizing algorithm that tries to find the best possible tree structure (i.e., topology). These phylogenetic trees provide information about the degree of divergence (i.e., absolute or relative time)

Ivana Vancurova and Yan Zhu (eds.), *Immune Mediators in Cancer: Methods and Protocols*, Methods in Molecular Biology, vol. 2108, https://doi.org/10.1007/978-1-0716-0247-8_27, © Springer Science+Business Media, LLC, part of Springer Nature 2020

between biological entities since their last common ancestor. By tracing gene sequences on these trees, researchers can infer ancestral states along the nodes of the phylogeny (i.e., hypothesized sequences in ancestors). Furthermore, comparisons among biological entities (e.g., genes, species) can be done using most statistical analyses by adding a correction for the underlying phylogenetic structure.

When reading a phylogenetic tree, its topology (i.e., the relative arrangement of terminal tips and their internal nodes through connecting branches) allows us to infer groupings or clades in which two or more tips (i.e., taxa) are connected to a common ancestor (i.e., a close shared node). These ancestors are inferred to have ancestral phenotypic or molecular states that, in most cases, are now lost due to extinction. The connecting lines between nodes of the tree are referred as branches, and their length represents an estimate of the genetic distance between connecting taxa, tips or clades [4]. If a tree is given a polarity, such phylogeny is said to be rooted by assigning a branch that connects the closest relative to an outgroup outside the group of interest (i.e., ingroup). A tree without polarity is said to be unrooted. The branch length units of a phylogeny can be relative (e.g., sequence divergence) or absolute (e.g., millions of years). Likewise, if the branch lengths (i.e., distances) of a phylogeny are the same from the root to each of the terminal tips, the phylogeny is said to be ultrametric.

Most phylogenetic analyses strive to have fully resolved (i.e., completely bifurcating) trees and well-supported topologies (e.g., high confidence on the presence of connecting nodes) using bootstraps or other measures of accuracy [1]. Toward these goals, the following steps are usually carried out before any phylogenetic tree reconstruction is done. First, a careful collection of sequence data from samples, whose origins can be traced back to their biological source (*see* **Note 1**), should be performed before any analysis. Second, a correct identification or annotation of the sequences should be confirmed to avoid mixing paralogous, pseudogenes or chimeric sequences, so that only orthologous sequences (*see* **Note 2**) or, if the interest is to analyze gene duplications, paralogous sequences are used in any downstream phylogenetic analyses without ambiguity. Third, most sequences include variations in length as result of nucleotide or amino acid insertions and deletions (indels), so a sequence alignment is a prerequisite before the phylogeny estimation. Sequence alignment is, on its own, a computational rigorous process in which gaps (i.e., spaces) are introduced along the sequences in the dataset to maximize homology [5]. With the aligned sequences, a model of molecular substitution is determined, which is necessary for the calculation of the probabilities of change between nucleotides or amino acids along the branches of the phylogeny. Finally, the evolutionary tree can be estimated from the optimal alignment and substitution models.

In sum, a phylogenetic tree represents a visual and statistical representation of the evolutionary diversification of a section of the Tree of Life. Most researchers will find these phylogenetic trees useful, as these hypotheses promote further comparative analyses among biological entities (e.g., sequences, individuals, genes, species). The objective of this chapter is to present commonly used methods to reconstruct molecular phylogenies using chemokine receptors as an example. However, the processes outlined here can be applied to other genes and phenotypic datasets. Likewise, the bulk of data retrieval and management is done through open-source software. For this reason, I will provide a brief introduction about the installation and management of packages in the *R* environment [6]. Then, the actual workflow starts from getting sequences from the NCBI or other public sequence archives, followed by sequence alignment, model estimation of molecular evolution, and phylogenetic tree reconstruction. I would like to emphasize that the software and procedures indicated here are one of many commonly used methodologies based on freely and commercially available programs. When pertinent, I will provide citations for alternative methods and relevant software.

2 Materials

For this chapter, I used a published list of chemokine receptors published by Bachelerie et al. [7]. This list is by no means exhaustive or complete, but it serves to guide the automatic retrieval of those protein and nucleotide sequences from the NCBI database. It is important to note that only sequences with UniProt [8] and NCBI accession numbers can be retrieved if sequence comparisons are requested. I deliberately included the installation of software as part of the Methods section because this chapter, in essence, aims to provide a hands-on practice for users with little or no familiarity with the *R* environment.

3 Methods

3.1 R *Installation*

R is a computing language and free software environment designed for statistical analyses with a graphics interphase [6]. Its computer requirements tend to be minimal, and *R* is distributed as precompiled binary executables. This software is also available in the three main base platforms: Windows, OS X (Mac), and Linux. Most users get *R* from the Comprehensive R Archive Network (CRAN), which hosts the source code, precompiled versions, installation instructions, and many basic manuals:

```
http://cran.r-project.org/
```

Once *R* is installed in a computer, the user can run the environment in the *R* console, which provides some basic information about the current version of *R* installed, computer platform, and working directory. If no additional packages have been installed, the base library includes essential commands such as reading/writing files, handling databases, standard statistical analyses, plotting, and other environment control functions. There are alternative ways to install and manage *R*, which might be more accessible to certain users (*see* **Note 3**).

3.2 R-Package Management

The *R* environment allows an expansive modularity with >18,000 free software packages available at public repositories including Bioconductor, GitHub, and the Comprehensive R Archive Network (CRAN). The *R* environment provides an easy installation of packages from the web by typing the following function in the *R* console (notice the punctuation, *see* **Note 4**):

```
install.packages("DESIRED_PACKAGE_NAME")
```

The name of the package can be found in the CRAN and a "mirror repository" should be selected. The location of the "mirror repository" should be the physically closest to the user, but most packages can be installed from any "mirror repository" with enough speed. It is important to note that CRAN regularly updates the repository, and it is up to the package developers to keep theirs current. Some functions in *R* packages might become deprecated in newer versions, and some entire packages are archived (i.e., disappear) from CRAN if not maintained by their developers. In those instances, the user can download the desired package using the *R*-package "devtools" [9]:

```
install.packages("devtools")
library(devtools)
devtools::install_version("ggplot2",
 version = "0.9.1",
 repos = "http://cran.us.r-project.org")
```

With "devtools" is also possible to install packages hosted in GitHub that are not currently available in CRAN. GitHub is a web-based hosting site where many software developers deposit working and recent updates of their computer code. Packages can be installed as follows:

```
library(devtools)
install_github("DEVELOPER_GITHUB_NAME/R_PACKAGE_NAME")
```

Some *R* packages used for phylogenomics, sequence retrieval, gene annotation, and gene ontology enrichment can be accessed and downloaded through Bioconductor [10, 11]. To install packages from this repository, the user can follow these instructions:

```
install.packages("BiocManager")
library(BiocManager)
BiocManager::install("DESIRED_PACKAGE_NAME",
 version = "VERSION_NUMBER")
```

3.3 Installation of R Packages Used for Phylogenetics and Sequence Manipulation

For the methods described here, the user needs to install the following *R*-packages: "annotate" [12], "ape" [13, 14], "phangorn" [15], and "rentrez" [16]:

```
BiocManager::install("annotate") # Using R environments for
annotation
install.packages("ape") # Analyses of Phylogenetics
and Evolution
install.packages("phangorn") # Phylogenetic
Reconstruction and Analysis Package
install.packages("rentrez") # Using R to access the
NCBI eUtils API
```

As noticed above, I added comments (i.e., text not read or run by *R*) preceded from a "#" sign.

The citation of most *R*-packages can be obtained within *R* with few commands (*see* **Note 5**).

3.4 Retrieval of Protein Sequences from Chemokine Receptors Using an Accession Number

For this example, I will work on CXCL chemokine involved in neutrophil trafficking.

1. Retrieve the human CXCL1 protein that has an accession number: P09341 and assign it to an object called "Human_CXCL1" using the *R*-packages "annotate" and "rentrez":

```
library(annotate)
Human_CXCL1 <- annotate::getSEQ("P09341")
[1]
"MARAALSAAPSNPRLLRVALLLLLLVAAGRRAAGASVATELRCQCLQTLQGIHPKNIQSV
NVKSPGPHCAQTEVIATLKNGRKACLNPASPIVKKIIEKMLNSDKSN"

library(rentrez)
Human_CXCL1 <- annotate::entrez_fetch(db = "protein",
 id = "P09341",
 rettype = "fasta")

Human_CXCL1 # to check what is in this object
[1]  ">sp|P09341.1|GROA_HUMAN RecName: Full=Growth-regulated
alpha protein; AltName: Full=C-X-C motif chemokine 1;
AltName: Full=GRO-alpha(1-73); AltName: Full=Melanoma
growth stimulatory activity; Short=MGSA; AltName:
Full=Neutrophil-activating protein 3; Short=NAP-3;
```

```
Contains: RecName: Full=GRO-alpha(4-73); Contains: RecName:
Full=GRO-alpha(5-73); Contains: RecName: Full=GRO-alpha
(6-73); Flags:
Precursor\nMARAALSAAPSNPRLLRVALLLLLLVAAGRRAAGASVATELRCQCLQTLQ
GIHPKNIQSVNVKSPGPHCA\nQTEVIATLKNGRKACLNPASPIVKKIIEKMLNSDKSN\n
\n"
```

2. Carry out an automatic BLAST (Basic Local Alignment Search Tool) query [17] using the standard protein search setting (i.e., protein sequence query against the NCBI protein database) using the "BLASTP" option for our given protein:

```
CXCL_df <- annotate::blastSequences
("MARAALSAAPSNPRLLRVALLLLLLVAAGRRAAGASVATELRCQCLQTLQGIHPKNIQS
VNVKSPGPHCAQTEVIATLKNGRKACLNPASPIVKKIIEKMLNSDKSN",
 hitListSize = "500", program =
"blastp",
 timeout=100, as= "data.frame")
```

With these commands, the "blastSequences" function of the *R*-package "annotate" will look for 500 entries (hitListSize = `"500"`), using "blastp," with a time out of 100 s and return as a data frame object. These results are assigned to an object called "`CXCL_df`" and different columns in this object can be retrieved by their name. To see the names of the columns in this object use the following command:

```
names(CXCL_df)
```

We are interested in the columns with sequences (i.e., `Hsp_qseq`), so these can be obtained by typing `CXCL1_df $Hsp_qseq`. Similarly, we are interested in these sequence annotations, which can be seen by typing `CXCL_df$Hit_def` and `CXCL_df$Hit_id`:

```
CXCL1_df$Hsp_qseq
CXCL_df$Hit_def
CXCL_df$Hit_id
```

3. Construct and write a *.txt file with an annotated data frame that would include species names, accession numbers, and sequences with the retrieved sequences. These files serve as references for later analyses or any other searches that the user might need to perform with those retrieved sequences:

```
CXCL_for_use_df <- subset(CXCL_df, select = c(Hit_def,
Hit_id, Hsp_qseq))
write.table(CXCL_for_use_df, file =
"CXCL_results_500_aminoacids.txt", sep = "\t")
```

4. Read this saved file as follows (the user should make sure that the working directory is the same as the one that contains the *.txt file, *see* **Note 6**):

```
CXCL_for_use_df <-
read.table("CXCL_results_500_aminoacids.txt", header = TRUE,
 sep = "\t", stringsAsFactors = FALSE)
```

5. Construct a file in fasta format that can be used for sequence alignments:

```
CXCL_definitions <- CXCL_for_use_df$Hit_def
extract_names_1_function <- function(x){
sub(".*\\[(.*)\\].*", "\\1", x, perl=TRUE)}
taxa_names_seq <- extract_names_1_function(CXCL_definitions)
taxa_names_seq <- gsub(" ", "_", taxa_names_seq)

CXCL_accession_numbers <- CXCL_for_use_df$Hit_id
extract_names_2_function <-
function(x){sub(".*\\|(.*)\\|.*$", "\\1",
CXCL_accession_numbers, perl=TRUE)}
taxa_accession <-
extract_names_2_function(CXCL_accession_numbers)

taxa_fasta_name <- paste0(">",taxa_names_seq, "_",
taxa_accession)

# construct fasta entries

taxa_fasta_seq_vector <- paste0(taxa_fasta_name, "\n",
CXCL_for_use_df$Hsp_qseq)
```

6. Remove repeated sequences that have the same accession number:

```
taxa_fasta_seq_vector_2 <-
taxa_fasta_seq_vector[!duplicated(taxa_accession)]
taxa_fasta_seq_vector_2 <- taxa_fasta_seq_vector_2
[!is.na(taxa_fasta_seq_vector_2)]
```

7. Remove entries with extraneous annotations (e.g., "synthetic_-construct", "Chain_A,"):

```
taxa_fasta_seq_vector_2 <- taxa_fasta_seq_vector_2
[!grepl("synthetic_construct|Chain_A",
taxa_fasta_seq_vector_2)]
```

8. Write a file in fasta format (*see* **Note** 7) with sequences that include the annotation for the species of origin and the corresponding accession numbers:

```
writeLines(taxa_fasta_seq_vector_2, "CXCL_aminoacid.fasta")
```

3.5 Retrieval of Protein Sequences Using a List of Accession Number for Chemokine Receptors

The accession numbers for the chemokine proteins are listed on Table 1 in Bachelerie et al. [7].

1. Retrieve amino acid sequences as vectors using "annotate," by providing a list of accession numbers for human and mouse into data frames:

```
library(annotate)
receptor_names <- c("CXCL1", "CXCL2", "CXCL3", "CXCL4",
"CXCL4L1", "CXCL5", "CXCL6", "CXCL7", "CXCL8", "CXCL9",
"CXCL10", "CXCL11", "CXCL12", "CXCL13", "CXCL14", "Cxcl15",
"CXCL16", "CXCL17", "CCL1", "CCL2", "CCL3", "CCL3L1",
"CCL3L3", "CCL4", "CCL4L1", "CCL4L2", "CCL5", "Ccl6", "CCL7",
"CCL8", "Ccl9", "CCL11", "Ccl12", "CCL13", "CCL14", "CCL15",
"CCL16", "CCL17", "CCL18", "CCL19", "CCL20", "CCL21", "CCL22",
"CCL23", "CCL24", "CCL25", "CCL26", "CCL27", "CCL28", "XCL1",
"XCL2", "CX3CL1")

human_access_numbers <- c("P09341", "P19875", "P19876",
"P02776", "P10720", "P42830", "P80162", "P02775", "P10145",
"Q07325", "P02778", "O14625", "P48061", "O43927", "O95715",
"NA", "Q9H2A7", "Q6UXB2", "P22362", "P13500", "P10147",
"P16619", "P16619", "P13236", "Q8NHW4", "Q8NHW4", "P13501",
"NA", "P80098", "P80075", "NA", "P51671", "NA", "Q99616",
"Q16627", "Q16663", "O15467", "Q92583", "P55774", "Q99731",
"P78556", "O00585", "O00626", "P55773", "O00175", "O15444",
"Q9Y258", "Q9Y4X3", "Q9NRJ3", "P47992", "Q9UBD3", "P78423")

mouse_access_numbers <- c("P12850", "P10889", "Q6W5C0",
"Q9Z126", "NA", "P50228", "NA", "Q9EQI5", "NA", "P18340",
"P17515", "Q8R392", "P40224", "O55038", "Q6AXC2", "Q9WVL7",
"Q8BSU2", "Q8R3U6", "P10146", "P10148", "P10855", "P10855",
"NA", "P14097", "NA", "NA", "P30882", "P27784", "Q03366",
"Q9Z121", "P51670", "P48298", "Q62401", "NA", "NA", "NA",
"NA", "Q9WUZ6", "NA", "O70460", "O89093", "P84444", "O88430",
"NA", "Q9JKC0", "O35903", "Q5C9Q0", "Q9Z1X0", "Q9JIL2",
"P47993", "NA", "O35188")

human_genes_df <-
data.frame(name=character(),sequence=character(),stringsAs
Factors=FALSE)
mouse_genes_df <-
data.frame(name=character(),sequence=character(),stringsAs
Factors=FALSE)

for(i in 1:length(human_access_numbers)) {
human_gene_name <- paste0(">human_",receptor_names[i],"_",
human_access_numbers[i])
mouse_gene_name <- paste0(">mouse_",receptor_names[i],"_",
```

```
mouse_access_numbers[i])
if(!human_access_numbers[i] == "NA") {
 Sys.sleep(2)
 human_CXCL_name <- human_gene_name
 human_CXCL <-
try(annotate::getSEQ(human_access_numbers[i]), silent =
TRUE)
 if(!class(human_CXCL) == "try-error"){
 one_human_gene_df <-
data.frame(name=human_CXCL_name,sequence=human_CXCL,strings
AsFactors=FALSE)
 human_genes_df <- rbind(human_genes_df,
one_human_gene_df)
 cat("\n retrieved human gene: ", human_CXCL_name, "\n")
 }
 }
if(!mouse_access_numbers[i] == "NA") {
 Sys.sleep(2)
 mouse_CXCL_name <- mouse_gene_name
 mouse_CXCL <-
try(annotate::getSEQ(mouse_access_numbers[i]), silent =
TRUE)
 if(!class(mouse_CXCL) == "try-error"){
 one_mouse_gene_df <-
data.frame(name=mouse_CXCL_name,sequence=mouse_CXCL,strings
AsFactors=FALSE)
 mouse_genes_df <- rbind(mouse_genes_df,
one_mouse_gene_df)
 cat("\n retrieved mouse gene: ", mouse_CXCL_name, "\n")
 }
 }
 }
```

The user should notice that using this approach requires the computer system to pause for 2 s (i.e., `Sys.sleep(2)`) so the automatic retrieval does not cause NCBI servers to return an error.

2. Create a fasta file ready for alignment with the resulting data frame objects:

```
human_sequence_vector <- paste0(human_genes_df$name, "\n",
human_genes_df$sequence)
mouse_sequence_vector <- paste0(mouse_genes_df$name, "\n",
mouse_genes_df$sequence)
human_mouse_sequence_vector <- c(human_sequence_vector,
mouse_sequence_vector)
```

3. Write this file in fasta format (*see* **Note 7**) with sequences that include the annotation for the organism of origin (i.e., mouse or human) and the accession numbers:

```
writeLines(human_mouse_sequence_vector,
"CXC_human_mouse_aminoacid.fasta")
```

3.6 Retrieval of Nucleotide Sequences from Chemokine Receptors

I will continue with the same CXCL1 chemokine example, but I will do a protein sequence query to obtain its matching nucleotide sequence from the NCBI database.

1. Retrieve a nucleotide sequence that corresponds to the human CXCL1 protein, which has the following accession number: P09341. With the retrieved nucleotide sequences, assign them to an object call "Human_CXCL1" in fasta format using "annotate":

```
library(annotate)
CXCL1_nucleotide_df <- annotate::blastSequences
("MARAALSAAPSNPRLLRVALLLLLLVAAGRRAAGASVATELRCQCLQTLQGIHPKNIQS
VNVKSPGPHCAQTEVIATLKNGRKACLNPASPIVKKIIEKMLNSDKSN",
 hitListSize = "20", program = "tblastn",
 timeout=100, as= "data.frame")
```

   In this search, we used the "TBLASTN" option (i.e., protein sequence query against the translated NCBI nucleotide database) to obtain nucleotide sequences.

2. From the resulting sequence hits, we see that the object on the "`CXCL1_nucleotide_df`" includes a list of sequences that can be sorted by their highest bit-score (i.e., `CXCL1_nucleotide_df$Hsp_bit-score`). In this case, the best-score nucleotide sequence corresponds to human CXCL1 mRNA transcript with an accession number: BT006880. This sequence can be retrieved following the same procedure for sequence retrieval as illustrated for proteins (see Subheading 3.4):

```
Human_CXCL1_nucleotide <- annotate::getSEQ("BT006880")
Human_CXCL1_nucleotide
[1]
"ATGGCCCGCGCTGCTCTCTCCGCCGCCCCCAGCAATCCCCGGCTCCTGCGAGTGGCACTG
CTGCTCCTGCTCCTGGTAGCCGCTGGCCGGCGCGCAGCAGGAGCGTCCGTGGCCACTG
AACTGCGCTGCCAGTGCTTGCAGACCCTGCAGGGAATTCACCCCAAGAACATCCAA AGTG
TGAACGTGAAGTCCCCCGGACCCCACTGCGCCCAAACCG AAGTCATAGCCACACTCAAG
AATGGGCGGAAAG CTTGCCTCAATCCTGCATCCCCCATAGTTAAGAAAATCATCGAAAA
GATGCTGAACAGTGACAAATCCAACTAG"
```

3. Carry out automatic BLAST queries using the standard nucleotide search setting (i.e., nucleotide sequence query against the NCBI nucleotide database) using the "BLASTN" option for our given nucleotide:

```
CXCL_df <- annotate::blastSequences
("ATGGCCCGCGCTGCTCTCTCCGCCGCCCCCAGCAATCCCCGGCTCCTGCGAGTGGCA
CTGCTGCTCCTGCTCCTGGTAGCCGCTGGCCGGCGCGCAGCAGGAGCGTCCGTGGCCAC
TGAACTGCGCTGCCAGTGCTTGCAGACCCTGCAGGGAATTCACCCCAAGAACATCCAAA
GTGTGAACGTGAAGTCCCCCGGACCCCACTGCGCCCAAACCGAAGTCATAGCCACACTC
AAGAATGGGCGGAAAGCTTGCCTCAATCCTGCATCCCCCATAGTTAAGAAAATCATCGA
AAAGATGCTGAACAGTGACAAATCCAACTAG",
 hitListSize = "500", program =
"blastn",
 timeout=100, as= "data.frame")
```

With these commands, the "blastSequences" function of "annotate" will look for 500 entries (hitListSize = "500"), using "blastn," with a time out of 100 s and return as a data frame object. The retrieved sequences would be on `CXCL1_df$Hsp_qseq` and their associated annotations on `CXCL_df$Hit_def` and `CXCL_df$Hit_id`.

4. Construct and write a *.txt file with an annotated data frame that would include species, accession numbers, and sequences with the retrieved sequences:

```
CXCL_for_use_df <- subset(CXCL_df, select = c(Hit_def,
Hit_id, Hsp_qseq))
write.table(CXCL_for_use_df, file =
"CXCL_nucleotide_df.txt", sep = "\t")
```

5. Read the information of this file back into *R* for later processing with the following commands:

```
CXCL_for_use_df <- read.table("CXCL_nucleotide_df.txt",
header = TRUE,
 sep = "\t", stringsAsFactors = FALSE)
```

6. Construct a file in fasta format that can be used for alignments:

```
CXCL_definitions <- CXCL_for_use_df$Hit_def
extract_names_1_function <-
function(x){sub(".*\\[(.*)\\].*", "\\1", x, perl=TRUE)}
taxa_names_seq <- extract_names_1_function(CXCL_definitions)
taxa_names_seq <- gsub(" ", "_", taxa_names_seq)

CXCL_accession_numbers <- CXCL_for_use_df$Hit_id
extract_names_2_function <-
function(x){sub(".*\\|(.*)\\|.*$", "\\1",
CXCL_accession_numbers, perl=TRUE)}
taxa_accession <-
extract_names_2_function(CXCL_accession_numbers)

taxa_fasta_name <- paste0(">",taxa_names_seq, "_",
```

```
taxa_accession)

# construct fasta entries

taxa_fasta_seq_vector <- paste0(taxa_fasta_name, "\n",
CXCL_for_use_df$Hsp_qseq)
```

7. Remove repeated sequences that have the same accession number:

```
taxa_fasta_seq_vector_2 <-
taxa_fasta_seq_vector[!duplicated(taxa_accession)]
taxa_fasta_seq_vector_2 <- taxa_fasta_seq_vector_2
[!is.na(taxa_fasta_seq_vector_2)]
```

8. Perform sequence clean-up by simplifying entry names (e.g., removing "PREDICTED:_", ",_mRNA"):

```
taxa_fasta_seq_vector_2 <- gsub("PREDICTED:_", "",
taxa_fasta_seq_vector_2, fixed = TRUE)

taxa_fasta_seq_vector_2 <- gsub("-", "",
taxa_fasta_seq_vector_2, fixed = TRUE)
taxa_fasta_seq_vector_2 <- gsub("(", "",
taxa_fasta_seq_vector_2, fixed = TRUE)
taxa_fasta_seq_vector_2 <- gsub(")", "",
taxa_fasta_seq_vector_2, fixed = TRUE)
taxa_fasta_seq_vector_2 <- gsub(",", "",
taxa_fasta_seq_vector_2, fixed = TRUE)
taxa_fasta_seq_vector_2 <- gsub("mRNA", "",
taxa_fasta_seq_vector_2, fixed = TRUE)
taxa_fasta_seq_vector_2 <- gsub("__", "_",
taxa_fasta_seq_vector_2, fixed = TRUE)
```

9. Remove entries with extraneous annotations (e.g., "Synthetic_construct"):

```
taxa_fasta_seq_vector_3 <-
taxa_fasta_seq_vector_2[!grepl("Synthetic_construct",
taxa_fasta_seq_vector_2)]
```

10. Write the final file in fasta format with species names and accession numbers for sequence alignments:

```
writeLines(taxa_fasta_seq_vector_3,
"CXCL_nucletotide_out.fasta")
```

These files can be modified by the user using a text editor, if further annotations should be incorporated.

3.7 Alignment of Amino Acid or Nucleotide Sequences from Chemokine Receptors

The files that contain the gene sequences in fasta format need to be aligned before the phylogeny can be estimated. Alignment is an iterative process that introduces gaps or spaces so each position along the matrix of sequences represent a homologous character (i.e., same nucleotide or amino acid position). This process can be achieved using sequence aligners that include command, online and GUI-based programs. We will use CLUSTAL OMEGA (online) [18, 19] and SeaView (GUI-based) [20]. For this example, we will use these files: "`CXC_human_mouse_aminoacid.fasta`," "`CXCL_nucletotide_out.fasta`," and "`CXCL_diversity_nucleotide_human.txt`." This latter file was created using the same procedure for nucleotide retrieval (*see* Subheading 3.6).

3.7.1 CLUSTAL OMEGA

To use this web application, the user needs to follow these steps.

1. Using a web browser, access the CLUSTAL OMEGA page: https://www.ebi.ac.uk/Tools/msa/clustalo/ and select the type of sequence format (i.e., PROTEIN, DNA or RNA).
2. The sequences could be pasted or uploaded. In our example, we paste directly the sequences into the web application.
3. Select "Pearson/FASTA" as the output format. The fasta format will preserve the long names associated with our sequences.
4. We have the option to provide an email contact to receive a file with the aligned sequences. In this case, we would click on submit and wait until the sequences are aligned.
5. After the alignment process is finished, check and download the aligned sequences. In this step, a new window will appear and we will copy and paste our alignment in a text document. Save this file with a pertinent name, e.g., `CXC_human_mouse_aminoacid_aligned_CLUSTAL.fasta`.

3.7.2 SeaView

This software is an open-source multiplatform GUI program for molecular phylogeny analyses and alignment [20]. It is provided freely and the user needs to download, install, and run the program with these steps:

1. SeaView is available from: http://doua.prabi.fr/software/seaview. This program can run in many platforms including: OS X (Mac), Windows, and Linux; SeaView source code is also available. The user should choose the platform that corresponds to their computer.
2. Once running, Seaview allows user to "drop" their unaligned sequences (e.g., fasta or txt files) and then the alignment function can be call.
3. Seaview can use different aligners including CLUSTAL OMEGA (default) or MUSCLE [21]. In this exercise, we use

MUSCLE by changing the option from the tab menu: Align > Alignment Options > muscle.

4. Start the alignment algorithm by selecting from the tab menu: Align > Align All.
5. After the alignment is completed, it can be inspected visually and saved as fasta file (i.e., *.fst).

For a detailed use of SeaView, the users are referred to its manual and website.

3.8 Determining the Best Model of Molecular Evolution for Aligned Chemokine Receptors

For this procedure, we will use the files: "`CXC_human_mouse_aminoacid_CLUSTAL_aligned.fasta`" and "`CXCL_diversity_nucleotide_human_MUSCLE.txt`." We will not use the file: "`CXCL_nucletotide_CLUSTAL_aligned.fasta`" because this alignment showed little diversity to do any meaningful phylogenetic tree inference.

3.8.1 Amino Acid Alignments

We would estimate the substitution models for the amino acid alignments while estimating a phylogenetic tree using RAxML 8.2.9 (Randomized Axelerated Maximum Likelihood) [22]. These procedures are provided in Subheading 3.9.1.

3.8.2 Nucleotide Alignments

For these type of data, we will use jModelTest2 [23]. This program provides an extensive statistical selection of models of nucleotide substitution, which are usually required to estimate phylogenetic trees. The software is provided freely and the user needs to download and install the program. For detailed use of this software, the users are referred to the jModelTest2 manual.

1. This program is available at: https://github.com/ddarriba/jmodeltest2. This program is written in Java and it can be used in most platforms that allow to execute a Java Runtime Environment (JRE). As indicated by the authors, jModelTest2 also depends on third-party binaries (e.g., PhyML [24]). In most cases, these software dependencies are installed with jModelTest2.
2. To execute the program, the user should start the java session by clicking on the file "jModelTest.jar." The alignment file can be in fasta format, which is loaded by clicking on the tab menu: File > Load DNA alignment. We can choose the location of our file (e.g., `CXCL_diversity_nucleotide_human_MUSCLE.txt`) and, if successful, the jModelTest2 console will show the number of sequences loaded and the number nucleotide sites.
3. Select the number of models to test and computer processors to be used during model evaluation. The user should click on the tab menu: Analysis > Compute likelihood scores. An interactive menu will provide with options on the number of

processors and likelihood settings. In most cases, the default options are recommended (see the jModelTest2 manual for details). To run model analyses, the user needs to click on "Compute Likelihoods." A new pop-up window will appear indicating the models being computed in real time.

4. After the model evaluations are done, compute the best model by selecting a model comparison method: Akaike Information Criterion (AIC), Bayesian Information Criterion (BIC), or performance-based decision theory (DT) calculations. For this exercise, we select AIC by clicking on the tab menu: Analysis > Do AIC calculations and selecting AICc (click on "Use AIC correction") and then on "Do AICc calculations." The results would be presented in the jModelTest2 console and those can be copied to a text file.
5. Explore the output and search for "Model selected." For our alignment file, the model selected was TrN+G (Tamura and Nei [25] with gamma rate variation) with the corresponding partition of "010020." In the output, we can also see some empirical values for the gamma parameter (i.e., G or gamma shape = 2.1300) and base frequencies: freqA = 0.2620, freqC = 0.2842, freqG = 0.2438 and freqT = 0.2099). The user should notice that these base frequencies are not equal (i.e., ~0.25).

3.9 Phylogenetic Inference Using Aligned Sequences in RAxML

The core of most phylogenetic procedures consists in the estimation of the phylogenetic tree and obtaining the support values for the nodes on that tree topology. In this exercise, we will use a maximum likelihood (ML) approach with a commonly used program: RAxML 8.2.9 [22]. Most programs that infer phylogenetic trees require installation. The instructions to do such installations and computer requirements are indicated on the RAxML website: https://github.com/stamatak/standard-RAxML.

3.9.1 Trees Inferred from Amino Acid Alignments

For this analysis, we will follow this procedure:

1. Run RAxML after compiling the software that uses the multicore processor architecture, which is common in most computers (see RAxML manual and website for details). To run the phylogenetic reconstruction, place the file with aligned sequences in the same folder with the compiled RAxML program. Here, I provide an example for this program execution:

```
raxmlHPC-PTHREADS-SSE3 -T 2 -m PROTGAMMAAUTO -N 3 -s
MY_ALIG.fasta -p 12345 -n TEST
```

These commands include the following arguments: -T corresponds to the number of threads that the user want to run and it should be at least 2, but no more than the physical cores of the computer. The -m argument corresponds to the model of substitution. In this case, we chose "PROTGAMMAAUTO" that indicates that the best-fitting model for amino acid substitution would be selected automatically while the tree estimation is running using a Bayesian Information Criterion (BIC). The -N argument corresponds to the number of alternative runs on distinct starting trees. The -s argument corresponds to the name of the alignment file in fasta format. The -p argument corresponds to any random number seed for the parsimony inferences. The argument -n corresponds to the name of the output file. For OS X (Mac), a "terminal" console is opened (for Windows users, *see* **Note 8**) to run the RAxML analyses with the following commands:

```
./raxmlHPC-PTHREADS-SSE3 -T 10 -m PROTGAMMAAUTO -N 3 -s
CXC_human_mouse_aminoacid_aligned_MUSCLE.fasta -p 12345 -n
CXC_raxml_trees
```

After the analysis is finished, the user can read the information about the model of amino acid substitution selected for our protein alignment, e.g., in this case the model was "JTT" [26]. The program will also output the information about the run, the location of the inferred repetitions, and the best -scoring ML tree. The format of the trees is "newick" which can be visualized later (see Subheading 3.11).

2. Estimate the support of nodes in this ML phylogeny by running 100 bootstraps. To run this analysis, we add the argument -b with a random seed number (e.g., 123476), changing the number of replicates to -N 100, and the name of the output file -n CXC_raxml_boot_trees. We run again these commands in a "terminal" console:

```
./raxmlHPC-PTHREADS-SSE3 -T 10 -b 123476 -m PROTGAMMAAUTO -N
100 -s CXC_human_mouse_aminoacid_aligned_MUSCLE.fasta -p 12345
-n CXC_raxml_boot_trees
```

These boostrap trees lack branch lengths, but the user can change this option (*see* **Note 9**).

3.9.2 Trees Inferred from Nucleotide Alignments

For this analysis, we will follow this procedure.

1. As indicated for amino acid sequences, run RAxML after compiling the software to allow the use of multicore processors. To run the analyses with our aligned nucleotide sequences, we placed the file with sequences in the same folder with compiled RAxML application. An example of the commands is the following:

```
raxmlHPC-PTHREADS-SSE3 -T 2 -m GTRGAMMA -N 3 -s
MY_ALIG.fasta -p 12345 -n TEST
```

These commands include the following arguments: -T corresponds to the number of threads that the user want to run and it should be at least 2, but no more than the physical cores of the computer. The -m argument corresponds to the model of nucleotide substitution. In this case, "GTRGAMMA" indicates one of the many models supported by this software (see RAxML manual for information about models). The -N argument corresponds to the number of alternative runs on distinct starting trees. The -s argument corresponds to the name of the nucleotide alignment file in fasta format. The -p argument corresponds to any random number seed for the parsimony inferences. The argument -n corresponds to the name of the output file. For OS X (Mac), the RAxML analysis is run (for Windows users, *see* **Note 8**) with the following commands:

```
./raxmlHPC-PTHREADS-SSE3 -T 10 -m GTRGAMMA -N 10 -s
CXCL_diversity_nucleotide_human_MUSCLE.fasta -p 12345 -n
CXC_nucleotide_raxml_trees
```

The users should notice that we chose "GTRGAMMA," which corresponds to GTR + Optimization of substitution rates + GAMMA rate heterogeneity. This model is more complex than the TrN+G selected by jModelTest2, but GTR+G approximates well TrN+G. However, the user can override complex models by using arguments such as "--JC69," "--K80," or "--HKY85" (see RAxML manual for information). The program will also output the information about the run, the location of the inferred repetitions, and the best -scoring ML tree. The format of this tree is "newick" which can be visualized later (see Subheading 3.11).

2. Estimate the support of nodes in this ML phylogeny by running 100 bootstraps. To run this analysis, we add the argument -b with a random seed number (e.g., 123476), changing the number of replicates to -N 100, and the name of the output file -n CXC_nucleotide_raxml_boot_trees. We run again these commands in a "terminal" console:

```
./raxmlHPC-PTHREADS-SSE3 -T 10 -b 123476 -m GTRGAMMA -N 100
-s CXCL_diversity_nucleotide_human_MUSCLE.fasta -p 12345 -n
CXC_nucleotide_raxml_boot_trees
```

These boostrap trees lack branch lengths, but the user can change this option (*see* **Note 9**).

3.10 Phylogenetic Inference Using Aligned Sequences in R

We can also estimate phylogenetic trees within the *R* environment. For this purpose, we can use the *R*-packages "ape" [13, 14] and "phangorn" [15]. This last package provides a series of tools to estimate trees from amino acid and nucleotide alignments. All these procedures start by reading the alignment file:

```
library(ape)
library(phangorn)

CXC_aminoacid <- phangorn::read.phyDat(file =
"CXC_human_mouse_aminoacid_aligned_MUSCLE.fasta",
 type ="AA",
 format = "fasta")

CXC_nucleotide <- phangorn::read.phyDat(file =
"CXCL_diversity_nucleotide_human_MUSCLE.fasta",
 type ="DNA",
 format = "fasta")
```

3.10.1 Trees Inferred Using Distance-Based Methods

For this type of trees, we need to infer a matrix of distances and the model that best fits our data. From the previous sections (see Subheading 3.9), we found that the CXC amino acid data were best fit with a JTT model, while the nucleotide data were best fit with a TrN+G model. For distance-based methods, "phangorn" allows many amino acid models including JTT, but only two for nucleotide models: "JC69" for equal base frequencies [27] and "F81" for empirical base frequencies [28]. Based on the output of jModelTest2, we found that the frequency of bases was unequal suggesting that the model "F81" is preferred. Likewise, we also know that the gamma parameter (i.e., the G in TrN+G was 2.1300) and this can be added with the argument "shape = 2.13." To estimate these distances-based trees, we will use the Neighbor Joining [29] method that results in unrooted trees:

```
distance_CXC_aminoacid  <-  phangorn::dist.ml(CXC_aminoacid,
model = "JTT")
distance_CXC_nucleotide  <-  phangorn::dist.ml(CXC_nucleotide,
model = "F81", shape = 2.13)

NJ_tree_CXC_aminoacid <-
phangorn::NJ(distance_CXC_aminoacid)
NJ_tree_CXC_nucleotide <-
phangorn::NJ(distance_CXC_nucleotide)

# save these trees to files

ape::write.tree(NJ_tree_CXC_aminoacid, file =
"NJ_tree_CXC_aminoacid.tree")
ape::write.tree(NJ_tree_CXC_nucleotide, file =
"NJ_tree_CXC_nucleotide.tree")
```

3.10.2 Trees Inferred Using Maximum Likelihood

We can also optimize an input tree using a maximum likelihood approach in *R*. For this purpose, we assign an object that will include the alignment, a starting tree, and the parameters for the optimization using ML. For this initial tree, we can use the NJ tree inferred on the previous section with the following commands:

```
##### For the CXC amino acid alignment

fit_CXC_aminoacid  <-  phangorn::pml(NJ_tree_CXC_aminoacid,
data = CXC_aminoacid)
fitJTT <- update(fit_CXC_aminoacid, model = "JTT", k = 4,
inv = 0.2)
fitJTT_opt <- phangorn::optim.pml(fitJTT ,
 optInv = TRUE,
 optGamma = TRUE,
 rearrangement = "stochastic",
 control = pml.control(trace = 0))

# we can see some of the parameters associated with this
tree

fitJTT_opt

# loglikelihood: -18278.72

# unconstrained loglikelihood: -2786.529
# Proportion of invariant sites: 3.465281e-05
# Discrete gamma model
# Number of rate categories: 4
# Shape parameter: 2.570192
# Rate matrix:

# save this tree to file

ape::write.tree(fitJTT_opt$tree, file =
"JTT_tree_CXC_aminoacid.tree")

# calculate 100 bootstraps and save file

fitJTT_opt_bs <- phangorn::bootstrap.pml(fitJTT_opt,
bs=100, optNni=TRUE, multicore=TRUE)
ape::write.tree(fitJTT_opt_bs, file =
"JTT_tree_CXC_aminoacid_boot.tree")

### For the CXC nucleotide alignment

fit_CXC_nucleotide  <-  phangorn::pml(NJ_tree_CXC_nucleotide,
data = CXC_nucleotide)
fitTrNG <- update(fit_CXC_nucleotide, k=4)
fitTrNG_opt <- phangorn::optim.pml(fitTrNG,
 model = "TrN",
 optInv = FALSE,
 optGamma = TRUE,
 rearrangement = "stochastic",
```

```
control = pml.control(trace = 0))

### we can see some of the parameters associated with this tree

fitTrNG_opt

# loglikelihood: -6621.57

# unconstrained loglikelihood: -5050.672
# Discrete gamma model
# Number of rate categories: 4
# Shape parameter: 2.060177

# Rate matrix:
# a c g t
# a 0.000000 1.000000 3.420504 1.000000
# c 1.000000 0.000000 1.000000 2.416139
# g 3.420504 1.000000 0.000000 1.000000
# t 1.000000 2.416139 1.000000 0.000000

# Base frequencies:
# 0.2611841 0.2863102 0.2431908 0.209315

### save this tree to file

ape::write.tree(fitTrNG_opt$tree, file =
"TrNG_tree_CXC_nucleotide.tree")

### calculate 100 bootstraps and save file

fitTrNG_opt_bs  <-  phangorn::bootstrap.pml(fitTrNG_opt,
bs=100, optNni=TRUE, multicore=TRUE)
ape::write.tree(fitTrNG_opt_bs, file =
"TrNG_tree_CXC_nucleotide_boot.tree")
```

For windows users, the "multicore" argument of the function "bootstrap.pml" cannot be used (*see* **Note 10**). Likewise, the values for bootstraps derived from "phangorn::bootstrap.pml" should be taken with caution (*see* **Note 11**).

3.11 Visualizing Phylogenetic Trees

The last part of most phylogenetic analyses is the visualization of the resulting phylogenies and preparing figures as *.jpg or *.pdf. There is many GUI visualization software (*see* **Note 12**), but the *R*-environment provides enormous flexibility in phylogenetic trees display and manipulation. For this reason, I included a simple approach using the "ape" and "phangorn" *R*-packages to print and save trees.

1. Plot the phylogenies inferred from amino acid alignments with the following code:

```
#### Read RAxML trees in R and assign them to objects:

human_mouse_CXC_tree <-
ape::read.tree("RAxML_bestTree.CXC_raxml_trees")
human_mouse_CXC_boostrap_trees <-
ape::read.tree("RAxML_bootstrap.CXC_raxml_boot_trees")

# best tree with bootstrap values:

phangorn::plotBS(tree = midpoint(human_mouse_CXC_tree),
 BStrees = human_mouse_CXC_boostrap_trees,
 p = 50,
 type = "phylogram",
 bs.col = "blue",
 cex = 0.9)
title("RAxML 100 bootstrap replicates based on aligned CXC
amino acid")
add.scale.bar(cex = 0.7, font = 2, col = "red")

#### Read NJ tree in R and assign them to objects:

human_mouse_CXC_NJ_tree <-
ape::read.tree("NJ_tree_CXC_aminoacid.tree")
plot(human_mouse_CXC_NJ_tree, type = "unrooted", main=" NJ
CXC aminoacid", cex = 0.9)
add.scale.bar(cex = 0.7, font = 2, col = "red")

#### Read ML tree in R and assign them to objects:

human_mouse_CXC_ML_tree <-
ape::read.tree("JTT_tree_CXC_aminoacid.tree")
human_mouse_CXC_ML_boot_tree <-
ape::read.tree("JTT_tree_CXC_aminoacid_boot.tree")

# best tree with bootstrap values:

phangorn::plotBS(tree = midpoint(human_mouse_CXC_ML_tree),
 BStrees = human_mouse_CXC_ML_boot_tree,
 p = 50,
 type = "phylogram",
 bs.col = "blue",
 cex = 0.9)
title("ML 100 bootstrap replicates based on aligned CXC
```

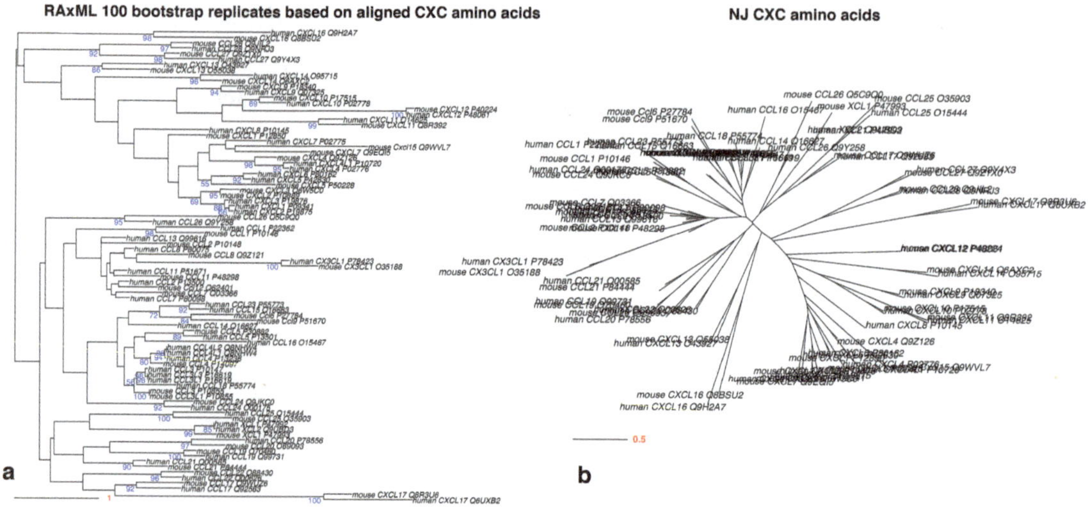

Fig. 1 Phylogeny of chemokine proteins from human and mouse as listed on Table 1 from Bachelerie et al. [7]. (**a**) Maximum Likelihood (ML) phylogeny inferred from the amino acid sequences aligned using MUSCLE with RAxML. The values at the nodes are ML bootstrap percentages ≥50%. (**b**) Neighbor Joining (NJ) phylogeny inferred from the amino acid sequences aligned using MUSCLE with the "phangorn" *R*-package

```
amino acid")
add.scale.bar(cex = 0.7, font = 2, col = "red")
```

These commands will allow the user to see the image of the trees (Fig. 1). The following arguments of the function "plotBS" of "phangorn" are indicated: "tree" indicates the phylogenetic tree on which edges the bootstrap values would be plotted (note: this tree is unrooted, so the "midpoint" function was used to perform a midpoint rooting); "BStrees" indicates the object with a list of trees that would be used to estimate the boostrap values; "p" indicates the minimal support percentage that would be plotted on the tree and values > 75 for ML trees are usually considered meaningful; "type" indicates the tree configuration to plot (i.e., "cladogram", "phylogram", or "unrooted"); "bs.col" indicates the color of bootstrap support labels; and "cex" indicates the relative size of the label font. The user can get more information about the function "plotBS" by typing: ?plotBS (*see* **Note 13**). We also added a title to the plot with the function "title" and a scale bar with "add.scale.bar."

We can save the plot image to a *.pdf file with the following commands:

```
# Open a pdf file and save tree plot:

pdf("human_mouse_CXC_boostrap_aminoacid_tree.pdf",
```

```
width=10, height=10)

phangorn::plotBS(midpoint(human_mouse_CXC_tree),
 human_mouse_CXC_boostrap_trees,
 p = 50,
 type = "phylogram",
 bs.col = "blue",
 cex = 0.9)
title("RAxML 100 bootstrap replicates based on aligned CXC
amino acid")
add.scale.bar(cex = 0.7, font = 2, col = "red")

plot(human_mouse_CXC_NJ_tree, type = "unrooted", main=" NJ
CXC aminoacid", cex = 0.9)
add.scale.bar(cex = 0.7, font = 2, col = "red")

phangorn::plotBS(tree = midpoint(human_mouse_CXC_ML_tree),
 BStrees = human_mouse_CXC_ML_boot_tree,
 p = 50,
 type = "phylogram",
 bs.col = "blue",
 cex = 0.9)
title("ML 100 bootstrap replicates based on aligned CXC
amino acid")
add.scale.bar(cex = 0.7, font = 2, col = "red")

dev.off()
```

2. With a similar procedure, plot the trees based on the nucleotide alignments (Fig. 2) with the following code:

```
#### Read RAxML trees in R and assign them to objects:

nucleotide_CXC_tree <-
ape::read.tree("RAxML_bestTree.CXC_nucleotide_raxml_trees")
nucleotide_CXC_boostrap_trees <-
ape::read.tree("RAxML_bootstrap.CXC_nucleotide_raxml_boot_
trees")

# best tree with bootstrap values:

phangorn::plotBS(tree = midpoint(nucleotide_CXC_tree),
 BStrees = nucleotide_CXC_boostrap_trees,
 p = 50,
 type = "phylogram",
 bs.col = "blue",
 cex = 0.9)
title("RAxML 100 bootstrap replicates based on aligned CXCL
nucleotide sequences")
```

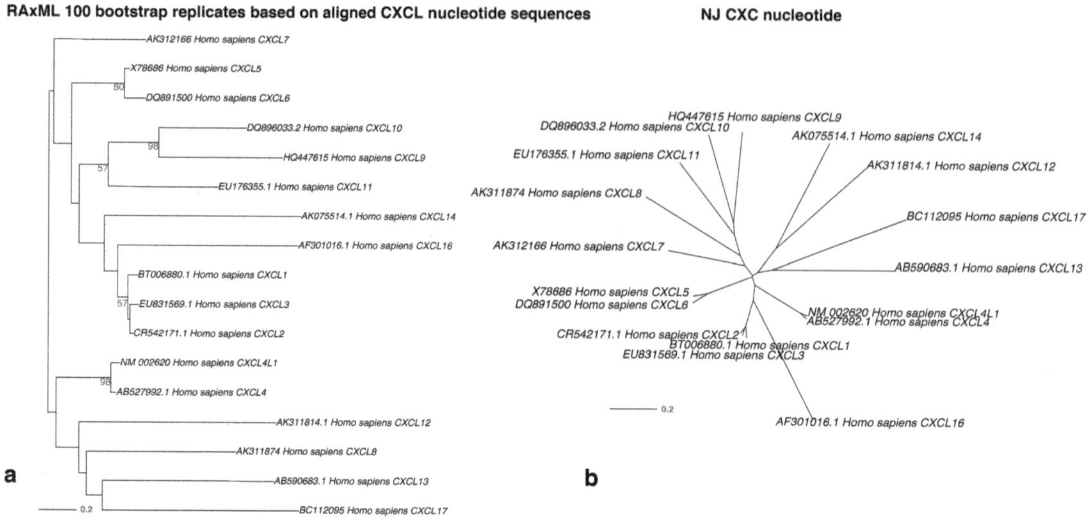

Fig. 2 Phylogeny of CXCL proteins from human specimens. (**a**) Maximum Likelihood (ML) phylogeny inferred from the nucleotide sequences aligned using MUSCLE with RAxML. The values at the nodes are ML bootstrap percentages $\geq$50%. (**b**) Neighbor Joining (NJ) phylogeny inferred from the nucleotide sequences aligned using MUSCLE with the "phangorn" *R*-package

```
add.scale.bar(cex = 0.7, font = 2, col = "red")

#### Read NJ tree in R and assign them to objects:

nucleotide_CXC_NJ_tree <- ape::read.tree("NJ_tree_CXC_nucleo
tide.tree")
plot(nucleotide_CXC_NJ_tree, type = "unrooted", main=" NJ CXC
nucleotide", cex = 0.9)
add.scale.bar(cex = 0.7, font = 2, col = "red")

#### Read ML tree in R and assign them to objects:

nucleotide_CXC_ML_tree <-
ape::read.tree("TrNG_tree_CXC_nucleotide.tree")
nucleotide_CXC_ML_boot_tree <-
ape::read.tree("TrNG_tree_CXC_nucleotide_boot.tree")

# best tree with bootstrap values:

phangorn::plotBS(tree = midpoint(nucleotide_CXC_ML_tree),
 BStrees = nucleotide_CXC_ML_boot_tree,
 p = 50,
 type = "phylogram",
 bs.col = "blue",
 cex = 0.9)
title("ML 100 bootstrap replicates based on aligned CXC
nucleotide")
```

```
add.scale.bar(cex = 0.7, font = 2, col = "red")

### Open a pdf file and save tree plot:

pdf("human_CXCL_nucleotide_boostrap_tree.pdf", width=10,
height=10)
phangorn::plotBS(tree = midpoint(nucleotide_CXC_tree),
 BStrees = nucleotide_CXC_boostrap_trees,
 p = 50,
 type = "phylogram",
 bs.col = "blue",
 cex = 0.9)
title("RAxML 100 bootstrap replicates based on aligned CXCL
nucleotide sequences")
add.scale.bar(cex = 0.7, font = 2, col = "red")

plot(nucleotide_CXC_NJ_tree, type = "unrooted", main=" NJ
CXC nucleotide", cex = 0.9)
add.scale.bar(cex = 0.7, font = 2, col = "red")

phangorn::plotBS(tree = midpoint(nucleotide_CXC_ML_tree),
 BStrees = nucleotide_CXC_ML_boot_tree,
 p = 50,
 type = "phylogram",
 bs.col = "blue",
 cex = 0.9)
title("ML 100 bootstrap replicates based on aligned CXC
nucleotide")
add.scale.bar(cex = 0.7, font = 2, col = "red")
dev.off()
```

The resulting pdfs with the tree plots can be seen in the working directory (*see* **Note 6**). The user is encouraged to explore more and change parameters for better tree inferences and presentation (*see* **Note 14**).

4 Notes

1. Most errors in phylogenetic estimations are due to mistakes derived from human oversights, which, in turn, derive from mislabeled samples, chimeric sequences, and poor-quality input data. All researchers should spend time to check the quality of their input data (if these sequences derive from PCR products, Next-Gen experiments or other sources). An easy and quick approach is to "BLAST" (https://blast.ncbi.nlm.nih.gov/Blast.cgi) the unknown sequence against the NCBI database. Most times, this sequence will match a sequence already present and the annotation or source can be verified.

2. Orthologous genes are those makers whose similarities (i.e., homology) are the result of speciation so that the history of the gene reflects the history of the species being compared. Most phylogenetic analyses are derived from homologous markers, whose sequences have been aligned to maximize homology at the level of nucleotide or amino acid site positions. If some parts of the alignment are "unalignable" or ambiguous, the user can exclude such sites by deleting or excluding those parts from the final alignment matrix before the tree estimation.
3. Some users find that the interaction with *R* console is cumbersome. In this case, *RStudio* constitutes an alternative software for integrated development and management of the environment for *R*. The desktop version of *RStudio* is free and can be found here:

```
https://www.rstudio.com/products/RStudio/
```

4. The punctuation in coding and writing scripts is very important. The use of quotation marks [" "], periods [.], colons [:], and spaces is commonly overseen by first-time users of *R*. One example is the use of curvy quotation marks [""] instead of straight quotation marks [" "]. *R* will only accept straight quotation marks, while it will throw errors if curvy quotation marks [""] are used instead.
5. To cite *R*-packages, libraries need to be installed and then loaded in the *R* environment as follows:

```
install.packages("devtools")
library(devtools)
citation("devtools") # a function for getting the
information about citation

To cite package 'devtools' in publications use:

 Hadley Wickham, Jim Hester and Winston Chang (2019). devtools:
Tools to Make Developing R Packages Easier. R
package
 version 2.0.2. https://CRAN.R-project.org/package=devtools

A BibTeX entry for LaTeX users is

 @Manual{,
  title = {devtools: Tools to Make Developing R Packages
Easier},
 author = {Hadley Wickham and Jim Hester and Winston
Chang},
 year = {2019},
```

```
note = {R package version 2.0.2},
url = {https://CRAN.R-project.org/package=devtools},
}
```

6. The working directory is usually defined by the user by giving its path:

```
setwd("MY_WORKING_FOLDER_PATH")
```

The path can also be set within the *R* console tabs as follows: Misc > Change Working Directory. Then, the user can select the folder with the files to be analyzed. If the user wants to know the current working directory, he/she should type:

```
getwd()
```

7. The fasta (also known as FASTA/Pearson) format is a text representation of nucleotide or amino acid sequences. To reconstruct this type of format in *R*, the first line starts with the ">" symbol preceded by a summary text about the sequence such as its accession number, species origin, or other descriptive. The second line will include the actual sequence of nucleotides or amino acids. See examples below:

```
>Pan_troglodytes_NP_001502.1
MARAALSAAPSNPXXXXXXXXXXXXXXXXXXXXXXSVATELRCQCLQTLQGIHPKNIQSVN
VKSPGPHCAQTEVIATLKNGRKACLNPASPIVKKIIEKMLNSDKSN

>Homo_sapiens_chemokine_CXC_motif_ligand_1_BC011976.1
ATGGCCCGCGCTGCTCTCTCCGCCGCCCCCAGCAATCCCCGGCTCCTGCGAGTGGCACTGC
TGCTCCTGCTCCTGGTAGCCGCTGGCCGGCGCGCAGCAGGAGCGTCCGTGGCCACTGAACT
GCGCTGCCAGTGCTTGCAGACCCTGCAGGGAATTCACCCCAAGAACATCCAAAGTGTGAAC
GTGAAGTCCCCCGGACCCCACTGCGCCCAAACCGAAGTCATAGCCACACTCAAGAATGGGC
GGAAAGCTTGCCTCAATCCTGCATCCCCCATAGTTAAGAAAATCATCGAAAAGATGCTGAA
CAGTGACAAATCCAACT
```

8. Opening a console for programing in most platforms could be cumbersome. For OS X (Mac), this can be called by finding the "terminal" application in Applications > Utilities and clicking on the "terminal" application. For Windows, the user needs to call the command prompt. A simple approach is to create a small batch file using "NotePad" or any other text editor. This file should include the RAxML commands in one line and the "pause" command in the next line:

```
raxmlHPC-PTHREADS-SSE3.exe -T 10 -m GTRGAMMA -N 10 -s
CXCL_diversity_nucleotide_human_MUSCLE.fasta  -p 12345  -n
CXC_nucleotide_raxml_trees
pause
```

This file is saved as a batch file (with a ".bat" file name extension) in the same folder with the RAxML executable (e.g., raxmlHPC-PTHREADS-SSE3.exe) and the input data file (CXCL_diversity_nucleotide_human_MUSCLE.fasta). To run the RAxML analysis on Windows, the user should double-click on the *.bat file.

9. The user can add the argument: -k which specifies that the bootstrapped trees should be saved with branch lengths. However, these analyses would take longer to run.

```
# for amino acids
./raxmlHPC-PTHREADS-SSE3 -T 10 -b 123476 -m PROTGAMMAAUTO -N
100 -s CXC_human_mouse_aminoacid_aligned_MUSCLE.fasta -p 12345
-n CXC_raxml_boot_trees

# for nucleotides
./raxmlHPC-PTHREADS-SSE3 -T 10 -b 123476 -m GTRGAMMA -N 100
-s CXCL_diversity_nucleotide_human_MUSCLE.fasta -p 12345 -k
-n CXC_nucleotide_raxml_boot_trees
```

10. A note from the *R*-package "phangorn" says: "Unfortunately the multicore package does not work under windows or with GUI interfaces ("aqua" on a mac)." The user should use this argument as "multicore = FALSE."
11. I noticed that some of the bootstrap values provided by the function "phangorn::bootstrap.pml" appear to be inflated (i.e., higher than expected) if compared with those obtained using RAxML. Therefore, I recommend using RAxML for bootstrap estimation.
12. GUI tree visualizing software: FigTree v1.4.3 (http://tree.bio.ed.ac.uk/software/figtree/); Mesquite v3.6 [30] (https://www.mesquiteproject.org/). More flexible tools for tree drawing are provided in the *R*-package "ggtree" [31].
13. Every *R*-package has a pdf manual usually found in CRAN, but the user can find the information for most functions by typing: ?NAME_FUNCTION within the *R* environment. This action will open a window where the user can read the main arguments required to run such function and, in most cases, a small example of this function's usage. However, the library that includes such function needs to be loaded first (e.g., library ("ape")) before we can read the manual.
14. The estimation of phylogenetic trees is a well-established field in comparative biology. The *R* environment is an ever-growing ecosystem, and many packages are published every day while others become obsolete or superseded by newer, faster, and more flexible ones. In spite of this, *R* keeps its spotlight by its

core accessibility to most biologists interested in sequence manipulation and phylogenetics. Like *R*-packages, phylogenetic programs also evolve toward faster, more flexible, and accommodating applications amenable for larger and more complex molecular data. The most successful programs are those that are kept current with the increasing computer capabilities in processing power. Likewise, most phylogenetic programs are adapting to genomic/proteomic levels of data that can only be handled with automatization. To keep up with this dynamism, users are encouraged to visit the following online resources and archives:

The CRAN Task View—Phylogenetics, Especially Comparative Methods: Given the size of CRAN (April 2019: 14086 available packages), this website provides a specialized collection of links to current *R*-packages related to phylogenetics and comparative methods.

https://cran.r-project.org/web/views/Phylogenetics.html

Bioconductor—This web-archive provides an easy access to tools and software for the analysis and comprehension of high-throughput genomic data. Bioconductor archives many *R*-packages not available in CRAN:

https://www.bioconductor.org/

References

1. Felsenstein J (2004) Inferring phylogenies. Sinauer Associates, Sunderland, MA
2. Gluckman P, Beedle A, Hanson M (2009) Principles of evolutionary medicine, 1st edn. Oxford University Press, Inc., New York
3. Garland T, Bennett AF, Rezende EL (2004) Phylogenetic approaches in comparative physiology. J Exp Biol 208:3015–3035
4. Baum D (2008) Reading a phylogenetic tree: the meaning of monophyletic groups. Nat Educ 1(1):190
5. Rosenberg M (2008) Sequence alignment: methods, models, concepts, and strategies. University of California Press, Berkeley, CA
6. R_Core_Team (2019) R: a language and environment for statistical computing. R Foundation for Statistical Computing, Vienna. https://www.r-project.org/
7. Bachelerie F, Ben-Baruch A, Burkhardt AM, Combadiere C, Farber JM, Graham GJ, Horuk R, Sparre-Ulrich AH, Locati M, Luster AD, Mantovani A, Matsushima K, Murphy PM, Nibbs R, Nomiyama H, Power CA, Proudfoot AEI, Rosenkilde MM, Rot A, Sozzani S, Thelen M, Yoshie O, Zlotnik A (2014) International Union of Pharmacology. LXXXIX. Update on the extended family of chemokine receptors and introducing a new nomenclature for atypical chemokine receptors. Pharmacol Rev 66(1):1–79. https://doi.org/10.1124/pr.113.007724
8. Bateman A, Martin MJ, O'Donovan C, Magrane M, Apweiler R, Alpi E, Antunes R, Ar-Ganiska J, Bely B, Bingley M, Bonilla C, Britto R, Bursteinas B, Chavali G, Cibrian-Uhalte E, Da Silva A, De Giorgi M, Dogan T, Fazzini F, Gane P, Cas-Tro LG, Garmiri P, Hatton-Ellis E, Hieta R, Huntley R, Legge D, Liu WD, Luo J, MacDougall A, Mutowo P, Nightin-Gale A, Orchard S, Pichler K, Poggioli D, Pundir S, Pureza L, Qi GY, Rosanoff S, Saidi R, Sawford T, Shypitsyna A, Turner E, Volynkin V, Wardell T, Watkins X, Watkins CA, Figueira L, Li WZ, McWilliam H, Lopez R, Xenarios I, Bougueleret L, Bridge A, Poux S, Redaschi N, Aimo L, Argoud-Puy G, Auchincloss A, Axelsen K, Bansal P, Baratin D, Blatter MC, Boeckmann B, Bolleman J, Boutet E, Breuza L, Casal-Casas C, De Castro E, Coudert E, Cuche B, Doche M, Dornevil D, Duvaud S, Estreicher A, Famiglietti L, Feuermann M, Gasteiger E, Gehant S, Gerritsen V, Gos A, Gruaz-Gumowski N, Hinz U, Hulo C, Jungo F, Keller G, Lara V, Lemercier P, Lieberherr D,

Lombardot T, Martin X, Masson P, Morgat A, Neto T, Nouspikel N, Paesano S, Pedruzzi I, Pilbout S, Pozzato M, Pruess M, Rivoire C, Roechert B, Schneider M, Sigrist C, Sonesson K, Staehli S, Stutz A, Sundaram S, Tognolli M, Verbregue L, Veuthey AL, Wu CH, Arighi CN, Arminski L, Chen CM, Chen YX, Garavelli JS, Huang HZ, Laiho KT, McGarvey P, Natale DA, Suzek BE, Vinayaka CR, Wang QH, Wang YQ, Yeh LS, Yerramalla MS, Zhang J, UniProt C (2015) UniProt: a hub for protein information. Nucleic Acids Res 43(D1):D204–D212. https://doi.org/10.1093/nar/gku989

9. Wickham H, Hester J, Chang W (2019) devtools: tools to make developing R packages easier. R package version 2.0.2. https://cran.r-project.org/package=devtools
10. Huber W, Carey VJ, Gentleman R, Anders S, Carlson M, Carvalho BS, Bravo HC, Davis S, Gatto L, Girke T, Gottardo R, Hahne F, Hansen KD, Irizarry RA, Lawrence M, Love MI, MacDonald J, Obenchain V, Oles AK, Pages H, Reyes A, Shannon P, Smyth GK, Tenenbaum D, Waldron L, Morgan M (2015) Orchestrating high-throughput genomic analysis with bioconductor. Nat Methods 12 (2):115–121. https://doi.org/10.1038/nmeth.3252
11. Gentleman RC, Carey VJ, Bates DM, Bolstad B, Dettling M, Dudoit S, Ellis B, Gautier L, Ge YC, Gentry J, Hornik K, Hothorn T, Huber W, Iacus S, Irizarry R, Leisch F, Li C, Maechler M, Rossini AJ, Sawitzki G, Smith C, Smyth G, Tierney L, Yang JYH, Zhang JH (2004) Bioconductor: open software development for computational biology and bioinformatics. Genome Biol 5 (10):16. https://doi.org/10.1186/gb-2004-5-10-r80
12. Gentleman R (2019) annotate: annotation for microarrays. R package version 1.60.1
13. Paradis E, Schliep K (2018) ape 5.0: an environment for modern phylogenetics and evolutionary analyses in R. Bioinformatics 35:526–528
14. Paradis E (2012) Analysis of phylogenetics and evolution with R, 2nd edn. Springer, New York
15. Schliep KP (2011) phangorn: phylogenetic analysis in R. Bioinformatics 27(4):592–593
16. Winter DJ (2017) rentrez: an R package for the NCBI eUtils API. The R Journal 9 (2):520–526
17. Camacho C, Coulouris G, Avagyan V, Ma N, Papadopoulos J, Bealer K, Madden TL (2009) BLAST plus: architecture and applications. BMC Bioinformatics 10:9. https://doi.org/10.1186/1471-2105-10-421
18. Sievers F, Wilm A, Dineen D, Gibson TJ, Karplus K, Li WZ, Lopez R, McWilliam H, Remmert M, Soding J, Thompson JD, Higgins DG (2011) Fast, scalable generation of high-quality protein multiple sequence alignments using Clustal Omega. Mol Syst Biol 7:6. https://doi.org/10.1038/msb.2011.75
19. Goujon M, McWilliam H, Li WZ, Valentin F, Squizzato S, Paern J, Lopez R (2010) A new bioinformatics analysis tools framework at EMBL-EBI. Nucleic Acids Res 38: W695–W699. https://doi.org/10.1093/nar/gkq313
20. Gouy M, Guindon S, Gascuel O (2010) SeaView version 4: a multiplatform graphical user interface for sequence alignment and phylogenetic tree building. Mol Biol Evol 27 (2):221–224. https://doi.org/10.1093/molbev/msp259
21. Edgar RC (2004) MUSCLE: multiple sequence alignment with high accuracy and high throughput. Nucleic Acids Res 32 (5):1792–1797. https://doi.org/10.1093/nar/gkh340
22. Stamatakis A (2014) RAxML version 8: a tool for phylogenetic analysis and post-analysis of large phylogenies. Bioinformatics 30 (9):1312–1313. https://doi.org/10.1093/bioinformatics/btu033
23. Darriba D, Taboada GL, Doallo R, Posada D (2012) jModelTest 2: more models, new heuristics and parallel computing. Nat Methods 9 (8):772–772. https://doi.org/10.1038/nmeth.2109
24. Guindon S, Dufayard JF, Lefort V, Anisimova M, Hordijk W, Gascuel O (2010) New algorithms and methods to estimate maximum-likelihood phylogenies: assessing the performance of PhyML 3.0. Syst Biol 59 (3):307–321. https://doi.org/10.1093/sysbio/syq010
25. Tamura K, Nei M (1993) Estimation of the number of nucleotide substitutions in the control region of mitochondrial-DNA in humans and chimpanzees. Mol Biol Evol 10 (3):512–526
26. Jones DT, Taylor WR, Thornton JM (1992) The rapid generation of mutation data matrices from protein sequences. Comput Appl Biosci 8 (3):275–282
27. Jukes TH, Cantor CR (1969) Evolution of protein molecules. In: Munro HN (ed) Mammalian protein metabolism. Academic Press, New York, pp 21–132
28. Felsenstein J (1981) Evolutionary trees from DNA sequences: a maximum likelihood approach. J Mol Evol 17(6):368–376

29. Saitou N, Nei M (1987) The neighbor-joining method—a new method for reconstructing phylogenetic trees. Mol Biol Evol 4 (4):406–425
30. Maddison WP, Maddison DR (2018) Mesquite: a modular system for evolutionary analysis. Version 3.51. http://www.mesquiteproject.org/
31. Yu GC, Smith DK, Zhu HC, Guan Y, Lam TTY (2017) GGTREE: an R package for visualization and annotation of phylogenetic trees with their covariates and other associated data. Methods Ecol Evol 8(1):28–36. https://doi.org/10.1111/2041-210x.12628

Chapter 28

Generation of IL17RB Knockout Cell Lines Using CRISPR/Cas9-Based Genome Editing

Olivia Hu, Alessandro Provvido, and Yan Zhu

Abstract

CRISPR/Cas9-based genome editing is an inexpensive and efficient tool for genetic modification. Here we present a methodological approach of establishing interleukin-17 receptor B (IL17RB) knockout cell lines using CRISPR/Cas9-mediated genomic deletion. IL17RB gene encodes for a cytokine receptor that specifically binds to IL17B and IL17E and overexpressed in various cancers. The method involves CRISPR design, CRISPR cloning, delivery of CRISPR clone into cells, and verification of IL17RB gene deletion by deletion screening primer design, genomic DNA extraction, and polymerase chain reaction (PCR). Similar approaches can be used for generating mammalian cell lines with gene knockout for other genes of interest.

Key words CRISPR/Cas9, Genomic deletion, Gene knockout, Interleukin-17 receptor B

1 Introduction

*C*lustered *R*egularly *I*nterspaced *S*hort *P*alindromic *R*epeat (CRISPR) system, an adaptive immune system in bacteria, has been modified for genome editing [1–3]. Engineered CRISPR systems contain two components: a CRISPR-associated endonuclease (Cas protein) and a guide RNA (gRNA or sgRNA), a short synthetic RNA composed of a scaffold sequence necessary for Cas-binding and a ~20 nucleotide spacer defining the genomic target to be modified [4]. Bioinformatics tools have been developed to identify a unique genomic target in comparison to the rest of the genome which presents immediately adjacent to a *P*rotospacer *A*djacent *M*otif (PAM) [5]. The canonical PAM is the sequence 5′-NGG-3′, where "N" is any nucleobase followed by two guanine ("G") nucleobases. When the gRNA spacer sequence shares substantial homology with the target DNA, Cas9 will cleave the locus, resulting in a double-strand break (DSB) within the target DNA (∼3–4 nucleotides upstream of the PAM sequence) which is repaired through two general mechanisms: nonhomologous end joining (NHEJ) and homology-directed repair (HDR) [6]. NHEJ is

Ivana Vancurova and Yan Zhu (eds.), *Immune Mediators in Cancer: Methods and Protocols*, Methods in Molecular Biology, vol. 2108, https://doi.org/10.1007/978-1-0716-0247-8_28, © Springer Science+Business Media, LLC, part of Springer Nature 2020

efficient but often causes small nucleotide insertions or deletions (indels) in the target DNA that result in amino acid deletions, insertions, or frameshift mutations leading to premature stop codons within the open reading frame (ORF) of the targeted gene. On the other hand, HDR is less efficient but repairs with high fidelity [5, 7]. Ever since its adaption for mammalian genome editing, CRISPR has been used for a wide range of applications such as knockout target genes through NHEJ or knock-in genes through FDR to facilitate gene function studies [8].

IL17RB is a cytokine receptor that specifically binds to IL17B and IL17E [9]. It has been shown to be involved in inflammatory diseases and cancers. IL-17RB has been found overexpressed in breast [10], gastric [11], pancreatic [12], prostate [13], and thyroid [14] cancer tissues. Here, we present a protocol to generate interleukin-17 receptor B (IL17RB) knockout cell lines using CRISPR/Cas9-based genomic deletion. Similar approaches can be used to generate knockout cell lines of any gene of interest.

2 Materials

2.1 CRISPR Constructs Design

1. Plasmid pX330 (addgene ID 42230; *see* **Note 1**).
2. Oligonucleotide for single guide RNA (sgRNA) on IL17RB (*see* **Note 2**).
3. BbsI_HF with NEB Buffer 2.1.
4. PCR purification kit.
5. T4 DNA ligase.
6. DH5α competent cells (*see* **Note 3**).
7. Plasmid miniprep kit.

2.2 Transfection, Selection, and Limiting Dilution for Single-Cell Clone Plating

1. U2OS cells.
2. DMEM complete medium: Dulbecco's Modified Eagle Medium supplemented with 10% fetal bovine serum and 100 μg/mL penicillin/streptomycin.
3. Opti-MEM (1×) medium (Thermo Fisher Scientific, *see* **Note 4**).
4. Lipofectamine 2000 (*see* **Note 5**).
5. pEGFP plasmid (*see* **Note 6**).
6. 250 mg/mL Geneticin (G418) stock (*see* **Note 7**).
7. Cell culture dishes: diameter 60 and 100 mm.
8. Cell culture plates: 96-well, 24-well, and 6-well.
9. Hemocytometer.
10. CO_2 incubator: set to 5% CO_2 and 37 °C.

2.3 Genomic DNA (gDNA) Extraction and Polymerase Chain Reaction (PCR)

1. DNA QuickExtraction kit (Lucigen, *see* **Note 8**).
2. Screening primers (*see* **Note 9**).
3. Phusion Flash master mix (*see* **Note 10**).
4. Thermocycler.
5. Nanodrop analyzer.

3 Methods

3.1 CRISPR Constructs

1. pX330 digestion
   4 μL 10× NEB Buffer 2.1.
   X μL pX330 (5 μg).
   2 μL BbsI (NEB).
   Y μL H_2O to 40 μL final volume.
   (a) Keep at 37 °C for 2 h (*see* **Note 11**).
   (b) Purify linearized plasmid with PCR purification kit.
2. Annealing of pair of oligos (20 μL total):
   2 μL 10× T4 DNA ligase buffer.
   2 μL oligo 1 (100 μM).
   2 μL oligo 2 (100 μM).
   14 μL H_2O.
   (a) Heat at 95 °C for 5 min and leave the tube on the heat block until it cools down to room temperature.
   (b) Dilute the annealed oligo 1:250.
3. Ligation for sgRNA cloning
   X μL pX330 BbsI digested vector (100 ng).
   2 μL annealed oligo duplex (1:250 dilution).
   2 μL 10× DNA ligase buffer.
   1 μL T4 ligase.
   Y μL H_2O to 20 μL final volume.
   Keep at room temperature for 2 h.
4. Transformation
   (a) Take 2 μL of ligation product from **step 3** and transform into 50 μL of DH5α competent cells.
   (b) Pick single colonies from the plate and grow them overnight in 2 mL LB with 100 μg/mL ampicillin at 37 °C.
   (c) Prepare plasmids with plasmid miniprep kit and verify the insertion of sgRNA sequence with U6 sequencing primer.

3.2 Transfection of CRISPR Constructs and Selection

1. Seed 1.5×10^6 U2OS cells into a 60 mm cell culture dish containing 10 mL DMEM complete media the day before transfection.
2. Transfect U2OS cells with CRISPR constructs together with pEGFP plasmid.
   (a) Add 9 μL Lipofectamine 2000 to a 1.5 mL microcentrifuge tube containing 300 μL Opti-MEM medium, mix well by pipetting, and incubate the solution at room temperature for 5 min.
   (b) Add two CRISPR constructs (2 μg each) and pEGFP (250 ng) into another 1.5 mL microcentrifuge tube containing 300 μL Opti-MEM medium and mix well by pipetting.
   (c) Transfer solution from **step (a)** into the microcentrifuge tube from **step (b)**. Mix well by pipetting and incubate the mixture at room temperature for 15 min.
   (d) During incubation, aspirate the medium in the 60 mm cell culture dish with U2OS cells and replace with 2.4 mL fresh complete DMEM.
   (e) Add solution from **step (c)** dropwise into the 60 mm cell culture dish with U2OS cells from **step (d)**.
   (f) Shake the plate gently and incubate the cells at 37 °C with 5% CO_2 for 12 h.
3. Replace the medium with 3 mL DMEM containing G418 (final concentration 500 μg/mL; 6 μL of G418 stock in 3 mL DMEM; *see* **Note 7**).
4. Incubate the cells at 37 °C with 5% CO_2 for 72 h (*see* **Note 12**).

3.3 Limiting Dilution for Single-Cell Clone Plating

1. Wash the 10 mm dish with 2 mL phosphate-buffered saline (PBS) for 5 s.
2. Aspirate the PBS.
3. Add 1 mL trypsin to dissociate the cells from the plate.
4. Incubate the dish at 37 °C for 1 min.
5. Add 5 mL DMEM to deactivate trypsin and resuspend the dish using sterile serological pipette.
6. Transfer 14 μL mixture from the dish to hemocytometer for cell counting.
7. Based on cell counting, transfer 100 cells into a 50 mL falcon tube containing 30 mL DMEM (*see* **Note 13**).
8. Resuspend the mixture and pour the mixture evenly in a 10 mm dish.
9. Use a multichannel pipette to aliquot 150 μL mixture from **step 8** into each well of two 96-well plates.

10. Incubate the 96-well plates in 37 °C with 5% CO_2.
11. Examine cell growth in each well daily and mark the wells containing a single colony (*see* **Note 14**).

3.4 Screening for CRISPR/Cas9-Edited Cell Clones

1. Prepare duplicate plate for cells from single colonies.
   (a) Allow the single colony to grow up to 70–80% confluence in the 96-well.
   (b) Aspirate the media from the well (original well) with the single colony.
   (c) Add one drop (15–20 μL) of trypsin into the well and incubate at 37 °C for 1–3 min. Check under the microscope to make sure that cells are detached.
   (d) Aliquot 150 μL DMEM into a well in a new 96-well plate (duplicate well).
   (e) Transfer 50 μL DMEM from well from **step** (**d**) (duplicate well) into the well from **step** (**c**) (original well), and gently pipette up and down to stop trypsinization.
   (f) Transfer 50 μL of the cell mixture from **step** (**e**) back into the well from **step** (**d**) (duplicate well).
   (g) Add fresh 150 μL of DMEM to the well from **step** (**c**) (original well).
   (h) Mark both original and duplicate wells with the same clone number.
   (i) Repeat the **steps** (**b**)–(**g**) for all the wells that contain single colonies.
   (j) Incubate both original and duplicate plates in 37 °C with 5% CO_2.
2. Genomic DNA (gDNA) extraction.
   (a) Examine cells in duplicate plates for the cell confluence to reach 80–90%.
   (b) Aspirate media from the well.
   (c) Add 50 μL of Lucigen DNA QuickExtraction solution. Resuspend the solutions by gently pipetting up and down.
   (d) Transfer the 50 μL of mixture to a PCR tube.
   (e) Run the sample in thermocycler with the following program: 65 °C for 5 min, 68 °C for 15 min, 98 °C for 2 min.
   (f) Measure the gDNA concentration using nanodrop analyzer.
3. Polymerase chain reaction (PCR) verification of CRISPR/Cas9-edited cell clones (*see* **Note 15**).
   (a) Set up PCR reaction with two primer pairs (IL17RB uncut forward and reverse primers and IL17RB deletion forward and reverse primers) as following:

   10 μL 2× phusion flash master mix.

1 μL forward primer (10 μM).
1 μL reverse primer (10 μM).
X μL genomic DNA (100 ng).
Y μL H_2O to total volume 20 μL.

(b) Run samples in thermocycler with the following program:
Denaturation at 98 °C for 10 s, then 34 cycles of denaturation at 98 °C for 1 s, annealing at 60 °C for 5 s, extension at 72 °C for 15 s, plus an additional extension at 72 °C for 1 min.

(c) Run PCR products in 1% agarose gel and visualize the PCR products.

4 Notes

1. Plasmid pX330 is used here for the co-expression of sgRNA and SpCas9 (Ran et al.). Other constructs may be utilized depending on preference and equipment availability. For example, a construct with an antibiotic selection marker or a GFP will facilitate the selection of positive clones. Most of those constructs can be obtained from Addgene.org.
2. There are many freely available software platforms and bioinformatics tools to facilitate the design of guide RNAs (gRNAs) for the CRISPR/Cas system. Please check individual website for details. You can also design sgRNAs manually. The goal is to identify the target sequences that have minimal off-targets in the genome upstream of a PAM sequence. Here we use the CRISPR Design tool from Zhang Lab, MIT. Two pairs of sgRNAs are designed to target exons 3 and 4 of IL17RB gene:

   Exon 3 (F: 5′-CACCGTTGTAACAGGTTCTACTCGG-3′; R: 5′-AAACCCGAGTAGAACCTGTTACAAC-3′).
   Exon 4 (F: 5′-CACCGGGCCTTCAACAAGCGGATGC-3′; R: 5′-AAACGCATCCGCTTGTTGAAGGCCC-3′).

   This strategy will create two double-strand breaks at IL17RB locus, leading to about 3 kb deletion in IL17RB genome. This genomic deletion approach allows simplified screening process through conventional PCR to identify gene knockout clones. Designed oligonucleotides can be synthesized by any preferred vendor. Schematic deletion and validation strategies is shown in Fig. 1.
3. DH5α chemically competent cells are used here for heat-shock transformation. Any other chemically competent cells or electrocompetent cells can be used for clone and propagate constructs.
4. Serum medium should not be used if Opti-MEM is not available.

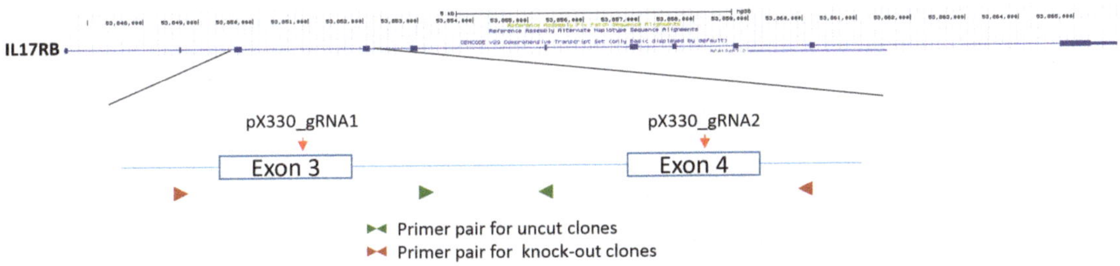

Fig. 1 Schematic deletion and validation strategies for IL17RB knockout. Two sgRNAs are designed and cloned to make two CRISPR constructs (pX330_gRNA1 and pX330_gRNA2). When they are delivered to cells, they will result in double-strand breaks on exon 3 and exon 4 of IL17RB gene respectively. This will lead to ~3 kb deletion in IL17RB locus. Two pairs of primers (uncut; green) and (KO; red) are also designed to detect the non-deletion and the deletion amplicon

5. Different transfection reagents need to be tested to ensure high transfection efficiency for each cell line. Alternatively, electroporation can be carried out if the equipment is available. In either case, transfection conditions need to be optimized for each cell line with a reporter construct beforehand.
6. pEGFP is used as a reporter construct to co-transfect with CRISPR constructs to make sure the transfection is done successfully. In addition, since pX330 does not contain a selection marker but pEGFP contains neomycin-resistant marker, co-transfection of pEGFP allows Geneticin selection to enrich the cells transfected with CRISPR constructs.
7. Dose response curve for Geneticin (G418) needs to be determined for each cell line beforehand. Typically, 200–800 μg/mL of Geneticin are needed for mammalian cells selection.
8. DNA QuickExtraction kit listed here is efficient for genomic DNA extraction. But any other reagents may be utilized.
9. Two pairs of deletion screening primers are designed. One set of primers internal to the sequence to be deleted (uncut) and another set of primers upstream and downstream of the CRISPR cleavage sites (KO stands for knockout). All the primers need to be at least 100 bp from the predicted cleavage site in case a small indel at the target site interferes with the annealing, therefore affecting screening detection. The two pairs of primers used here are: IL17RB uncut (F: 5′-CCAAGATTGTGCTGCAAGGC-3′; R: 5′-AGACCCACAAAGACCCTCCA-3′) and IL17RB KO (F: 5′-TCAGCCAGCGCTAAGAAACA-3′; R: 5′-GCAGCA CATCATCCATGCTC-3′).
10. Phusion Flash master mix allows fast and accurate PCR reaction with extremely short PCR protocols. But any other PCR mix may be utilized.
11. Digestion product needs to be run on agarose gel to ensure complete digestion (~200 ng). If digestion is not complete,

add more enzyme and 1× buffer and incubate longer time. Then re-run the product to confirm complete digestion.

12. The purpose of G418 selection is to enrich the cells with CRISPR constructs transfection. Longer G418 treatment is not recommended here as neomycin-resistant gene is only transient expressed from co-transfected pEGFP plasmid.
13. The remaining cells from Subheading 3.3, **step 7** will be spun down with clinical centrifuge at 700 × *g* for 15 s. Half of the cells will be frozen down for future plating. The other half will be used for screening and primer validation.
14. Limiting dilution is used here for single-cell clone plating. Depending on cell type, plating needs to be optimized to reliably obtain approximately 50 cells per 96-well plate. For adherent cells, cells are also to be plated in a 100 mm dish at low concentration so that individual single-cell derived clones can be picked and later moved to 96-well plate. If a flow cytometer sorter is available, cells can be sorted individually into 96-well plate.
15. Primer validation needs to be done with the remaining cells from Subheading 3.3, **step 7** (*see* **Note 13**) during the incubation time that allows for single cell to proliferate and form single colony. Genomic DNA extracted from those cells as well as from parental cells will be used as templates for PCR reaction to validate and optimize PCR program for uncut and knockout/deletion PCR amplification. Representative results are shown in Fig. 2. Both biallelic and monoallelic deletion clones need to be validated with quantitative RT-PCR and western blot with standard procedures. Representative validation results are shown in Fig. 3.

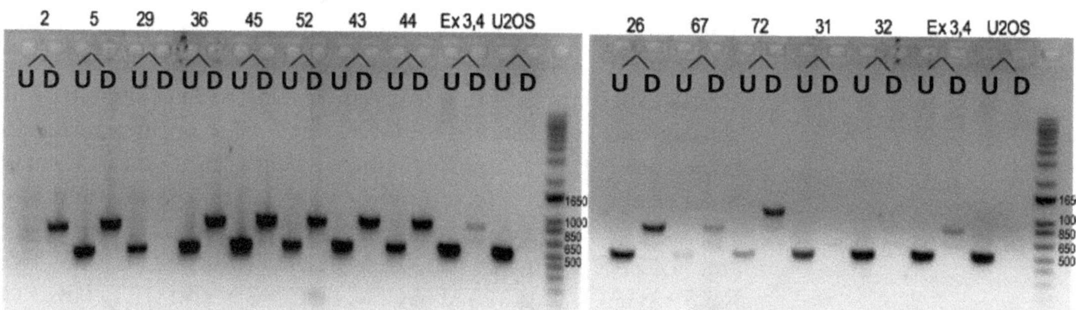

Fig. 2 Sample PCR results using genomic DNA from single clones as templates and uncut or knockout primers for PCR amplification. Genomic DNAs from parental U2OS cells (U2OS) and U2OS transfected with Crispr constructs (Ex 3, 4) were used as controls. Based on the prediction, clones without exon 3 and 4 deletion will yield ~600 bp PCR products using uncut primer pair and ~3.5 kb PCR products using knockout primer pair (will not be amplified with our program). Clones with deletion will have no PCR products using uncut primer pair and ~950 bp PCR products using knockout primer pair. Total 77 single clones were analyzed by genomic DNA PCR. In summary, Clone #29, 31, and 32 are wild type clones. Clone #2 is a homozygous clone. Clones #5, 26, 36, 45, 52, 43, and 44 are heterozygous clones. Clone #72 may be a heterozygous clone with additional DNA rearrangement

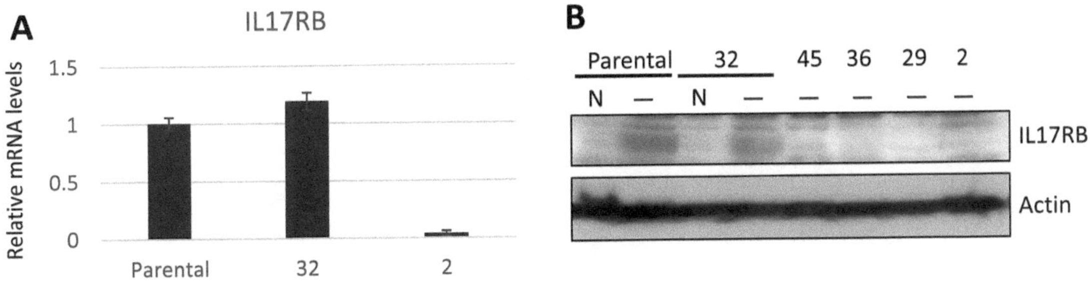

Fig. 3 Representative validation results for U2OS clones with IL17RB knockout. (**a**) Relative mRNA levels of Il17Rb in U2OS wild-type or IL17RB knockout clones by quantitative RT-PCR analysis. (**b**) Western blot analysis of different U2OS clones

Acknowledgment

This work was supported by St. John's University and NIH grant CA213426 to Yan Zhu.

References

1. Cong L, Ran FA, Cox D, Lin S, Barretto R, Habib N et al (2013) Multiplex genome engineering using CRISPR/Cas systems. Science 339(6121):819–823
2. Mali P, Yang L, Esvelt KM, Aach J, Guell M, DiCarlo JE et al (2013) RNA-guided human genome engineering via Cas9. Science 339 (6121):823–826
3. Terns MP (2018) CRISPR-based technologies: impact of RNA-targeting systems. Mol Cell 72(3):404–412
4. Gaj T, Gersbach CA, Barbas CF 3rd (2013) ZFN, TALEN, and CRISPR/Cas-based methods for genome engineering. Trends Biotechnol 31(7):397–405
5. Ran FA, Hsu PD, Wright J, Agarwala V, Scott DA, Zhang F (2013) Genome engineering using the CRISPR-Cas9 system. Nat Protoc 8 (11):2281–2308
6. Hsu PD, Zhang F (2012) Dissecting neural function using targeted genome engineering technologies. ACS Chem Neurosci 3 (8):603–610
7. Urnov FD, Rebar EJ, Holmes MC, Zhang HS, Gregory PD (2010) Genome editing with engineered zinc finger nucleases. Nat Rev Genet 11(9):636–646
8. Knott GJ, Doudna JA (2018) CRISPR-Cas guides the future of genetic engineering. Science 361(6405):866–869
9. Bie Q, Jin C, Zhang B, Dong H (2017) IL-17B: a new area of study in the IL-17 family. Mol Immunol 90:50–56
10. Alinejad V, Dolati S, Motallebnezhad M, Yousefi M (2017) The role of IL17B-IL17RB signaling pathway in breast cancer. Biomed Pharmacother 88:795–803
11. Bie Q, Sun C, Gong A, Li C, Su Z, Zheng D et al (2016) Non-tumor tissue derived interleukin-17B activates IL-17RB/AKT/beta-catenin pathway to enhance the stemness of gastric cancer. Sci Rep 6:25447
12. Wu HH, Hwang-Verslues WW, Lee WH, Huang CK, Wei PC, Chen CL et al (2015) Targeting IL-17B-IL-17RB signaling with an anti-IL-17RB antibody blocks pancreatic cancer metastasis by silencing multiple chemokines. J Exp Med 212(3):333–349
13. Eiro N, Fernandez-Gomez J, Sacristan R, Fernandez-Garcia B, Lobo B, Gonzalez-Suarez J et al (2017) Stromal factors involved in human prostate cancer development, progression and castration resistance. J Cancer Res Clin Oncol 143(2):351–359
14. Ren L, Xu Y, Liu C, Wang S, Qin G (2017) IL-17RB enhances thyroid cancer cell invasion and metastasis via ERK1/2 pathway-mediated MMP-9 expression. Mol Immunol 90:126–135

Chapter 29

Engineering Mutation Clones in Mammalian Cells with CRISPR/Cas9

Zijun Huo, Jian Tu, Dung-Fang Lee, and Ruiying Zhao

Abstract

CRISPR, *C*lustered *R*egularly *I*nterspaced *S*hort *P*alindromic *R*epeat, as a powerful genome engineering system has been widely accepted and employed in gene editing of a vast range of cell types. Comparing to zinc finger nucleases (ZFNs) or transcription-activator-like effector nucleases (TALENs), CRISPR shows less complicated process and higher efficiency. With the development of different CRISPR systems, it can be used not only to knock out a gene, but also to make precise modifications, activate or repress target genes with epigenetic modifications, and even for genome-wide screening. Here we will describe the procedure of generating stable cell lines with a knock-in mutation created by CRISPR. Specifically, this protocol demonstrated how to apply CRISPR to create the point mutation of R249 to S249 on *TP53* exon 7 in human embryonic stem cells (hESC) H9 line, which includes three major steps: (1) design CRISPR system targeting *TP53* genomic region, (2) deliver the system to H9 hESC and clone selection, and (3) examination and selection of positive clones.

Key words CRISPR, Genome editing, Precision gene editing, gRNA design, Donor vector, Stable cell line validation, Southern blot

1 Introduction

It has been a long journey of searching for precision genome editing methods. The emergence of ZFNs for the first time provides a method to produce a double-strand break at any desired DNA locus [1]. Later, the arising of TALENs provides a better tool for cutting and thereby editing specific genomic loci [2–5]. Still, the approach requires considerable amount of work, requiring a new pair of TALEs for each target. In 1993, CRISPR was first discovered as a structure with multiple copies of repeated sequences in microbes [6], later proved to be an adaptive immune system in bacteria [7–9]. A decade later, it is suggested as current name CRISPR, clustered regularly interspaced palindromic repeats [10]. It composes with tandem repeated sequences separated by spacers, and a group of Cas proteins serve as the nuclease. In effect,

Ivana Vancurova and Yan Zhu (eds.), *Immune Mediators in Cancer: Methods and Protocols*, Methods in Molecular Biology, vol. 2108, https://doi.org/10.1007/978-1-0716-0247-8_29, © Springer Science+Business Media, LLC, part of Springer Nature 2020

Cas proteins work as programmable restriction enzymes cut DNA at 3 nucleotides upstream of the proto-spacer adjacent motif (PAM) sequences [11]. Soon after Cas9 was proven to cleave DNA in vitro, CRISPR is predicted to be repurposed for genome editing in other organisms [12, 13]. With the discovery of Cas proteins, a small RNA transcribed from a sequence immediately adjacent to the CRISPR locus called trans-activating CRISPR RNA (tracrRNA) and processed CRISPR RNA (crRNAs) have been shown required for specific DNA locus recognition [14]. To reprogram Cas9 with custom-designed spacers to cut any target site [15], people found fusing crRNA and tracrRNA to a single guide RNA (sgRNA) could direct Cas9 function [16]. Especially, Zhang group modified the original sgRNA and found a full-length fusion of sgRNA efficiently cut desired DNA loci in vivo [17]. Briefly, CRISPR systems contain two components: a guide RNA and a CRISPR-associated endonuclease (Cas proteins). Through the design of guide RNAs specific to the DNA locus of interest, CRISPR system can be freely used in any cells.

In this chapter, the steps of the generation of a CRISPR produced point mutation on *TP53* R249 locus in hESC H9 line will be described. First of all, design and generate guide RNA and corresponding donor vector targeting *TP53* genomic locus. Second, deliver these plasmids to H9 cells and following with selection and validation. Clone verification process contains several approaches, including PCR, sequencing, and southern blot. Selected clones need the excision of selection cassette from genome to minimize the impact of exogenous DNA on the insertion locus. This procedure has been used to precisely modify genes in various cell lines, as showed in many publication [18, 19].

2 Materials

2.1 gRNA Cloning

1. pX335-U6-Chimeric_BB-CBh-hSpCas9n (D10A) (Addgene, Plasmid no. 42335).
2. BbsI (BpiI) (New England BioLabs).
3. T4 DNA Ligase (New England BioLabs).
4. LB Agar.
5. 50× TAE.
6. Agarose.
7. DNA ladder mix (Goldbio).
8. QIAquick gel extraction kit (Qiagen).
9. QIAprep spin miniprep kit (Qiagen).
10. PCR machine.

2.2 T7 Endonuclease I Assay

1. OneTaq® Quick-Load 2× Master Mix (New England BioLabs).
2. NEB buffer 2 (New England BioLabs).
3. T7 endonuclease I (New England BioLabs).
4. Human embryonic kidney (HEK) 293T cells (ATCC).
5. Dulbecco's modified Eagle medium (DMEM) with high glucose (Life Technologies).
6. FBS.
7. L-Glutamine solution (GenDEPOT, cat. no. CA009-010).
8. Penicillin/streptomycin solution.
9. Lipofectamine 3000 (Life Technologies).
10. Opti-MEM (Thermo Fisher Scientific).

2.3 Donor Vector Cloning

1. OneTaq® Quick-Load 2× Master Mix (New England BioLabs).
2. pGEM-T Easy (Promega).
3. DpnI (New England BioLabs).
4. EcoRI (New England BioLabs).
5. BamHI (New England BioLabs).
6. NotI (New England BioLabs).
7. pFrt-PGK-EM7-NeoR-bpA-Frt (Addgene, Plasmid no. 22687).

2.4 H9 Human Embryonic Stem Cell (H9 hESC) Culture

1. hESC line H9 (WiCell Institute).
2. Matrigel.
3. DMEM/F12.
4. StemMACS™ iPS-Brew XF (Miltenyi Biotec).
5. Accutase Cell Detachment Solution (Corning).
6. hESC medium: DMEM/F12 with 20% KnockOut Serum replacement (Life Technologies), 1% Gibco GlutaMax (Life Technologies), 1% NEAA (Corning), 0.0007% β-mercaptoethanol (Sigma), and 10 ng/mL FGF2 (EMD Millipore).
7. Type A Gelatin from porcine skin (Sigma-Aldrich).
8. 0.1% Gelatin solution (wt/vol): To prepare 1 L of 0.1% (wt/vol) gelatin solution, dissolve 1 g of gelatin powder in 1000 mL distilled H_2O. Autoclave the solution, then filter with the 0.22 μm filter to eliminate any impurity.
9. Filter unit (500 mL, 0.22 μm).

2.5 Cell Electroporation

1. Embryo Max Electroporation Buffer (Millipore).
2. Electroporation Cuvettes (Bio-Rad).

3. Bio-Rad Gene PulserXcell System (Bio-Rad).
4. NEO-resistant MEFs, CF6Neo Irradiated, Neomycin Resistant (MTi GlobalStem).
5. G418 Sulfate Solution.
6. ROCK inhibitor Thiazovivin (Millipore Sigma).

2.6 PCR and Southern Blot Validation

1. Easy DNA gDNA purification kit (Life Technologies).
2. PCR DIG Probe Synthesis Kit (Roche).
3. Depurination solution: 250 mM HCl. Mix 20.80 mL of (37%) HCl solution with deionized water and make final volume to 1 L.
4. Denaturation solution: 0.5 M NaOH, 1.5 M NaCl. Dissolve 20 g NaOH and 87.75 g NaCl in a 1 L glass beaker containing 700 mL of deionized water. Mix well and make final volume to 1 L with deionized water.
5. Neutralization solution: 0.5 M Tris–HCl (pH 7.5), 1.5 M NaCl. Add 87.75 g NaCl to 500 mL 1.0 M Tris–HCl (pH 7.5) to a 1 L glass beaker. Mix well and add deionized water to a total volume of 1 L.
6. 20× SSC.
7. DIG wash and block buffer set (Roche).
8. Low stringency buffer: 0.1% SDS, 2× SSC. Add 1 g SDS and 100 mL 20× SSC buffer to deionized water, mix well, and adjust volume to 1 L.
9. High stringency buffer: 0.1% SDS, 0.5× SSC. Add 1 g SDS and 25 mL 20× SSC buffer to deionized water, mix well, and adjust final volume to 1 L.
10. Anti-Digoxigenin-AP, Fab fragments (Roche).
11. CDPstar chemiluminescent substrate (Roche).
12. Nylon membranes.
13. Hybridization bags.

2.7 FNF Cassette Removal

1. pCAGGS-flpE-puro (Addgene, # 20733).
2. Puromycin (RPI).

3 Methods

3.1 Design and Generate the CRISPR Plasmids to Target Your Gene of Interest

To make the precise modification of the gene of interest, homology-directed repair (HDR) is a good method to choose. In order to employ HDR in gene editing, a DNA repair template with the desired alteration, the gRNA and Cas9 nickase have to be introduced to your cell of interest at the same time. The DNA repair

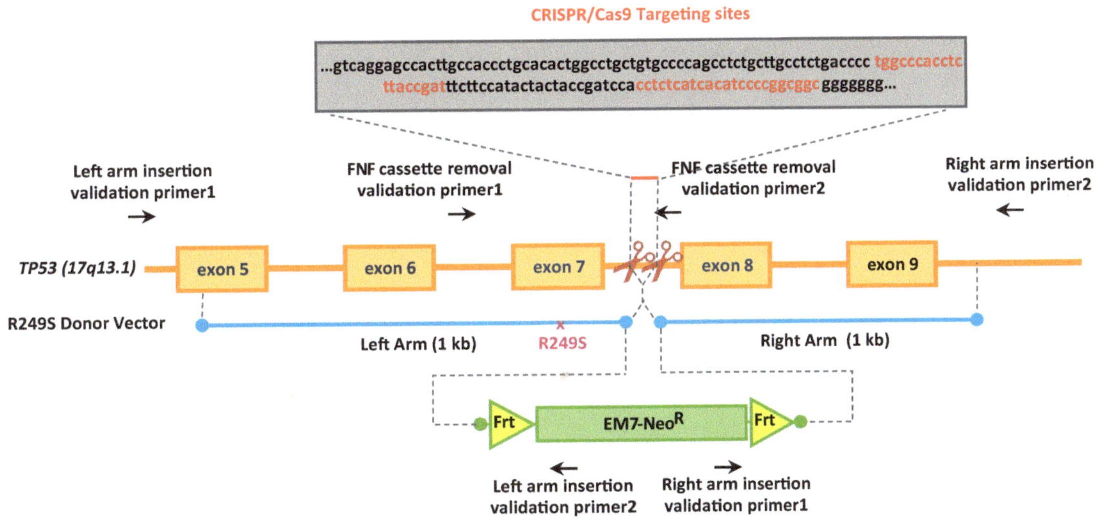

Fig. 1 Schematic diagram of CRISPR/Cas9 design for creating R249S mutation on *TP53*. The gRNA targeting loci are depicted and sequences are in red in the top box. The donor vector consists of the left homology arm (with p53 R249S mutation), right homology arm, and a FNF cassette. Gene-specific primers are designed for validation of the left arm and right arm insertion and FNF cassette removal

template is also named donor vector, which contains left and right homology arms and selection marker for picking up positive cells. The desired DNA alteration needs to be located within the homology arms, along with its upstream and downstream sequences. Figure 1 illustrates the design of donor vector and gRNAs to generate the point mutation that convert Arginine 249 to Serine 249 on *TP53* exon 7.

3.1.1 CRISPR Target Sites Selection, Guide RNA (gRNA) Design and Making

1. Searching CRISPR target sites for your gene of interest using the website: https://benchling.com/crispr. Import your target regions by type in the official gene symbol or transcript ID, or entry your own sequence. After define parameters, such as "single guide" or "pair guide," the website will analyze the gene or sequence you entered, then produce a list of guide oligoes each with its on-target and off-target scores. For instance, the official gene symbol of human p53 is *TP53* and its reference transcript ID is NM_000546.5. Click "Design CRISPR Guides" and select "Paired guides" to design gRNA sequence binding to sense and antisense strand. Choose the gRNA sequence with both higher on-target and off-target scores (*see* **Notes 1** and **2**). Two pairs of gRNA were selected for targeting *TP53*R249 locus (Fig. 1), and are shown in Table 1. Add BbsI enzyme sequence (5′-caccg-gRNA sense-3′; 5′-aaac-gRNA antisense-c-3′) to the gRNA oligoes for subsequent cloning convenience.

Table 1
gRNA oligoes for targeting p53/R249 locus

Oligo name	Sequence (5′–3′)
gRNA1 sense	*caccg*tggcccacctcttaccgat
gRNA1 antisense	*aaac*atcggtaagaggtgggccac
gRNA2 sense	*caccg*cctctcatcacatccccggcggc
gRNA2 antisense	*aaac*gccgccggggatgtgatgagaggc

2. Generate gRNA-expressing pX335 construct.
   (a) After received oligoes from commercial vendors, resuspend them at a concentration of 20 μM in sterile DNase/RNase-free ddH_2O.
   (b) Prepare 50 μL of the oligo duplex mixture by mixing 5 μL of 10× NEB buffer 2, 2 μM of forward and reverse oligo each in sterile DNase/RNase-free ddH_2O.
   (c) Boil 1 L water in a glass beaker on the heating block. Incubate the tube of the oligo duplex mixture in the boiling water for 5–8 min. Turn off the heater and let the temperature of the gRNA duplex mixture gradually down to room temperature, which usually takes 4–6 h. The annealed gRNA duplex can be kept at 4 °C for later use (*see* **Note 3**).
   (d) Digest 6 μg of pX335 vector with BbsI, then run the digested vector on a 0.8% (wt/vol) agarose gel. Cut and extract the digested vector from the agarose gel with a gel extraction kit. Ligate the purified vector with annealed gRNA duplex in a mixture of 1 μL annealed gRNA oligo, 0.5 μL digested vector, 1 μL 10× NEB T4 DNA ligase buffer, 1 μL NEB T4 DNA ligase, and 6.5 μL ddH_2O. Incubate the ligation mixture at room temperate for 1 h or 16 °C overnight. Following with transformation of gRNA-vector ligation product into DH5α competent cells.
3. Validate the pX335-gRNA construct.

   Pick up antibiotic-resistant clones, culture them, isolate plasmids by using the miniprep kit, and check gRNA insertion with Sanger sequencing. The sequencing primer for this particular construct is: 5′-TGCATATACGATACAAGGCTGTTAG-3′.

3.1.2 Test gRNA Targeting Efficiency Using T7 Endonuclease 1 Assay

1. Plate HEK293T cells in 6 cm cell culture dishes using DMEM + 10% FBS + 1% L-Glutamine + 1% P/S medium.
2. Start the transfection until cells reach 50% confluence. Prepare the transfection mixture with 3 μg pX335-gRNA plasmid in 300 μL of Opti-MEM I reduced-serum medium. Mix the DNA cocktail with 10 μL Lipofectamine 3000 as describe by manufacturer protocol.

3. Harvest cells at 48 h after transfection and isolate genomic DNA using genomic DNA extraction kit.
4. Amplify fragments bracketing gRNA targeted region using primers (5′-TGTAAAACGACGGCCAG TGCCTCCCCTG CTTGCCACAG-3′ and 5′-CAGGAAACAGCTATGACCGGG AGCAGTAAGGAGATTCC-3′). Run 10 μL PCR product on 2% agarose gel to make sure one single fragment as the predicted size (*see* **Note 4**).
5. Reannealing 13.6 μL PCR product with 1.6 μL NEB buffer 2 using the cycle in Table 2 to generate heteroduplex DNA.
6. Add 0.4 μL NEB buffer 2 and 0.2 μL T7 endonuclease I to the heteroduplex DNA mixture and digest at 37 °C for 30 min. Run the digested product on a 2% agarose gel. Multiple cleavage bands should be present below the original PCR product if gRNA can target the designed region (Fig. 2). Choose the gRNA pair with the highest cleavage efficiency for future step.

Table 2
Reannealing program

Temperature (°C)	Time
95	5 min
95–85	−2 °C/s
85–25	−0.1 °C/s
25	10 min

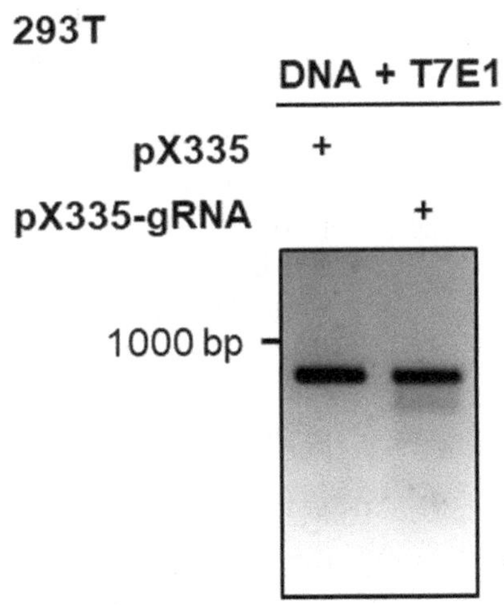

Fig. 2 Representative result of T7E1 assay. The right lane shows T7E1 assay performed after transfection of the gRNA vectors, while the left lane shows negative control after transfection of empty vectors

3.1.3 Donor Vector Design and Synthesis

1. As shown in Fig. 1, the left and right homology arms are at up- and downstream of the gRNA targeting site, respectively. Both arms have been designed about 1 kb long, flanking several *TP53* exons and introns (*see* **Note 5**). Using the H9 hESC genomic DNA as template and the specific primers amplify homology arms (Fig. 1). The left arm primers are 5′-GAA TTCCGCGTCCGCGCCATGGCCATCTACAAGCAGT CAC AG-3′ and 5′-GAATTCAGGCCAGTGTGCAGGGTGGCAAG TGGCTCCTGACCT-3′. The right arm primers are 5′-GGA TCCGCTGTGCCCCAGCCTCTGCTTGCCTCTGACCCCT GG-3′ and 5′-GCGGCCGCCAGGCTAGGCTAAGCT ATGAT GTTCCTTAGATTAGG-3′. After confirming the PCR product on a 0.8% agarose gel, cut and extract the band from the agarose gel with a gel extraction kit. Ligate it with a pGEM-T Easy vector according to manufacturer's protocol. Incubate the ligation mixture at room temperate for 1 h or 16 °C overnight. Following with transformation of pGEM-T vector ligation product into DH5α competent cells.
2. Generate the R249S mutation in the left arm/pGEM-T construct by PCR using the primers: 5′-TGCATGGGCGGCATG AACCGGAGTCCCATCCTCACCATC-3′ and 5′-GATGGT GAGGATGGGACTCCGGTTCATG CCGCCCATGCA-3′. Digest the PCR product using DpnI at 37 °C for 2 h and then transform digestion product into DH5α cells.
3. Pick up antibiotic-resistant clones, culture them, isolate plasmids by using the miniprep kit, and send for Sanger sequencing to validate the point mutation.
4. Digest the left homology arm/pGEM-T construct with EcoRI and right homology arm/pGEM-T construct with BamHI and NotI to get the left and right arm fragments. At the first time digest the pFrt-PGK-EM7-NeoR-bpA-Frt (pFNF) vector with EcoRI, then ligate the left arm fragment with this digested pFNF vectors using T4 ligase. Following with transformation of ligation product into DH5α competent cells. Isolate plasmids and confirm the successful insertion of left arm in the pFNF vector. Next, digest this left arm containing pFNF vector with BamHI and NotI, then ligate with right arm fragment, flowing with transformation and confirmation. The end pFNF plasmid should contain both left arm and right arm with desired DNA modification.

3.2 Deliver gRNA and Donor Vector into the Target Cells

1. Maintain H9 hESCs in StemMACS™ iPS-Brew XF medium on Matrigel-coated plates for 2 weeks to reach its optimal condition for electroporation.

   Making Matrigel coating plates: Thaw Matrigel aliquots for at least 3–4 h on ice or at 4 °C overnight. Dilute Matrigel at a 1:50 ratio in DMEM/F12 medium. Add 4 mL diluted Matrigel into a 10 cm plate and gently shake the plate until the plate is evenly covered. Leave the Matrigel-coated plate at room temperature for 30 min and then remove any remaining Matrigel by aspiration before plating cells. Otherwise, keep Matrigel inside plates and place at 4 °C overnight. The plate is ready to use the next day.

2. On day 1, prepare MEF feeder cells coated culture dishes.
   (a) Making gelatin-coated culture dishes for MEF feeder cells. Use 5 mL 0.1% gelatin solution to cover a 10-cm plate, put into a 37 °C incubator for at least 15 min. Before use, aspirate off the gelatin and seed cells immediately. For a long time storage, more solution should be used. Gelatin-coated plates can remain in a 37 °C incubator for up to 7 days before use.
   (b) Prepare MEF feeder cells plated culture dishes. The maintenance of clonal H9 ESCs requires supporting from MEF feeder cells. Thaw a cryo vial of NEO-resistant MEFs and plate them onto four to six gelatin-coated 10-cm plates. The dilution of MEFs seeding on culture dishes should be determined by the frozen cell concentration or according to the provided protocol. Incubate overnight at 37 °C and allow cells to attach.
3. On day 2, perform the electroporation transfection of H9 hESCs.
   (a) H9 hESCs are grown in StemMACS™ iPS-Brew XF medium on one 10 cm Matrigel-coated dish at 80–90% confluency. Remove the medium and wash with 5 mL 1× DPBS. Replace the DPBS with 1 mL Accutase and incubate at 37 °C for 3–5 min. Resuspend cells in 10 mL DMEM/F12 medium and centrifuge the cells at 1000 rpm, 4 °C for 5 min.
   (b) Aspirate and discard the supernatant. Resuspend cells in 10 mL Opti-MEM medium to remove remaining FBS, Accutase, etc. in the medium. Count cells and centrifuge 1×10^7 cells for each electroporation reaction at 1000 rpm, 4 °C for 5 min. Remove the supernatant and resuspend cells (1×10^7) in 600 μL Embryo Max electroporation buffer (EEB).
   (c) Mix 50 μg pFNF donor vector plasmid, 5 μg pX335-gRNA1 and 5 μg pX335-gRNA2 in a total volume of 50 μL. Then add this DNA mixture to cells/EEB suspension drop wise and mix well.
   (d) Transfer the cells/DNA/EEB mixture into electroporation cuvettes, and immediately perform electroporation at 300 V/500 μF.
   (e) Transfer transfection mixture into 12 mL hESC medium containing conical tube right after the electroporation.

Seed cells to six 10 cm MEF-coated dishes with different cell solution volumes (1, 1, 2, 2, 3, and 3 mL). Add hESC medium with 2 μM ROCK inhibitor to a final volume of 10 mL.

4. On day 3, check cells and replace with 10 mL fresh hESC medium with 50 μg/mL G418.
5. Change with fresh hESC medium plus 50 μg/mL G418 every 2–3 days for clone growth.
6. When clones are visible, remove the medium and rinse the cells twice with 5 mL 1× DPBS. Prepare Matrigel-coated 48-well plate, and add 500 μL hESC medium with 2 μM ROCK inhibitor to each well. Pick up every single clone using 200 μL pipet tips and plant to each well.

3.3 Validation of the Positively Modified Clones by PCR, Sanger Sequencing, and Southern Blot

3.3.1 Confirmation of Donor Vector Insertion at Correct Locus by PCR

1. When a single clone expands to 90% confluency in one well of 48-well plate, passage all cells to one well of 6-well plate. When the cells in one well of 6-well plate are 90% confluent, keep 10% of the cells for continuing culture, and extract genomic DNA from 90% of the cells using Easy-DNA gDNA purification kit following the manufacturer's protocol.
2. PCR amplify the inserted region with primers (5′-TGTAAAA CGACGGCCAGTCT AGCTCGCTAGTGGGTTGC-3′ and 5′-TCCAGACTG CCTTGGGAAA-3′ for the left arm, and 5′-GGGGAGGATTGGGAAGACAA-3′ and 5′-CAGGAAA CAGCTATGACCGCCCA GGAGGGTATAATGAGCTA-3′ for the right arm).
3. Run the PCR product on a 0.8% agarose gel using 1× TAE buffer until good separation is achieved. The single band at correct size (Fig. 3) indicates the precise insertion into the correct locus.

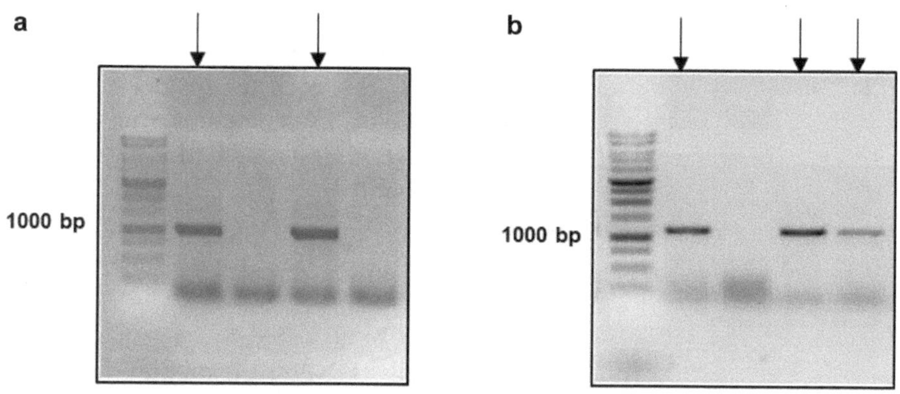

Fig. 3 Representative results of PCR validation of left homology arm and right homology arm insertion. Arrows indicate positive left arm insertion clones with a band around 1000 bp in panel (**a**), and positive right arm insertion with a band around 1200 bp in panel (**b**)

3.3.2 Sanger Sequencing

Pick positive clones according to above PCR results. Perform gel purification of the PCR products and send them for Sanger sequencing to confirm the knock-in point mutation in the selected clones. The primer for sequencing is 5′-TCCAGACTGCCTTGGG AAA-3′.

3.3.3 Southern Blotting

PCR and Sanger sequencing prove the presence of desired modification at the correct location; however, these assays are not able to exclude the possibility of multiple insertion of the donor vector. Southern blotting is the only method to identify single insertion clones.

1. Synthesize a probe that targets the neomycin region using primers 5′-ATGGGATCGGCCATTGAACAAGAT-3′ and 5′-TCAGAAGAACTCGTCAAGAAGGCG-3′ according to the instruction of PCR DIG Probe Synthesis Kit.
2. Digest 10 μg of genomic DNA from positive clones overnight at 37 °C water bath with *BamHI*. Load the digested products on a 0.7% agarose gel 100–150 V electrophoresis for 60 min to achieve a good separation.
3. Prepare the gel for transfer.
   (a) Wash the gel once for 10 min in the depurination solution with gentle shaking, then rinse the gel once with ddH_2O.
   (b) Wash the gel twice for 15 min each time in the denaturation solution with gentle shaking, then rinse the gel once with ddH_2O.
   (c) Wash the gel twice for 15 min each time in the neutralization solution with gentle shaking.
   (d) Rinse the gel once for 10 min in the 20× SSC buffer.
4. Set up the blot transfer "sandwich," and transfer DNA to the nylon membrane overnight in 2× SSC buffer. Disassemble the transfer "sandwich" the next day and mark the wells of the gel on the nylon membrane with a pencil.
5. Expose the wet membrane to UV light at 120 mJ energy to cross-link the membrane. Rinse the membrane briefly with ddH_2O.
6. Preheat the hybridization oven and pre-warm DIG Easy Hyb buffer at 42 °C. Place the membrane into a hybridization bag, fill with DIG Easy Hyb buffer, seal the bag around the membrane, and eliminate any air bubbles. Put the bag on the rotator in the hybridization oven, incubate for 30–60 min.
7. Add 4 μL of probe to a 1.5 mL Eppendorf tube containing 50 μL ddH_2O. Place the tube to boiling water bath for 5 min to denature the probe. Chill the denatured probe immediately on

ice for 2 min. Add the denatured probe to 13 mL pre-warmed DIG Easy Hyb buffer to make the hybridization buffer. Replace the DIG Easy Hyb buffer in the hybridization bag with probe-containing hybridization buffer and avoid making air bubbles. Incubate the membrane in the hybridization buffer at 42 °C in the oven with rotation overnight.

8. Stop the hybridization and prepare the membrane for signal detection.

   (a) Transfer the membrane onto a plastic tray the next day. Wash the membrane twice for 5 min each time with 100 mL low stringency buffer.

   (b) Preheat the high stringency buffer to 68 °C. Wash the membrane three times for 10 min each time in pre-warmed 100 mL high stringency buffer with gentle shaking.

   (c) Block the membrane at room temperature by incubation with 100 mL blocking solution for 30 min.

   (d) Incubate the membrane with 50 mL diluted Anti-Digoxigenin-AP solution (1:5000 diluted in blocking solution) for 30–60 min with gentle shaking.

   (e) Wash the membrane twice with 100 mL washing buffer.

9. Incubate the membrane with 20 mL detection buffer for 3 min. Pour off the detection buffer and add 1–2 mL CDPstar chemiluminescent substrate to cover the membrane. Use pipette to make the substrate distribute evenly on the membrane. Incubate the membrane at room temperature for 2 min. Remove excess chemiluminescent substrate and place the membrane into a film cassette. Expose the film.

10. Single band with the predicted size indicates there is no off-target insertion. Choose clones with single insertion for the following experiments (Fig. 4).

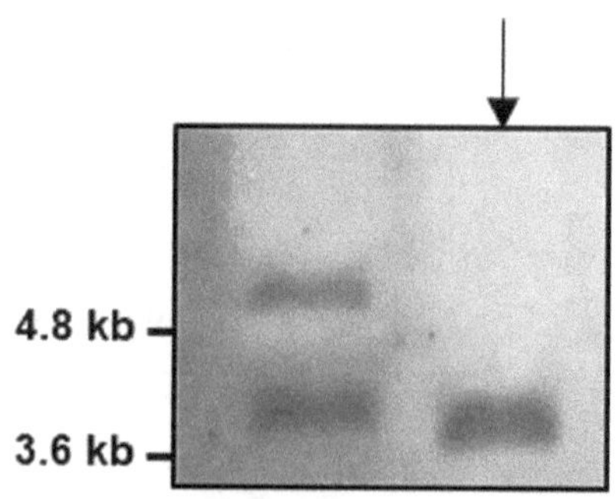

Fig. 4 Representative result of Southern blot. The right lane demonstrates a positive clone without off-target insertion

3.4 The FNF Cassette Removal

After examined by PCR, sequencing, and Southern blot, the correct clone will be picked for FNF cassette removal. In order to eliminate the risk that the FNF cassette affects normal gene function around the insertion locus, it is necessary to remove the cassette from the correct clone genome.

3.4.1 Express Flp Recombinase into Correct Clone Cells

1. Day 1, seed the picked H9 hESC clones into a Matrigel-coated 6-well plate, grow cells at 37 °C and 5% CO_2 overnight to reach 70% confluence at transfection.
2. Day 2, transfect the cells with 2 μg pCAGGS-flpE-puro plasmid each well of the 6-well plate using Lipofectamine 3000 reagent according to the manufacturer's protocol. The pCAGGS-flpE-puro plasmid will express Flp recombinase to excise neomycin-resistant cassette from the genome, at the same time expressing puromycin resistance to provide the selection opportunity.
3. Day 3, change cells with fresh hESC medium, and it is better to do this in the morning.
4. Day 4, 48 h after transfection, begin puromycin treatment at the dosage of 0.5 μg/mL (*see* **Note 6**). Only treat cells with puromycin for 2 days. At the end of puromycin treatment, cells without successful pCAGGS-flpE-puro plasmid transfection will be killed. Gently wash cells with medium once, replace with fresh hESC medium and continue culturing cells for 1–2 more days.
5. Day 6, prepare MEF feeder cells plated culture dishes. Thaw a cryo vial of MEFs and plate them onto four to six gelatin-coated 10-cm plates. The dilution of MEFs seeding on culture dishes should be determined by the frozen cell concentration or according to the provided protocol. Incubate overnight at 37 °C allow cells to attach.
6. Day 7, wash transfected and puromycin treated H9 hESC cells with 2 mL 1× DPBS, add 0.5 mL Accutase into each well, and incubate at 37 °C for 5 min. Neutralize cells with 2 mL fresh medium, and centrifuge cells at 1000 rpm for 5 min. Resuspend cells with 10 mL medium. Count cells and seed 500 cells to each MEF-coated 10 cm plate.
7. Change medium every 2–3 days until clones are visible. Pick up single clones using 200 μL tip to each well of Matrigel-coated 48-well plate.

3.4.2 Validation of Successful Removal of the FNF Cassette

1. When cells are confluent in 6-well plate, maintain 10% of the cells for continuing culture and extract genomic DNA from 90% of the cells using Easy-DNA gDNA purification kit.
2. Use primers flanking the CRISPR editing locus (Fig. 1) (5′-TGTAAAACGACGGCCAGTGCCTCCCCTGCTTG CCACAG-3′ and 5′-CAGGAAACAGCTAT GACCGGGAG-CAGTAAGGAGATTCC-3′) to perform PCR examination.

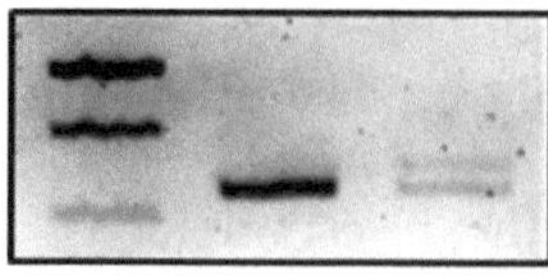

Fig. 5 Representative result of FNF cassette removal by PCR validation. The right lane shows a positive clone without FNF cassette. The upper band indicates the mutant allele with a Frt scar and the lower band indicates the WT allele without any genome editing

Run the PCR product on a 0.8% agarose gel until the separation is ideal. A 329 bp PCR fragment indicates a WT *TP53* allele without any genomic editing. A 363 bp product (329 + 34 bp Frt scar) indicates a mutant *TP53* allele with Frt insertion, which the majority of FNF cassette has been excised (Fig. 5). At this time the clone is ready to expand for future applications.

4 Notes

1. Several criteria need to be met when designing the gRNA. It is better to choose gRNA located in the intron region and avoid any splicing sequence to reduce the risk of unwanted change on the target DNA. Make sure not to include PAM sequence in the oligoes.
2. When using "https://benchling.com/crispr" for gRNA design, it provides multiple candidates to choose from. Oligoes with higher on- and off-target scores usually work better, but has exceptions. Start with several pairs of gRNA with the highest scores, and test their efficiency by T7 E1 assay before delivery into cells.
3. Cooling down the gRNA duplex mixture slowly is essential for annealing gRNA oligoes perfectly. After turning off the heater, the beaker can be covered to prevent fast temperature dropping.
4. The PCR product size could be variable depending on the genomic DNA region, the length around 500 bp is an optimal size for following steps.
5. The length of left and right homologous arms depends on the genomic region of your target gene; usually, the longer the gene, the longer the homology arms. Also, it tends to design longer homology arm for increasing homologous recombination efficiency. Typically, one side of homology arm is 500–1000 bp.
6. It is necessary to test the tolerance dosage of puromycin for your cell of interest. Generally, the dose is ranging between 0.5 and 2 μg/mL for mammalian cells.

References

1. Bibikova M et al (2001) Stimulation of homologous recombination through targeted cleavage by chimeric nucleases. Mol Cell Biol 21 (1):289–297
2. Zhang F et al (2011) Efficient construction of sequence-specific TAL effectors for modulating mammalian transcription. Nat Biotechnol 29(2):149–153
3. Miller JC et al (2011) A TALE nuclease architecture for efficient genome editing. Nat Biotechnol 29(2):143–148
4. Xu A et al (2018) Establishment of a human embryonic stem cell line with homozygous TP53 R248W mutant by TALEN mediated gene editing. Stem Cell Res 29:215–219
5. Zhou R et al (2018) A homozygous p53 R282W mutant human embryonic stem cell line generated using TALEN-mediated precise gene editing. Stem Cell Res 27:131–135
6. Mojica FJ, Juez G, Rodriguez-Valera F (1993) Transcription at different salinities of Haloferax mediterranei sequences adjacent to partially modified PstI sites. Mol Microbiol 9 (3):613–621
7. Mojica FJ et al (2005) Intervening sequences of regularly spaced prokaryotic repeats derive from foreign genetic elements. J Mol Evol 60 (2):174–182
8. Pourcel C, Salvignol G, Vergnaud G (2005) CRISPR elements in Yersinia pestis acquire new repeats by preferential uptake of bacteriophage DNA, and provide additional tools for evolutionary studies. Microbiology 151 (Pt 3):653–663
9. Bolotin A et al (2005) Clustered regularly interspaced short palindrome repeats (CRISPRs) have spacers of extrachromosomal origin. Microbiology 151(Pt 8):2551–2561
10. Jansen R et al (2002) Identification of genes that are associated with DNA repeats in prokaryotes. Mol Microbiol 43(6):1565–1575
11. Marraffini LA, Sontheimer EJ (2008) CRISPR interference limits horizontal gene transfer in staphylococci by targeting DNA. Science 322 (5909):1843–1845
12. Deveau H et al (2008) Phage response to CRISPR-encoded resistance in Streptococcus thermophilus. J Bacteriol 190(4):1390–1400
13. Horvath P et al (2008) Diversity, activity, and evolution of CRISPR loci in Streptococcus thermophilus. J Bacteriol 190(4):1401–1412
14. Deltcheva E et al (2011) CRISPR RNA maturation by trans-encoded small RNA and host factor RNase III. Nature 471(7340):602–607
15. Gasiunas G et al (2012) Cas9-crRNA ribonucleoprotein complex mediates specific DNA cleavage for adaptive immunity in bacteria. Proc Natl Acad Sci U S A 109(39): E2579–E2586
16. Jinek M et al (2012) A programmable dual-RNA-guided DNA endonuclease in adaptive bacterial immunity. Science 337 (6096):816–821
17. Cong L et al (2013) Multiplex genome engineering using CRISPR/Cas systems. Science 339(6121):819–823
18. Tu J et al (2018) Generation of human embryonic stem cell line with heterozygous RB1 deletion by CRIPSR/Cas9 nickase. Stem Cell Res 28:29–32
19. Huo Z et al (2019) Generation of a heterozygous p53 R249S mutant human embryonic stem cell line by TALEN-mediated genome editing. Stem Cell Res 34:101360

Index

Ivana Vancurova and Yan Zhu (eds.), *Immune Mediators in Cancer: Methods and Protocols*, Methods in Molecular Biology, vol. 2108, https://doi.org/10.1007/978-1-0716-0247-8, © Springer Science+Business Media, LLC, part of Springer Nature 2020

G

H

I

L

M

N

O

P

FSC
www.fsc.org
MIX
Papier | Fördert gute Waldnutzung
FSC® C083411

Kolibri 360 GmbH
Ferdinand-Jühlke-Straße 7
99095 Erfurt, Deutschland
produktsicherheit@kolibri360.de